THE HISTORICAL EMERGENCE OF THE I

ESSAYS ABOUT ONE CHAPTER IN THE HISTORY OF THE SOUL

With 13 pictures in full color

WOLFGANG GIEGERICH

DUSK OWL BOOKS
London, Ontario, Canada

Cover design by
Michael Mendis
24 Blackfriars Street
London, Ont. N6H 1K6
Canada

ISBN: 978-1-9992266-1-9

7xxx

THE HISTORICAL EMERGENCE OF THE I

Table of Contents

Chapter Two

The Western Soul's Historical Project of the Development of the "I". A few selected aspects 135

Chapter Three

Chapter Four

Sources and Abbreviations

For frequently cited sources, the following abbreviations have been used:

CW: Jung, C. G., *Collected Works.* 20 vols. Ed. Herbert Read, Michael Fordham, Gerhard Adler, and William McGuire. Trans. R. F. C. Hull. Princeton: Princeton University Press, 1957–1979. Cited by volume and, unless otherwise noted, by paragraph number.

GW: Jung, C. G., *Gesammelte Werke*, 20 vols., various editors, Olten and Freiburg im Breisgau: Walter-Verlag, 1971–1983. Cited by volume and, unless otherwise noted, by paragraph number.

Letters: Jung, C. G., *Letters.* 2 vols. Ed. Gerhard Adler. Bollingen Series XCV: 2. Princeton: Princeton University Press, 1975.

MDR: Jung, C. G., *Memories, Dreams, Reflections.* Rev. ed., Ed. Aniela Jaffé. Trans. Richard and Clara Winston. New York: Vintage Books, 1989. Cited by page number.

Erinn.: *Erinnerungen, Träume, Gedanken von C.G. Jung*, ed. by Aniela Jaffé, Zürich and Stuttgart (Rascher) 1967.

CEP: Giegerich, W., *Collected English Papers*, 6 vols. New Orleans, LA 2005 ff. (Spring Journal Books), now London and New York, 2020 (Routledge).

Transl. modif.: Appearing at the end of a citation, this indicates that I modified the particular quotation from the *Collected Works* in order to bring the English translation a bit closer to the wording and spirit of Jung's original German text.

Introduction

The importance of history for psychology

The topic of this book, the historical emergence of the I, involves two main concepts, the I and the soul's historicity. What the nature of the I is, what different senses of I must be distinguished, what the I's psychological implications and effects are, and, furthermore, why I speak in the first place of the I rather than of the ego (which so far has been the standard term of psychological work in the English language), will, I hope, be adequately and sufficiently elucidated in the following essays.

The same applies to the second central notion, the perhaps surprising idea that, and why, the I is a historical acquisition and not a constant, naturally given with the existence of humans. It is the purpose of this book to trace the historical origin of the I in such away that we can ourselves, as it were, witness its emergence from what preceded it, participate in the birth pangs through which it came about, and see its further development.

This Introduction does therefore not need to devote any space and additional effort to introducing these two notions.

There is, however, one general and fundamental topic that does need some discussion. This is the role and significance of the concept of history as such for the soul, as well as the relation of history to psychology.

It is well known that it was mature Jung's point-blank thesis that "without history there can be no psychology, and certainly no psychology of the unconscious" (*MDR* p. 205f.), a statement in which we are well advised to translate the term "the unconscious" by "the objective soul". This bold and apodictic statement runs absolutely counter to the generally prevailing standpoint of psychology and psychotherapy, which proceeds from the tacit assumption that the "psychic apparatus" of people, and its psychic "organs", that the internal dominating factors, desires, emotions, mechanisms, and potentials were *basically* the same at all times and differed only due to circumstance and to the particular individuality of people. This assumption is fully in accordance with the stance of the natural sciences and medicine and expressive of a naturalistic point of view. And as long as psychology restricts itself to mean the study of 'the behavior of the human organism' (as it has been defined at times), i.e., of the *psyche* of people, the exclusion within it of a historical perspective is of course justified. Not so in a psychology in the true sense of the word, a psychology *with* soul and of the objective soul.

At numerous times I have in my writings documented the importance of history as constitutive for Jung's understanding of psychology. I have shown that, according to him, in former ages the soul used to be outside, and that the fact that it is now inside, in ourselves, is an absolutely novel situation and at the same time the *sine qua non* of the possibility and actual emergence of modern psychology (*CW* 10 § 158 ff.). I have pointed to Jung's idea that there is in history a general "metamorphosis of the gods" and that "the gods die from time to time" (*CW* 9i § 22); that likewise symbols die and are then only of historical significance because then their meaning has been born out of them (*CW* 6 § 816); that Jung accordingly insisted that we cannot turn the wheel backwards and return to a symbolism that is gone, because it no longer expresses our psychological condition (*CW* 18 § 632). All this shows that Jung was convinced that a *historical gulf* separates us and our psychological condition from that of former ages. For the same reason, for example, during earlier ages of the Christian aeon it needed no *sacrificium intellectus* to believe in miracles, as Jung pointed out, and the report of the birth, life, death, and resurrection of the Redeemer could in those days still pass as biography, whereas for us today the object of belief is no longer inherently convincing (*Letters 2*, p. 485, to Tanner, 12 Feb 1959).

Jung provided us with a graphic image of the historical obsolescence of a whole mode of being-in-the-world, an image paradigmatic for the rupture between the pre-modern and the modern world, namely in the figure of an old *laibon* (medicine man) whom he had met in Uganda. With the arrival in East Africa of the English as ruling power, this *laibon*, Jung tells us, had lost his *raison d'être* because now "the English knew better" and the divine voice which before had counseled the tribe through the *laibon's* dreams was no longer needed, the value of life now laying wholly in *this* world (*MDR* p. 265).

I have also referred to Jung's idea that the population living at a given time consists of different historical layers, in the sense that only a few people have actually reached the level of consciousness of their own historical time and that many other persons belong psychologically, as far as the structure of their consciousness is concerned, to earlier centuries rather than to their actual time (see *CW* 11 § 463). Jung's own dream of the multi-storied house (*MDR* p. 158f.) represented for him the conception that the individual psyche, too, consists of historical layers within itself. Essential works of Jung's, such as his study of the dogma of the Trinity and *Answer to Job* (both in *CW* 11), show the historical-psychological approach in action. The fact *that* the sense of history was of crucial significance for Jung's understanding of psychology can therefore be considered as established.

But is this view justified? Is "history" indeed indispensable for psychology? There has been a powerful voice within the wider field of the Jungian tradition that passionately objected and that systematically rejected history as constitutive for psychology, even dismissing the historical perspective in psychology as "historical literalism". This was the voice of James Hillman, the founder of the Jungian school of "archetypal psychology". He insisted that the ancient gods, for example the Greek god Zeus, are still alive just as in former times and that they are unchanged, namely, timeless or eternal presences. Accordingly he tried to interpret even such decidedly modern phenomena as modern science and technology in terms of the gods or archetypal images, specifically as the manifestation of the fact that such specific archetypal forces as Apollo or Hercules have become the dominants of consciousness.

So we have two totally contrary positions concerning the topic of history and psychology. As always in such a case of fundamental stances there can be no decision as to which one is right and which one is wrong. Both are in themselves possible and legitimate positions. What can and needs to be investigated is another question, the question of *what is at stake* with the inclusion or not-inclusion of the sense of history (or better: of historicity) in the very concept of psychology? What does the concept of historicity do to and make possible for psychology? And conversely, what happens to psychology if it is conceived without a sense of history as intrinsic to it? These questions can best be examined by comparing and contrasting the two radically opposite standpoints.

I will start my comparison of these two fundamental points of view by presenting a quotation from Jung that highlights the figure of thought that underlies his historical sense of the soul's life. It is a quotation that in its own context refers to individual, personal psychology, but the structure described applies equally to collective or cultural psychology. Talking about the frequent confusion between cause and effect in the psychological explanations of neurotic disorders, he states as his view that the actual cause of neurosis is that

> ... consciousness is faced with a situation and task to which it is not equal. It does not understand how its world has altered and what attitude it would have to assume in order to be adapted again (*GW* 9i § 61, my transl.).

The first thing to be noted is that the logic of this conception is that of a two-place relation. There are two separate empirical structures: consciousness, and the world in which it finds itself. The position that repudiates the "category" of history for psychology operates only with a one-place system. For it there is only consciousness together with the *consciousness-internal* question of which archetypal structure prevails in it. Any kind of "relation" that can come into play for the second view is again consciousness-internal, namely consciousness's relation, or lack of relation, to its own dominants, to the archetypal structures, the archetypal images, to "the Gods". The "Gods" or archetypes may be others to consciousness in some sense, but certainly not empirical others. They belong to the ideal or transcendent sphere, which makes one's relationship to them fundamentally subjective and vertical. The relation that Jung has in mind is, by contrast, a horizontal one. Really existing consciousness finds itself *in* a given real situation, *in* a "world" all around it. It is *faced* with something real vis-à-vis itself, a given condition or task (not simply determined or dominated internally by some "factor").

A psychic disorder is according to Jung's dictum due to the fact that a discrepancy has arisen between the two structures. Consciousness and the situation or world are no longer in alignment; consciousness is no longer adapted to the world. It finds itself alienated from the real situation in which it lives and to which it is inevitably exposed. It stands helplessly and without comprehension before the situation with which it is faced.[1] For the approach of archetypal psychology, psychic health and disorders are due to consciousness's good or bad archetypal perspectives, to too much or too little senex / puer / Great Mother / hero / anima, or what have you, to one-sidedness, a monotheistic stance, or to a binary opposition mindset, etc.

The discrepancy in Jung's scheme has the additional feature that the two structures are not simply two positions existing alongside each other on the plane of empirical reality, each one by itself. Rather, there is an intrinsic connection between them, inasmuch as the new situation or altered world ipso facto represents a task for consciousness. Consciousness is essentially challenged, called to the fore. There is an inescapable necessity to become adapted again. And if it refuses to respond to this call to duty then it gets into a contradiction with *itself*, since the task of adaptation to the new situation is *its very own inner necessity*, not something imposed upon it by some other force. Through the intrinsic connection between consciousness and its world the at first merely objective, factual discrepancy is doubled into a subjective, psychological self-contradiction, self-dissociation. And this self-dissociation is what we call a neurosis and what produces all sorts of symptoms. If the task were merely imposed from outside, then the refusal to shoulder it would, probably or certainly, lead to bad

1 Of course, a real neurosis is more than mere helplessness or not understanding. It is the result of the *obstinate refusal* to adapt to the new situation and instead the regressive restoration of the old consciousness as irrenunciable.

practical consequences, to punishment by society or by nature, but not to self-contradiction. A rebel may be completely at one with himself.

This raises the question what it is that makes the adaptation to the altered world consciousness's own psychological duty. The answer is that the altered world referred to is more than the world in which consciousness "happens to find itself", more than the external physical and social environment. The latter may present us with tasks, but ones that remain *psychologically* irrelevant, merely external, although of course in practical regards and for our well-being of great importance. We need to listen to Jung's wording "how its world has altered", and underline "its". What this means becomes clear from the context of Jung's statement. Here he is criticizing the Freudian idea that sexuality is the essential ground of all disorders. With respect to this conception Jung introduces his view that cause and effect have been confused and that the real cause of psychic disorders is the lack of adaptation to an altered world, which secondarily may also have pathological consequences in the area of sexuality and the relation between the sexes.

If we stay strictly within the area of the personal psychology of the individual neurotic we may, for example, think of the "altered world" as the child's all of a sudden finding itself catapulted into puberty and the totally unexpected emergence in him of the nascent adult ego-personality. It is a real change that comes as a total surprise and as something completely new. Although not invited by the child but rather sprung on it, it is nevertheless *its own* altered world. And this is why the task of adapting to it is its own inner necessity.

By the same token, on the collective or cultural level "its world" (consciousness's own world) refers to the culturally apperceived and shaped world, such as the world of the hunter, of the agriculturalist, of scientific and technological civilization, of the industrialized world, to the world of social customs, societal institutions, the organization of the state, and, last but not least the world of a society's ruling ideas. It is always the world as man's own *home* in contrast to an externally given *factual* reality.

As early as 1912, Jung had already pointed out:

> We must never forget that the world is, in the first place, a subjective phenomenon. *The impressions we receive from these accidental happenings are also our own doing* (*CW* 4 § 400, Jung's italics).

Here we need to appreciate the dialectical contradiction at work in Jung's thought. What we *receive*, what truly *comes* to us from out there, is nevertheless our own *product*; it comes to us as always already produced (although not produced by the ego, nor by the individual, but by the non-ego, the suprapersonal objective soul). This far-reaching dictum of Jung's is echoed some years later by his other oft-quoted apodictic statement from his book on psychological types: "The psyche creates reality every day" (*CW* 6 § 78), which in turn has its echo in texts from Jung's late years ("All comprehension and all that is comprehended is in itself psychic, and to that extent we are hopelessly cooped up in an exclusively psychic world" [*MDR* p. 352]. "We are in truth so wrapped about by psychic images that we cannot penetrate at all to the essence of things external to ourselves" [*CW* 8 § 680]). In the "adaptation" quote, Jung clearly has *reality* in mind, the real world around us, but the world *as* psychological world, the soul's own world.

If consciousness's world as its own home has unexpectedly altered of its own accord, if what comes to us from outside as the impressions of a surprisingly different world, the *mind of people* with its habitual traditional form of consciousness and its inherited expectations and conceptions feels helplessly confronted *with its own home as* now alien, fundamentally incomprehensible (Jung had emphasized about consciousness that "it does not *understand* how its world has altered"). A good example in literature is the last line of a 19th century tragedy (*Maria Magdalene*) by Friedrich Hebbel, spoken by one of the main characters with total surrender: "*Ich verstehe die Welt nicht mehr*" ("I no longer understand the world").

I pointed out at first that the logic of Jung's dictum involves a two-position relation, the relation of two separate realities. It is that between the I or consciousness and a real other. Now, however, we need to add to this description the insight that on both sides of the relation we find one and the same soul, that of consciousness, and that of consciousness's other, the world.

Put another way, it is not a question of an isolated subject vis-à-vis a logically or structurally wholly other object (as in the modern subject/object split). The otherness is not one that is inherent in the mental system because its very syntax has a priori been *set up* in such a way that it assigns to the object the place of the other, as being beyond an unbridgeable gap. To be sure, there is real otherness here too that makes itself all too painfully felt, but this other is empirical and experiential otherness, otherness due to a fundamental historical transformation of the hitherto logically and even practically familiar world. Because it is *this familiar world* that has suddenly become absolutely unfamiliar and incomprehensible, it is and remains for consciousness emphatically "*its* world", its very own. Otherness does not imply the distance caused by a logically unbridgeable gap. It is not systemic. It implies only a practical psychic difficulty or plight caused by an empirical change in time, consciousness's incapability to understand, its unadaptedness.

Because the soul is on both sides of the relation, Jung's concept of psychological adaptation is truly psychological. It has nothing to do with any accommodation to socially imposed role models or other external demands. Adaptation is a necessity within the context of the soul's self-relation. Nevertheless, the soul's self-relation is a relation between itself as experiencing subject and itself as this subject's world, and thus as a real other, namely the soul's utterly surprising new self-definition. So we have here a dialectic of same and other.

The same becomes other to itself, which nevertheless remains what it had been: consciousness's own. It might be easy to confuse things at this point and think that same and other refer to consciousness or the subject vis-à-vis the world. Consciousness as such is not an empty vessel and the world not the content with which this vessel is filled. At first there is only One, the *world* the particular way it is apperceived and experienced. As long as the world is the familiar ego-syntonic world, consciousness does not exist separately as something in its own right; it *is* in this stage the experienced *world* and implicitly contained in, and an attribute of, the latter. It is only the surprising alteration or transformation of the before familiar world and the ensuing experience of the discrepancy between what it was used to and what now all of a sudden seems to prevail that forces consciousness to become explicit as something separate from the world. However, the now existing difference or discrepancy between Two[2] is not that of subject or consciousness as vessel, and world as content or object of consciousness. It is the conflict between the old hitherto familiar world with which the I is identified, and the new, altered and incomprehensible world. This alteration of the *world* and its duplication as obsolete but cherished familiar world, and rejected but real new world is what we call an event in the soul's historical life. Consciousness has here not yet become (and does not need to become) conscious *of itself* to experience the threat to its familiar world posed by a new world.

The soul's history is not like natural growth, not, for example, like the growth of a child's *body* or an acorn's sprouting and the sprout's getting bigger and finally developing into a mighty oak tree. There is change and transformation in such a case, too, but not through the opening up of a fundamental discrepancy between two, a conscious expectation and a factual utterly different reality. Natural change means that the previous condition goes totally under in its new form or is replaced by it. No self-alienation, self-dissociation, because nothing of the old situation is retained, and thus also no need for adaptation. Soul history is objective change, the objective soul's giving itself a new form, a new objectification or *real* presence, that catches subjective consciousness by surprise because consciousness stays faithfully, loyally, committed to and informed by the old condition of its world. Consciousness experiences the necessity of becoming adapted again to the altered world as an imposition.

Returning from here to the psychological theory that rejects history as intrinsic to psychology we have to state that in it there is no equivalent to this relation and dynamic. Being structurally a one-position theory, it is only concerned with explicit consciousness in isolation, with the subject. This may be an utterly surprising thesis since it was Hillman who demanded that psychology

2 This is actually a pleonasm since "Two" and "discrepancy" are one and the same thing.

move "from mirror to window", that is, from the individual's ultimately narcissistic introspection and self-exploration in the consulting room to the concern with the real world out there. Did he not, in his "Yellowing of the Work", declare that all kinds of "fermenting corruption" (that he diagnosed as plaguing psychology today) "may actually be how the psyche is yellowing into the cosmos"? It was Hillman who showed his own serious concern with the real world out there by proclaiming in the very first statement with which he opened his and Michael Ventura's book (with the same title) that "We've had a hundred years of psychotherapy and the world's getting worse"? Did he not want to bring imaginal psychology to such topics of public interest as city planning, architecture, the modern traffic situation, etc.? How then can I claim that his approach is even intrinsically worldless and solely concerned with subjective consciousness?

I admit this needs some explanation. In his Paris1989 lecture on the yellowing of the work Hillman announced that he had literally given up work in the consulting room and instead begun to become active in the public world, for example, by lecturing and getting active in the "men's movement". If we focus on his being one main figure in the men's movement of that time, in which the reading of or listening to poetry seems to have been one essential feature, we can say that his commitment to this movement has certainly nothing to do any more with introspection. But is it merely because of this a move into the *world*, into the cosmos, or not much rather the same old kind of devotion to the subjective consciousness of *people* with the only difference that it is now addressing a crowd instead of single individuals and remaining on the universal level of the imaginal or poetic (instead of one's concern with concrete personal details)? The minds of the participants are supposed to become more poetical through more contact with poetry and other imaginal material. Hillman himself declared in other contexts that in his work he was in general "out to affect vision". This means of course people's or our vision. The style of consciousness, the perspectives dominating our consciousness were the true focus of his psychological work. He emphasized rhetoric. He wanted us to develop what he called "animal sense" and "*aisthesis*" because then we would find the world alive. "Vision makes the world real; aisthesis makes it bearable; rhetoric makes it speakable ..." All this takes place solely on the human, all-too-human side, in subjective consciousness. In *us* something has to change. The world itself is not reached. Malgré lui, the world does not really figure in his scheme as something in its own right. There is no engagement of or interconnection with it. His work dwells on the ego-personality side. The logical place for the world (the "second position") in his psychology does not merely remain empty, but is on principle absent.

The fact that the world as a real other *does not matter* for archetypal or imaginal psychology comes out clearly through a comparison of Hillman's "the world's getting worse" with Jung's "[consciousness] does not understand how its world has altered". The first statement is a condemnation. The world is dismissed as being in the process of decline. Getting worse includes its having become soulless. The tacit implication is that this decline is *our* fault. We have forgotten the gods, we have not been soulful enough or too monotheistic, probably on account of having been dominated by the false or bad archetypal images. If *we* change, if we move from the modern abstract "universe" to "cosmos", from concept to *aisthesis* and animal sense, if we work on our vision and rhetoric, then and only then something might change for the better in the world, too. Ultimately, our task is to rescue the world. Man as the sole subject, indeed as Savior; the world as passive, if not dead object.

Jung's scheme, by contrast, assigns subjectivity to the world. *It* has changed. The change is *its* doing. We have no guilt (German *Schuld*). But instead we owe something to the altered world (*wir sind ihr etwas schuldig*), namely, to adapt to it. This requires that we learn to understand, truly comprehend it. *It* is the standard and measure for consciousness, for the new attitude that the latter has to assume to be once more attuned to it. We must allow *it* to teach us about its new form. *It* is man's psychopomp. The answer is already there; it lies in the altered world itself (as negative or "worsened" as it might appear). Consciousness has merely not understood it yet.

The problem is not the world, nor the subject or the consciousness of the human being(s) either, but the connection between the subject and its world, namely, the *lack* of adaptation to the world, consciousness's (perfectly natural) lagging behind in its comprehension of a surprise alteration. There is nothing wrong with the world, the alteration does not (in itself) mean decline or decay. All that happened is the world's radical form change, its historical movement and self-transformation *of its own accord*.

In other words, for Jung it is the *objective, autonomous soul* that is at work in the historical alteration of the world. He works with or in terms of the two-position logic of the psychological difference whose internal relation he once tried to capture in a simple ordinary-life image by referring to a small bank teller who, when he led a guest through his city, also showed him "his bank". The subject is dethroned. Not dethroned because it is subject to powerful archetypes, but because there is this real objective other of which *he* is a small part. The soul is precisely not in consciousness. It is not dependent on a particular soulful style or perspective of consciousness, on the anima being present in its thinking, on its vision being informed by poetic imagination, etc., as important as all this *subjectively* doubtlessly is. No, the real soul, the real negation,[3] is in the alteration of the world.

The bank teller is employed by his bank and has a subservient job to perform for it. In a similar way consciousness has a task, the task of adaptation to its world. And adaptation is more than one's work on consciousness and its images or vision. It means a real engagement with the other, a cognitive relation, a penetration of its innermost logic. We may think here of the Biblical Adam's *knowing* Eve his wife and she conceived (Gen. 4:1).

I mentioned earlier that the dictum of Jung's that I relied on in this Introduction referred only to personal psychology. I merely claimed that it can also directly be transferred to the collective or cultural sphere. Now I want to corroborate this claim and above all also the thesis that the soul is in the objective world and not in our consciousness, by citing late Jung's metaphor for the cultural predicament of the modern world, the metaphor of "the guest requesting admittance" and what Jung has to say about him.

> We have no dominants any more, they are in the future. Our values are shifting, everything loses its certainty, even *sanctissima causalitas* has

3 "Real negation" is the title of an as yet unpublished paper.

> descended from the throne of the axioma and has become a mere field of probability. Who is the awe-inspiring guest who knocks at our door portentously? Fear precedes him, showing that ultimate values already flow towards him. Our hitherto believed values decay accordingly and our only certain[t]y is that the new world will be something different from what we were used to.

A little later in the same letter Jung speaks of

> the intensity of our prejudice against the future, which we obstinately want to be as we expect it. *We* decide, as if we knew. (*Letters 2*, pp. 590 and 591, to Read, 2 September 1960.)

Jung does not resort to a value judgment, does not denounce the world as getting worse, despite his very clearly being aware of the decay of our hitherto believed values and, we could say, that the rug has psychologically been pulled out from under us. He remains on the descriptive level. Instead he looks at the situation from a strictly psychological point of view and sees in this fundamental, and as yet incomprehensible, change the arrival of a guest who, as guest, needs to be received into consciousness. (The metaphor of the guest confirms the soul connection between consciousness and its other, the "its" of the earlier phrase "how its world has altered".) This guest knocking at its door is in this passage his image for the objective, autonomous soul. For this reason we must not entertain prejudices against the future. Jung sees that our dominants and values are not to be found in the past, in what we were accustomed to and is so precious to us, but only in the future. And he warns against our obstinately holding on to and defending our old values and expectations. This defense would be a pure ego stance. It is not the world that needs to adapt to our ideas, but the other way around. The future, that is, the new world that will be very different from what we were used to, brings the new dominants to us as the awe-inspiring guest.

It is not without good reason that the words "our" and "we" in the statement about "our prejudice against the future" are used, which include the speaker, Jung. For with his unflinching rejection of a negative stance towards the future late Jung also courageously dismisses his own earlier deep-seated longing to cling at least to the *old form* of the mythic, the longing, still today so widespread among Jungians, for a recovery of myth and meaning, even if he had already in his early years fully understood that the old myths themselves (including the Christian "myth") had become obsolete.

Written long before Hillman's work, many ideas in Jung's quoted statement from the letter to Read could be read as an advance critique of Hillman's position. "*We* decide, as if we knew"! We "obstinately want [the future, the world] to be as we expect it". This applies very well to Hillman's response to the state of the world, to his offering the ego program of advocating, for the subjective mind, a psychological polytheism, Greek myths as well as Neoplatonic philosophy and Renaissance spirit, etc., i.e., the cherished old values and recipes. What remains excluded is a real other. An other that makes demands on us and that is precisely not the problem, but the answer,[4] not "bad" or "getting worse", but the advent of the guest, the manifestation of the objective, autonomous soul in its new shape. We can now even say that psychologically consciousness's moral disqualification of the new world as "getting worse" and as a "fallen world" is nothing but the refusal to *own* this world as truly *its* (*his*, *our*) world, or consciousness's stubborn dissociating itself from it. It is the refusal to let the knocking guest in and to accept him as the teacher from whom alone consciousness can learn what its attitude would have to be like to be able to make it be adapted to its world again. There *is* in this scheme no other world. The longing to return to and revive what once was, the dream of a new "renaissance" as an alternative to the awe-inspiring guest is illusionary.

Now we have become ready to see through Hillman's using the phrase of "historical literalism" as his slating attack on the focus of psychology on historical phenomena.

Before coming to this analysis, we need to see that this is a strange use of "literalism". Normally, this term refers to one's mistakenly reading *symbolic* texts like myths as reports about real people and happenings, identifying a *dream* father with the father in external reality, or taking a *metaphorically* meant expression at face value. It is a critique of one's understanding something. But in combination with "historical", literalism is used as a verdict

4 This is the same logic as in Jung's dictum about neurosis: "It is not what *is being* cured, but what cures us" (*GW* 10 § 361, my translation. The whole sentence is in italics in the original).

against the *text* itself, as it were, the historical material, and not the *understanding* of the text, namely against one's studying historical situations and conditions, customs and rituals, events or processes for the purpose of interpreting them psychologically.

What according to this view needs to be excluded from psychology is obviously the admission that there is something unchangeably real and inexorably *given* to the reflecting mind of the psychologist, to subjective consciousness, that cannot be completely dissolved and absorbed into the imaginal, i.e., into the mind's own *ideal* sphere, for example, through one's working with "likenesses" or "*epistrophê*". "Vision makes the world real; aisthesis makes it bearable; rhetoric makes it speakable", we have heard Hillman saying. The world does not *come* to us as real, it has to be *made* real by and in *our* vision.

It is the inexorable otherness and adamant reality of something outside subjectivity's own imaginings, or it is, to use a favorite phrase of Jung's, the "collision with reality", that threatens the very principle of imaginal psychology and its precious sovereignty. In other words, the formula "historical literalism" is a defense against imaginal psychology's having to acknowledge a really real other, the actually existing world as standard and measure given to it from outside its own subjectivity. It is an attempt to blind itself to its finding itself in a real historical situation that challenges consciousness, calling it to the fore: in the case of an unexpectedly *altered* world by demanding of consciousness its adaptation *to* this real other, and in the case of the psychological study of earlier historical phenomena by demanding that consciousness revises its possibly naive, possibly superficial and unpsychological cherished preconceptions of them. Ultimately, this means that this formula ("historical literalism") is imaginal psychology's *defense against the concept of the objective, autonomous soul.* The poetic mind wants to stay virginally untouched. The charge of "historical literalism" is sleeping beauty's hedge of thorns.

With this insight a first answer to our main question in this Introduction has already been given, an answer to the question what, both psychologically (for the soul) and for the constitution of psychology, is at stake with the inclusion of the sense of history in psychology's very definition, as it is to be found in Jung's dictum, "without history there can be no psychology, and certainly no psychology of the unconscious". On psychology's theoretical acknowledgment of history, that is, on its logical openness to a possible collision with reality, depends whether or not a psychology provides a place in its thinking for the *autonomous* or *objective soul* as something inexorably real, with which consciousness is unamenably *confronted* and to which it needs to *adapt* as *its* own world. Can it accept that *its own* world may at times have become a fundamentally *altered* world, and is it ready to accept this altered world as its one and only world, more than that, as its teacher? Does one's psychological theory truly allow for a second position in its logic, for "the bank" in addition to "the bank-tellers"? Or does it, as one-position scheme, stay encased in its subjectivity?

Jung's ideas about the arrival of the guest were laid down in a letter written during his last year of life. Another text written more than twenty years earlier gives voice to the same figure of thought, only in a very different context and with different emphases, showing that his thinking along this line of thought is more than an occasional and isolated instance. The text I have in mind was briefly mentioned at the beginning of this Introduction. It is contained in his seminar talk to the London Guild of Pastoral Psychology in 1939 on *The Symbolic Life*, specifically in § 632 of *CW* 18.

> What I have spoken of is, alas, to a great extent the past. We cannot turn the wheel backwards; we cannot go back to the symbolism that is gone. ... Doubt has killed it, has devoured it. So you cannot go back. I cannot go back to the Catholic Church. I cannot experience the miracle of the Mass; .... I know it is the truth, but it is the truth in a form in which I cannot accept it any more. I cannot say "This is the sacrifice of Christ," and see him any more. I cannot. It is no more true to me; it does not express my psychological condition. My psychological condition wants something else. I must have a situation in which that thing becomes true once more. I need a new form.

Just as we had read in the passage from his late letter that "Our hitherto believed values decay", we hear in the present quotation that "Doubt has killed it [the symbolism from the past], has devoured it." It has become obsolete, truly passé. A radical change has happened. Consciousness's world has altered. What is, however, different to the earlier idea as well as Jung's dictum about the necessity of adaptation to the altered world is that the inexorable other, the collision with reality, shows itself here only negatively, namely as an irrevocable loss, an emphatically repeated "I cannot", and a "not any more", which might even evoke in us the association of the "Nevermore!" of Poe's Raven. Instead of the painfully felt *presence* of a new world which remains completely ununderstandable, and instead of the insistent knocking of the guest at our door wanting to be admitted into consciousness, we have here only the expression of a need, a longing, a hoped-for future. But this is a semantic difference between the two statements and does not imply a difference of the basic thought structures.

If we think back to the dictum about the necessity for adaptation, we realize that Jung's "*I need* a new form" is, compared to the idea of the guest in his late letter, a deficient form of his thought. It expresses an *ego* demand and settles in the stance of waiting and hoping, like "Waiting for Godot" in the Theater of the Absurd. To correct it we need to say: There is nothing to wait for, to long for. The very point is that "the new form" *is* already present; the guest is already portentously knocking at consciousness's door. The truth in its new form is inherent and already at work in the inexorably real *altered* world that emerged as the result of the loss of the past symbolism, as the loss's own result. And the feeling of one's needing a new form, that is, of its still having to come or needing to be sought, is the defense mechanism of procrastination, of projecting the idea of a Savior (a "saving *new* form of truth") into the no-man's-land of a utopian future at the very time when the New is already standing right in front of consciousness's own door, demanding to be let in. It is the wrong way about: Not "*I* need ..." but *the guest* needs. And what he needs is to be allowed to teach consciousness about the appropriate attitude to be assumed so that it becomes at long last able to *understand* how concretely its world has altered and be adapted to it again.

It would be another crucial error if we thought that this understanding has to be the work of the ego, the subjective soul, our consciousness. It is not an ego achievement, and to see it as such would be absolutely counterproductive. It is not our intellectual effort that is required. Thinking back to the cited sentence from Gen. 4:1 about Adam's *knowing* Eve his wife and she conceived, we must not think that "Adam" would in our context refer to the subjective psyche. No, our consciousness has the position of "Eve", who *is being* known; our consciousness has to receive and *conceive*, whereas the adamantly real altered world corresponds to the penetrating Adam. *We* cannot, we do not have to *do* anything—except *owning* the altered world as *our own* (one and only) world and *receiving* it as the guest. It is the guest who will do the work.

- One point here is that he will *force* the necessary understanding upon consciousness. Real learning in psychological spheres is always learning the hard way, is *being* taught by the Real, by the objective soul.[5]
- A second point is: the guest will force this understanding on consciousness in the course of time. This being taught will take time, decades or maybe centuries. Patience is needed, both in the sense of our enduring the guest's painful work upon our consciousness and in the sense of allowing it to take

5 Our having to be the *passive* "victims" of the autonomous soul's work upon us has its place only in the psychological sphere of man's in-ness in the processes of the soul's logical life and the need of his "becoming adapted again". There is another sphere, that of psychology itself as a discipline, that is, the sphere of the psychologist's work of studying psychological phenomena from a reflective distance, and in it the human subject's *activity* has its place. In working with dreams, interpreting myths, fairy tales, historical or cultural phenomena with a view to gaining a psychological understanding of them by interiorizing them into themselves, the psychologist is called to the fore on his own responsibility. Here the labor of the concept is needed. The way I described things so far, passivity and activity are each unambiguously distributed among the two spheres. But it is more complicated. Each side has also its own opposite aspect. The soul's work upon us has to be answered by our courageously coming forward, as will, e.g., become apparent in chapter 1 on Luther. We cannot just sit down and keep passively waiting for the door to be opened like the "man from the country" did in Kafka's "Before the Law". Conversely, the psychologist's active thinking on his own responsibility has to be a truly *passive listening* to what the soul is saying about itself in the respective phenomenon studied. It is not the ego's activity. The subject doing the thinking, if it is to be a real psychologist's thinking, has to be an already "deceased one", to have "crossed over to the other side", as I put it elsewhere. I even compared it once to the activity of a "sleepwalker". In other words, passivity and activity are dialectically interlaced.

all the time *it* needs.

- And the third point is that the guest will force it not upon my or your personal consciousness, as our individual experience and insight, but upon the objective logical constitution of modern man's consciousness at large.

The first answer to our question of the importance of history for the constitution of psychology was that the notion of the objective, autonomous soul depends on the inclusion of a sense of history. There is a second answer to our main question. It is that it is the notion of history that brings interiority, our in-ness in the soul. The Jungian idea about the necessity of becoming adapted to the altered world thrusts us right between the old and the new, right into the soul's logical life, into the stream of events, into "the great battle between the present and the past or the future" (*CW* 18 § 279). According to a central axiom of Jung's we are surrounded by the objective soul on all sides. The soul is not in us, we are in it. And it, the soul, is the place where the action is.

This is what also forces us to retract part of Jung's statement, hinted at in the beginning, that in contrast to all former times when the soul was not on the inside, but outside, now and for modern psychology "everything lies *in the soul*; everything, so to speak, on the *side of the inner*" (*CW* 10 § 158, transl. modif.). No, *the soul* is still outside just as it has always been, and everywhere in pre-modern cultures.[6] What in our time is indeed inside, in us, is, on the one hand, our emotions, desires, impulses, our fantasies, ideas, ideals, and hopes, our likings and dislikes, our illusions and prejudices, and so on. But all this belongs to the private psyche and the personal unconscious, not to the soul. On the other hand, it is only the sedimented semantic contents of the now obsolete *former* soul, which in the *altered* world have sunken *into* the pri-

6 A neurosis with severe symptoms is an imitation of the *autonomous* soul *in little*, the subjectivized experience and thus toy version of one's being faced with an inexorable other within the encapsulation in the private sphere of the personal psyche, as if it were an external reality. Freud spoke of the *innere Ausland*, the internal foreign country. The fact that neurosis is an *imitation* and *subjectivization* of the autonomous soul as a real Other may explain why, according to the observation of Viktor Frankel and others, personal neuroses recede or go away when the individual is directly caught up in an actual war.

vate psyche's bottomless pit as the so-called (collective) unconscious, from where isolated, contextless fragments of them may at times surface in the form of archetypal or numinous dream images and visionary experiences.

History as psychological concept allows us to see the soul not as entity and agent behind the scene, but as actuosity, as life, ongoing process, as "formation, transformation", in short as history itself. Thus it makes itself felt as fundamentally *open future*, an unknown and unknowable future for and from the point of view of *each* present, that is, our present today just as well as each present in the past.[7] This is in contrast to the static idea of soul as timeless images, eternal gods or archetypes, and as *our* cultivation of a soulful, poetic vision and approach to life. Paradoxically, a psychology that is based on the concept of timeless images or archetypes is comparable to the natural sciences. For the latter, the so-called "laws of nature" are always the same; there can in principle not be anything new under the sun as well as of above the sun; only the phenomenology of nature is in constant flux

7 The process of history could be described in the following way:
1. Primary unity: The familiar ego-syntonic world. 2. The awe-inspiring guest's completely upsetting knock at the door, resulting in the lack of adaptation. 3. The guest's slowly forcing his way inside and decomposing the old mentality (the battle between the old and the new as the process of gradual adaptation and learning to understand). 4. A new primary unity, which as the end of the first process is at the same time phase 1 of a new process, which in turn shows that the phase with which I began here is itself already the last result of a preceding 4-phase process resulting in a state of harmonious adaptation experienced as oneness.

If one wishes to know what motivates the historical process, what and how one phase leads to the next, I would say that when consciousness has subjectively fully adapted to the altered world the adaptation is nevertheless not yet complete. It becomes complete only by objectifying itself, giving itself a real presence in the culture through produced cultural works, through new social forms, new explicit doctrines, etc. This externalized, objectified, and materialized form of the *subjective* newly adapted form of consciousness is not only different from what subjective consciousness had in mind, it also develops its own internal dynamic and independence (e.g., technology!) and so slowly turns into what Jung called the altered world, which in turn produces a discrepancy and makes a new adaptation necessary.

The further back in history we go, the longer the phases of primary unity lasted because life stayed so close to nature and the changes did not make a fundamental difference. But with time the alterations became so extensive and incisive that the process of history happens at much greater speed.

("Big Bang", the birth and dying of stars, the continental drift, ocean floors becoming the highest mountain chains, ice ages and interglacial periods, biological evolution, etc.). For archetypal or imaginal psychology the basic factors are likewise eternal; only how their effects show in different persons, at different times, in different cultures, and in the same person at different phases of their life is mutable, as is at the altars of which "gods" people choose to worship. People's behaviors, beliefs, feelings, and customs change. The soul itself, its nature and interest, remains the same.

That we should become soulful in our thinking style is certainly a very nice, indeed a *noble* program. But as program it is an ego project, not soul; educational, not psychological. What *it* is about is cultural refinement of the mind, the formation of subjective consciousness in the direction of what has been called (and criticized as) "the beautiful soul" (Schiller, Goethe, Hegel).[8] With all this we are concerned only with our self-education, and are cocooned in ourselves. We entertain our own "hobby". *We* decide, as if we knew. *We* assign the remedies, pretending to have the answers in our readily available tool chest filled with the old myths, the "Gods", and the imaginal as such, or also, e.g., with ideas of carefully selected "soulful" Neoplatonic philosophers and Renaissance poets.

Apropos "soulful": In response to the charge that his basic stance was nostalgic, Hillman once answered: "... we need to see ... that the nostalgia is a soul mood that can motivate reflective thought, and that without anima the thought becomes ineffective,

---

8 It needs, however, to be noted, as Greg Mogenson reminded me, that there is *another* style of soul-making that does not succumb to "the beautiful soul". For a discussion of it I refer the reader to Part 3 of my book *What is Soul?* entitled, "The Phenomenology of the Soul (2): The Soul as *subject*, style, and work (soul-making)". Almost simultaneously with the present book, another book of mine, *Working with Dreams*, is being published. The two books complement each other and together exemplify the two different psychological concerns. Whereas the present book is devoted to the reflection of man's in-ness in the historical process of the soul's logical life and the question of adaptation to his *world* if it has unexpectedly altered, *Working with Dreams* is an attempt to train the *mind* of the psychologist to read soul phenomena (in this case dreams) truly psychologically, from the perspective of soul, inwardizing them into themselves.

dry, barren". That without anima thought becomes dry and barren is well taken. No objection to that assertion. But apart from the fact that the idea of "soul mood" reveals that the *horizon* of this particular thought is solely the subjective psyche (moods are states of or in the ego-personality) and excludes any hint of the objective soul, the main critical point to be made here is that "anima" is used in a *preconceived fixed* sense. This is already apparent from the context ("nostalgia" and "soul mood"). Once Hillman reacted to my having put Hegel into the foreground with the statement, "Not Hegel; Whitman." Seen in the light of the notion of the present anima topic, this wholesale rejection sight unseen of Hegel implies, I would say, that Hillman is not willing to let himself *be told* by the altered world what "anima" means *now*, means in *it*, how the category of "anima" has redefined itself. He assumes he already knows what anima means and that its definition is timeless.

Could it not be that Hegel's rigorous thinking, his labor of the concept, is a paradigmatic exemplar of how *anima* appears in thought in the modern world and that as such his work might serve as a textbook from which to learn what the *now* necessary *sense* of "anima" is?[9] No, for archetypal and imaginal psychology the soul must not be alive. It must be static. The old definitions of categories like anima or soul or the "Gods" must be atemporal and eternal, immune to history, exempt from epochal transformations. No metamorphosis of "the gods" (consciousness's ruling dominants or categories) in the sense that they "die from time to time". Jung's idea of the "altered world" that needs one's new adaptation to it means, however, a revolutionary change of the very values, highest ideas, categories, and definitions. What else than the very definitions, values, supreme principles, and the logical constitution should be what is altered in a *psychological*, a *soul* sense of "altered world"?

With Jung we could say that clinging to the old sense of anima as a counter-program to the world's getting worse is a perfect example of "the intensity of our prejudice against the future, which we obstinately want to be as we expect it". There is no room for an

9 The fact that there is a new and other sense of anima makes it clear why there can be a form of soul-making not subject to the beautiful soul.

open future, for anything epochally new, unheard of, totally unsuspected. But if so, then psychology is a priori closed, only dealing with a *caput mortuum*, a hangover from the past (cf. *CW* 10 § 363). And would *that* not be what would truly deserves the charge "historical literalism"?

* * *

After this discussion of a crucial theoretical question about history and psychology a few simple comments about the following essays may be in place.

The first essay on young Luther's religious torments takes the reader right into the *present* of (or lying in) a historical past, the time around 1500 A.D., the present precisely in Jung's sense as "the great battle" between the past and the future and as the forceful intrusion of the awe-inspiring guest. We can see here in a concrete example how this battle fought itself out in the psyche of an exceptional individual, a "great man".

What was fought out and what resulted from this battle is the emergence and establishment of the I, a completely new and before unimaginable acquisition or "invention". It is that I that determined the modern Western world from the early-modern period onwards and that was what clearly set apart the Western world—its cultural-historical development and its characteristic form of being-in-the-world—as unique from both the spirit of its own ancient and medieval background *and* from the cultural traditions in other parts of the world (the Islamic world, India, the Far East, to mention only these).

The next two essays explore the same emergence of the I and focus likewise on the historical epoch of the transition from the ancient and medieval to the modern world, so that we can say that all three essays circumambulate the same chapter in the history of the Western soul. But both put another example of the manifestation of the revolutionary change at the center, the invention of linear perspective during the Renaissance. And the stage for this particular manifestion of the change is, other than in Luther's case, not the inwardness of the psyche, but the impersonal or suprapersonal (collective) sphere of the culture at large, and within this sphere the particular cultural domain of painting, the arts.

These two essays, dealing in part with the same topic, the invention of perspective and its psychological implications, overlap to some extent, but are different enough in their vista upon this development and the highlighted features of these processes to complement each other and enrich the understanding of the historical emergence of the I.

The final essay places the historical emergence of the I in the wider context of what it means for the development of *consciousness* as such by exploring Jung's ideas about what precisely 'truly being conscious' means, in particular his ideas about the fundamental shortcomings of the generally prevailing form of consciousness and consciousness's future potential inherent in its concept. The essay discusses what the necessary requirements and "ingredients" are for a possible further development of consciousness into its psychologically full-fledged form that fulfills its concept. ❦

The Introduction and chapters 2 and 4 were written in 2019. A shorter version of Chapter 2 was written for, and in a shorter version presented at, a seminar for Japanese Jungian professors of psychology. Chapter 1 on Luther dates back to 1999, when I delivered an earlier version as a lecture at the Graduate School of Education, Department of Clinical Psychology, Kyoto University. This version was published in Japanese translation by Prof. Toshio Kawai in my book *Shinwa to Ishiki* (Yungu Shinrigaku no Tenkai [Gîgerihhi Ronshû], vol. 3, Tokyo (Nihon Hyôron-sha) 2001. Between 2004 and 2010 it was also presented in a revised German version at my Neresheim seminars, at the Zürich C.G. Jung Institute and the München C.G. Jung Institute. The English version presented in this book includes all the later revisions. The first version of Chapter 3 was written in the early 1990s and in different expansions presented to Jungian colleagues at various occasions and also at the Zürich C.G. Jung Institute during the winter semester 2008/2009.

Chapter One

Young man Luther's terrible spells of religious anguish and the soul's construction of the modern[10] "I"

At the same time an incidental contribution to the theory of neurosis

As is well known, while as monk in the monastery, pre-Reformation Luther went through a long time of terrible qualms, severe anguish about his salvation caused by doubts up to the point of spiritual despair—his so-called '*Anfechtungen*'[11] (*vexationes* and *tentationes*)—until at long last he experienced a breakthrough that ultimately gave rise to the Reformation. In this paper I want to examine in detail and illuminate *psychologically* just *what* it was that was going on in those tribulations. But I must immediately make it clear that this cannot mean reducing religious experience and theological thinking to "nothing but" psychology and deriving the intellectual labor and achievement of a great man of cultural history from the personality of its author and the empirical facts of his biography. For instance, it cannot mean, in explain-

10 I have to caution the reader about the word "modern". It refers here to the *early-modern* (in German: *neuzeitliche*) period from the Renaissance and Reformation to around 1800 and needs to be distinguished from the emphatically "modern" age, the period starting with the Industrial Revolution, the end of classical metaphysics, and politically, after the time of Napoleon. I use "modern" in the title because "early-modern" had not yet been introduced.

11 Roland H. Bainton, *Here I Stand. A Life of Martin Luther*, New York (Mentor Books) 1955, p. 31, explains: "The word he used was *Anfechtung*, for which there is no English equivalent. It may be a trial sent by God to test man, or an assault by the Devil to destroy man. It is all the doubt, turmoil, pang, tremor, panic, despair, desolation, and desperation which invade the spirit of man."

ing his anguish, falling back on alleged traumatizing early childhood experiences, on the family constellation in which he grew up, and on possibly resulting character deformations. All this is something that Luther, as so many others, has been exposed to not only by analysts, but sometimes even by theologians. You must therefore not expect a *clinical* examination.

One really has to make up one's mind. Does one want a clinical approach, or a really psychological one that takes the concept of soul seriously? Psychology must not be confused with a subdivision of anthropology. Psychology is the study of "the soul" and not of man, of personality, of what goes on inside people. For psychology in the strict sense, the human being is not, in the metaphysical sense, the underlying substrate on or in which the soul is to be found as an attribute among other attributes. Psychology "is something broadly human, [...]. Nor, again, is it merely instinctual or biological. If it were, it could very well be just a chapter in a text-book of biology. It has an immensely important social and cultural aspect without which we could not imagine a human psyche at all", says Jung (*CW* 16 § 52), or, another time, "But psychology is neither biology nor physiology nor any science other than the knowledge of the soul" (*CW* 9/I § 63). The soul is a reality *sui generis*, not reducible to anything else. It is itself something, not merely an expression, appearance, reflection *of* something.

What this means is that nothing must be clipped off from the religious and theological dimension of Luther's experiences and thoughts. The religious character is here nothing inauthentic, behind which "actually" *something else* stands, e.g. a drive problem or a conflict of the son with his personal father; nor is it only the rationalization, sublimation, projection, mystification of that alleged "actual". Rather, the respective experience itself, exactly the way it is, is "the best possible formulation"[12] of what it is all about. It must be taken seriously in its content and substance.[13]

But this also means, conversely, that in Luther's experience we

12 I take this phrase from Jung who spoke of the symbol "as the best possible formulation of a relatively *unknown* thing, which for that reason cannot be more clearly or characteristically represented" (*CW* 6 § 815).

13 For an in depth discussion of this emphasis on content and substance see my "The Provenance of C.G. Jung's Psychological Findings", chapter VI in vol. I (*The Neurosis of Psychology*) of my Collected English Papers.

do not understand the religious in its turn religiously or theologically. We do not on our part reduce it once more to *something else*, namely now to ready-made entities presupposed to the experience itself as existing outside of it, such as God, devil, angels or other transcendent realities. Jung once expressed the principle of a truly psychological approach as follows: "In myths and fairy tales as in dreams the soul speaks about itself and the archetypes reveal themselves in their natural interplay as 'creation, transformation, eternal Mind's eternal recreation'" (*CW* 9/I § 400, transl. modif.). The soul speaks about itself, not about us, but also not about God or the world. So when Luther speaks of sin, justification, God, then for theology, to be sure, he is speaking precisely about these objects, e.g., about God. But not so for psychology, *if* it really is psychology. For psychology the soul expresses only itself in its talking of a God. It is similar to a sandplay picture in sandplay therapy: it represents a psychological image, a soul constellation, a picture of a particular moment in the soul's logical life with its internal tensions and differences, rather than being about toy figures and sand.

It is, mind you, a constellation "of *the soul*", a constellation which, as a whole, only gives expression *to itself* and refers to itself or points deeper into itself. It has *omne quo indiget* ("everything that it needs") in itself. It is thus not an expression of the state of mind of Luther as person (or an expression of anything else), not conditioned by causes lying in his biography or biology. And it is not about any objects, it has no referent. It is pure self-reference. The soul displays only itself. To exaggerate: the "religious qualms" that he experiences have nothing to do with Luther personally (that is exaggerated, because as a matter of course they did not exist completely without connection with his personality). It is the other way around. Luther is much rather placed into these religious qualms, as into the first immediacy of a new constellation. He is seized and taken hold of by this constellation as by one historical configuration of the soul's logical life. He is used by it and for it. He is the place of *its* manifestation (not the manifestation of *his* nature, of his *self*). He is the place where the dialectical life inherent in this particular configuration comes out into the open, frees itself to itself and brings about its resolution.

In seiner Seele kämpft, was wird *und* war,
Ein keuchend hart verschlungen Ringerpaar.

(His soul is the battlefield of what *was* and *will be*,
A pair of interlocked and panting wrestlers.)

(C.F. Meyer)

Although on first appearance it may look for us as if he, Luther, was the one who is battling, C.F. Meyer tells us that it is *they*, those two "wrestlers", the past and the future constitution of the soul, who fight their conflict out. Within his subjective psyche, but unbeknownst to him, the objective soul is trying to wriggle out of its old skin, and through this struggle, and as a result of it, to produce for itself an entirely unforeseen new self-definition as its new "skin". It has to be a painful struggle because there is no master plan and no antecedently known goal. The new is simply what happens to arise as result from the battle.

My exploration has two parts. I will first briefly present the phenomenology of Luther's religious qualms and thereafter in detail interpret it psychologically in many separate steps and in various aspects. Despite my rejection of the clinical approach, I will, to begin with, present Luther's struggles *as if* they were the struggles of a patient in analysis.

Part One of the Case History: The Symptoms

Luther's *Anfechtungen*

At the age of 22, Luther entered the monastery of the Augustinians in Erfurt. Why exactly is not clear. He had been in the middle of his academic studies (Law), had apparently been successful and seems to have been a cheerful and outward-looking student. In the monastery, however, he did not find the calm and deep inner peace that was promised by the status of a monk and which he probably had hoped for himself.[14] On the contrary, he was plunged

14 Only the initial period, the time of his novitiate, seems to have been free of inner turmoil.

into the deepest conflicts precisely by his resolute dedication to God, and these were not, as we might think, conflicts *between* the monastic and the worldly way of life or *between* his spiritual vows and the temptations of instinct and sensuality. The latter was not his problem. The renunciations that are imposed on those who want to live as Augustinian monks did not seem to cause him any difficulties. He had once and for all left the world behind, and thus the renunciation of the world was an accomplished fact. The world and worldly desires were simply no longer an issue for him. *They* could not plague him. No, the conflict was a genuine intra-monastic, a purely spiritual or intra-religious one. It is important to get that straight and not to lose sight of it.

The conflict was sparked off by the Mass, more specifically, when young Luther, having been ordained as priest, had to celebrate Mass. He was horrified by the thought that God, according to doctrine, becomes in fact present in human form at Mass. Every day the priest stands in the presence of the All High and the All Holy. How could he, Luther, a sinful man, face and hold his ground vis-à-vis the *holiness* of God?

In the Middle Ages, entry into a monastery was generally regarded as a return to innocence like that of a newly baptized child. For Luther, however, this return to innocence did not become an existentially felt truth. He stayed conscious of his essential state of sinfulness, not because of particular failings of his, but simply *as a human* confrontated with God. In view of the knowledge and deeply felt awareness of his own *absolute* unworthiness[15] and impurity over against God on the one hand and his recognition of God's *absolute* majesty on the other, he was thrown into a total panic and despair. He went through torments of hell that did not subside. He sought help from all the means provided by the medieval Church for such qualms.

He fasted, prayed and kept vigils far beyond what the rules demanded. But all devotions and good works were to no avail. As a measure of self-mortification, he also slept without the blanket

15 The unworthiness is *absolute* precisely because it is one that is not dependent or based on specific empirical offenses or faults, on evil deeds or omissions by the individual. It is the unworthiness (over against God) inherent in human *nature* as such.

granted to the monks in their unheated cells, and almost literally froze to death, but without being rewarded by the return of inner tranquillity. Obviously all these measures were not the way to obtain certainty that the just wrath of God would be soothed, that one could strike a deal with God about one's salvation or "justification". Even the Church's treasury of merit piled up by the superfluous merits of the righteous and the saints could not reach him, nor could the Church's established means of grace.

Luther had a very wise, experienced, and warm-hearted spiritual advisor, Dr. Staupitz, a man himself filled with a deep religious feeling. Dr. Staupitz was not unimportant for him, on the contrary, but as far as Luther's particular problem was concerned he was unable to really help him, neither by advice and arguments, nor by words of encouragement and consolation. The anguish of the sinful man, that is, man alienated from God, only became embedded deeper and deeper in Luther. The question Luther was driven by was: "How do I get a gracious God? How can I become just before God?" Even the Sacrament of Penance (extremely extensively made use of by him), which qua sacrament had to directly bring a real influx of grace, did not bring him this grace. The problem with it was that, in order to be forgiven, sins must be confessed, but that in order to be unreservedly confessed they must be completely and precisely recognized and remembered. Luther searched his conscience and memory most painstakingly for every small and smallest non-pious emotion and confessed extensively, once for up to six hours in one go, only to find out that the more meticulously he sought to win God, the more desperate he became. He had fallen into a dead end, a vicious circle: His conflict was on principle unsolvable.

For one thing, there was this problem: In spite of all his honest efforts, he could never be sure that he had detected within himself all the sins, all the secret impulses of the egoistic will. Memory plays tricks on you, and there is even a natural but often unconscious interest in yourself as sinful man to hide certain things from yourself. But if at any point something, even the slightest sin, had escaped him, then he could ipso facto not confess or repent of it, and then forgiveness was impossible, and all other efforts of his self-searching were also in vain. In addition, there was a second and much worse point: even if he had discovered absolutely every sinful emotion in himself, how could he be sure that his repentance was really authentic, that his will to satisfy God was really a total and pure one? For it was clear that man's sinful heart is not at all capable of the true repentance demanded of it, that repentance must much rather already come out of love for God in order to be perfect repentance. But God could only be loved by a heart which was not sinful, only by one which was already in God's grace. This, however, was precisely the very goal to be achieved through repentance and penance. Here we see how hopeless his situation was, because it was circular. Luther was trapped. Man's natural will was earthly, an eudemonistic will. A repentance, through which one only wants to avoid God's punishment and attain happiness, eternal beatitude, for oneself, in truth did not serve God at all, but only one's selfish will. Even piety could be a way in which man seeks only himself. But egoism or self-centeredness was the core of all sin; it was at bottom the very unbelief and ingratitude towards God.

But that is not all. A third still higher level of distress lay in the thought of the absolute majesty of God, which is above all human concepts and expectations of justice. God was so exalted that he was not bound by any rules, but could have chosen or condemned people to the status of election or damnation before all time, regardless of their merits or sins. This was expressed in the doctrine of predestination. With it, all efforts, all struggling to obtain the grace of God would be exposed as completely meaningless.

Luther's terrible disconcertment mounted to such a nightmarish state that the mere rustling of a leaf in the wind could throw him into fear and tremble. The battle he fought, or perhaps more correctly: the one that raged in him, must have been of tremendous might. Luther felt himself surrounded by demons, and when he speaks of hell, one can feel that for him it was not a place in the afterlife, but a living experience that he had already lived through in this life in his own inner being.

His despair drove him to the point that he hated God. The hatred of God rose in him because God, as Luther experienced him in such moments, demanded something on principle unfulfillable from man in order to punish him for not having fulfilled it. That was precisely the vicious circle. Was God only an unjust, cruel, arbitrary god who, on a whim, hardened the hearts of certain people and condemned them, thus from the outset giving them no chance at all, just as if he had his joy in their eternal torment? Was God, we might say, a sadistic God? *Theoretically*, such hatred could perhaps have brought Luther liberation from his crisis. In his hatred Luther could have completely turned away from God, turned against him. That would, to be sure, not have been the real *solution* to his conflict, but it would have been a de facto end of his suffering from it. As hateful, God would have been brought into the status of an external enemy, that is to say, Luther would have transformed an internal, intrapersonal conflict between a deeply felt demand or desire and his equally experienced own absolute incapability into a kind of interpersonal conflict between himself and God, however a God from whom he would in this case precisely have explicitly dissociated himself. He would thus have simply 'got out' of his conflict as one that was solely *his* own.

But his hatred did not have this separating effect. On the contrary, it pushed the conflict to its extreme. This was so because Luther, in spite of his hatred, held fast to his deepest longing as irrenunciably his own, namely the longing to be able to love God from the bottom of his heart. But this meant that his hatred of God was the absolute opposite extreme to what he actually wanted; it was the ultimate, even absolute sin: blasphemy, rebellion against the majesty of God. These blasphemous thoughts were torture for Luther, and he fought against them at the first moment when they tried to emerge in him, without being able to stop them. That was for him his being "*in morte et inferno*" (in death and in hell). "The fate of the damned in hell had to be like this: to be forced to have thoughts that were blasphemous and from which one was nonetheless not able to free oneself", Karl Holl says, describing Luther's feelings at that time.[16]

Luther told his spiritual guide Staupitz about these thoughts and feelings, and the latter's response was: "I don't understand it".

16 Karl Holl, *Gesammelte Aufsätze zur Kirchengeschichte I, Luther*, Tübingen (J.C.B. Mohr [Paul Siebeck]) ^{6}1932, p. 27, my transl.

Psychological Interpretation

Tragedy, not comedy. In my book *Der Jungsche Begriff der Neurose*[17] I developed the Jungian concept of neurosis on the basis of the neurosis that C.G. Jung himself had at the age of eleven and of which he said that it was from it that he learned what a neurosis is.[18] On his way home from school Jung had been pushed from behind by a classmate, so that he fell down and hit his head on the curb of the sidewalk. At the moment of the impact the thought flashed through his mind: "Now you won't have to go to school any more." He remained lying there longer than necessary and a little later was taken to the nearby house of two aunts of his. Since then, he repeatedly developed fainting spells as soon as he was supposed to go to school or study for school. Thanks to these fainting spells he could stay at home and pursue his games and hobbies and indulge in his dreams to his heart's content. Jung was once again able to enjoy the paradise of childhood, unmolested by all social demands and duties.

We see immediately that the disorder in Luther has a completely different character. I wrote in the referenced book about Jung's childhood neurosis that in it Jung had once again performed for himself the comedy of the paradise of childhood. In the case of Luther's disorder, one could not claim something analogous. In Jung's case, neurosis could take the form of comedy because in his case there was a strict separation between the symptoms, which were limited and only occasionally occurring fainting spells, on the one hand, and the "morbid gain" achieved through the symptoms (complete freedom from school and having to learn), on the other. On account of the splitting of the whole into two separate empirical phenomena, the gain was not amalgamated and burdened with the symptoms. It could be pure gain. Such a separation obviously does not exist with Luther. In his case, there is decidedly only a unified One, only one empirically visible phenomenon: the painful state of terrible feelings of unworthiness. Even if Luther pretended something in his "neurosis"

17 W. G., *Der Jungsche Begriff der Neurose*, Frankfurt/Main et al. (Peter Lang) 1999.
18 *MDR* p. 30 ff.

(let's call his condition neurosis for the moment), it was definitely a "tragedy", not a comedy. And if there should be any profit or triumph in it, then it must lie completely *concealed* in the suffering inside or behind him.

In fact, I maintain that seen from the outside this intolerable state went along with an inner gain, even triumph, however not on the empirical but on the psychological level. The gain consisted in the fact that in and by means of what was empirically *truly* unbearable, *psychologically* an absolute claim was realized, the claim of being called or destined to the highest. His absolutely miserable suffering was the very form in which the self-edification of the claim to his belonging *absolutely* to God took place. Completely independent of whether this claim could be shown to be obviously *empirically* fulfilled or whether, as in the case of Luther, one failed with it, this claim was *psychologically* fully established, even, and indeed precisely, in the case of its empirical failure. For the soul, only the *claim* as such, the concept, the mere idea, counts. The question of its positive-factual realization is irrelevant. The soul is, after all, the sphere of absolute negativity.

Here we come across a form of how the *psychological difference* shows itself. Two levels must be distinguished. What from its empirical-factual outside and *for* man as a person is in Luther's case nothing but utter pain, humiliation, failure, is, seen from the inside and *for* the "soul", highest triumph and greatest bliss. It is similar to what happens in a psychological complex, e.g. the mother complex. The "mother" as mental idea or concept triumphs just as much when sons or daughters want to distance themselves from the empirical mother by hating and constantly fighting with her as when they are tied to their mother's apron strings and fear to have to take a step away from her. For in hatred and argument "the mother" is just as much constantly edified and proves to be of absolutely importance as when she is obviously loved. Love or hate make no difference to "the mother". In both cases "she" as psychological complex and soul topic gets what she wants, the unconditional importance, the quasi divine worship that "she"—seen from "her" point of view—deserves.

It is therefore not *Luther*'s gain or triumph, but the triumph of *that claim itself*, that principle, which asserts itself in him and through him even and precisely by going *against* him, against his personal well-being. It is as if this process followed the motto of Emperor Ferdinand I: *fiat iustitia, et pereat mundus*. I said that it is "*precisely* in the case of his empirical failure" that the claim establishes itself as a reality. For it could not do this at all to the same extent if he succeeded with his project. This is because the claim obviously does not aim at empirical conditions or states of being. As an unconditional claim, it is also a claim *to* something *unconditional*, something that is fundamentally above the sphere of empirical factual conditions. In one's practical failure, and only in it, only in the way of negativity, can the proof be furnished that the soul is not at all concerned with pragmatic advantages or benefits, that it is fundamentally superior to all such natural needs and desires. And precisely in this lies the triumph. We can perhaps make the initially somewhat strange idea of the identity of (empirical) failure and (mental) triumph a little more accessible to ourselves by thinking of the example of anorexia nervosa. In empirical starvation and excessive loss of weight, sometimes to the point of literal death, the principle, the idea, of standing above all bodily needs triumphs—at the expense of the person in whom it triumphs.

In the neurosis of the eleven-year-old Jung it was not so clear that it was about an unconditional claim. True, it was also about something "metaphysical": about rescuing the idea of "childhood paradise" in the sense of the fundamental sympathetic oneness of man and nature and total freedom from any sense of responsibility and duty. But inasmuch as Jung's "morbid gain" was first of all quite earthly-practical in nature, the psychological essence of the gain had not yet been truly released into its own, come home to itself. The mental triumph was still adulterated and mixed up with the natural and practical, so that it could also be confused with a merely natural and factual benefit of the ego-personality, a practical advantage. "The soul", however, is *contra naturam*, counternatural, inhuman.

Luther, on the other hand (or more precisely: "the soul" in him) had clearly reached beyond the whole level of the merely-natural to the highest and absolute. By almost literally bringing himself even to the brink of physical death, the overcoming of nature (*not* of this or that natural thing or aspect, but the whole level of the natural as such, the naturalistic standpoint in general) was fully accomplished. And by *not* achieving in practical reality what he was seeking, the psychological-spiritual (ontological or logical) level of his aspiration was released into itself in full purity. On this level triumph was indeed *attained*. It was precisely the triumph of man's being, in his self-understanding, fundamentally above earthly-natural interests and states. He was in his humanity or his innermost essence a child of God and not only, as according to his external reality, a child of nature, of the earth, a child of his parents, not only "dust of the ground". It was precisely in the desperate feeling of being radically alienated from God that the claim to be actually, namely *in principle*, connected with God was established and solidified: to be allowed to understand oneself *from God*. To under'stand' oneself from God means, however, nothing other than that one stands oneself on the standpoint of God, that oneself has taken this standpoint. Could there be anything greater? Failure is the way in which the idea of *absolutely* belonging to God edifies itself.

Positedness. The psychic states into which Luther had gotten were not absolutely necessary from the point of view of empirical reality, but owed themselves to a making, a mise-en-scène. The questions with which Luther wrestled were not fundamentally new. The medieval Church offered both detailed theoretical answers and practical pastoral solutions for such problems and experiences. Numerous extremely pious monks and other believers had in the past already fallen into doubts and religious qualms. The theologians had long since answered the question of the salvation of sinful man in a differentiated way. From a psychological point of view we can also not assume that a fundamentally novel, radically different experience of God had happened to Luther for which medieval consciousness was completely unprepared. It is not the case that Luther simply was all of a sudden *exposed* to and *overwhelmed* by a wrathful God, a God who was absolutely unreachable in his holiness and majesty. Of course, from a purely empirical point of view, what happened to Luther did indeed *happen* to him. *He* did not want his despair, *he* did not seek it. On the contrary, he endeavored seriously, we may assume, to attain the grace of God.

But what happened *to him*, was in itself something arranged, posited, perhaps one may even say: it was somehow instigated. It was not an ill fate, the way all kinds of natural disasters, for example, earthquake catastrophes come upon us completely without our doing. Luther is himself complicit in what indeed *happened* to him.[19] He insisted on and immensely intensified the notion of the angry, unreachable absolutely holy God, the severe judge, and he manoeuvered himself ever deeper into this experience. In the whole course of events in this phase of Luther's life we sense a "will" at work that consistently aims for the attainment of the state of total despair. Only it is not his, Luther's, will, but the will of "the soul".

To the extent that this development is not *his* will, it befalls him as a *passively* suffering victim, completely against his own will. To the extent, however, that this course of events has the character of a "will" and a downright obsessive doing resulting from this will, it is arranged (in Alfred Adler's sense), staged. The

19 On this point, my position differs from that of archetypal psychology in general. Archetypal psychology is based on the idea of the *spontaneous event character* of the images, the archetypal fantasies, the gods, on their *happening* to us completely of their own accord. The only part that man has in this regard is to see how he can, secondarily, correctly deal with what has happened to him or is an image dominating his consciousness. What I have emphasized above, however, is the dialectic of happening-to (befalling) and staging (Adler's "*arrangement*", so to speak). Certainly, the images and archetypal fantasies that shape my consciousness happen to me. So far I agree with the theory of archetypal psychology. But that is only the one side. The other side, which Archetypal Psychology does not see, is that in the images that happen to me, and in the gods that befell man in former times, man is, albeit unconsciously, also himself always already in it, part and parcel of it: the images, the gods, the fantasies have to be seen through as having been produced, *made*. Soul-making! Unconsciousness does not mean uninvolvement, it does not mean innocence (this word in the psychological, not moral or legal sense). It is one and the same soul that creates the images (but creates them *as* primordial, *as* their own origin and in this sense *as not* created) and then also imposes them ("springs them") on itself (namely in the form of man's consciousness). The primordiality of the primordial or archetypal image must be taken seriously, but by no means at face value, literally. The latter would amount to superstition and mystification. Like all psychological phenomena images, too, are in themselves the dialectical unity of unpredictable surprise occurrence and active production, mise-en-scène, invention.

feeling of being accepted by God is systematically undermined and destroyed. All means of grace, which had always worked before in countless other cases of religious distress, are one after the other invalidated. The problem is incredibly exacerbated, radicalized in an extremist fashion. A spiritual excessiveness and unconditionality is at work here, which unerringly, albeit unconsciously for the person concerned, strives towards hopelessness with a "madness" that has method in it. This hopelessness is "intended", it is the very *purpose* of the whole mise-en-scène (even if only the first immediacy of this purpose), not simply a misfortune. The process in which Luther finds himself drives him into a dead end with methodical consistency. It is a process that, to say it with Nietzsche, "wants to get to the *end*".

The positedness of the whole problem is actually obvious from the outset. His going into a monastery alone and the unconditional devotion to God that goes with it reveals that from now on it should be primarily a matter of positedness and no longer of what is naturally present. For the monastic existence is an artificial one and explicitly segregated from the natural form of life. God is not a positive given to begin with, not a positivity, but something posited by "the soul". One's turning to God or gods generally expresses the desire to transcend the level of the purely pragmatic, or rather, in it the real fact expresses itself that this level has psychologically already been transcended. It shows that man understands (or wants to, or must) understand and experience himself from a completely different, not simply naturally given, practical level.

The positedness that occurred with the entry into monastic life is one thing. In Luther's case it was topped and became a second-level positedness, in that "he" (not he as ego, but as "soul") *within* the monastic existence pushed off from the monastic lifestyle the way it was given by the tradition. This monastic lifestyle, having always already been laid down and hallowed by tradition, and being as such culturally predetermined, was in truth nothing but a *second quasi "natural"* way of life. Inasmuch as Luther had entered the monastery as a whole person and once and for all left the world behind, that is to say left behind what before his becoming a monk used to be the natural way for him, the distinction between “the natural” and “overcoming nature” returns for him on the new level of monastic life itself.

1st stage opposition:	worldly life or **natural** life	—	monastic life or **nature overcome**		
2nd stage opposition:			monastic life as *second-stage* **“natural”** life	—	absolute God-man relation as *second-stage* **nature overcome**

For him, pious life as monk in the traditional sense now holds the place that worldly life used to hold prior to his entering the monastery. The monastic form of existence does not give him inner tranquillity, and this traditionally utmost form of piety proves for him not to be the truly highest and ultimate form of human existence. This is so because he has unwittingly already transcended it. A new, hitherto unsuspected dimension has de facto opened up for him, has in fact catapulted him onto a new, no longer medieval level, although his conscious awareness is still stuck in the old conventional expectations and thus lags unsuspectingly behind his new inner reality, behind the fact that his innermost feeling and standpoint *are already* irrevocably beyond them.

The fact that he does not find inner peace in the highest form of existence established so far is posited, is arranged. In the context of the medieval world, it would have been quite possible, even the most natural thing, to achieve peace of mind in the monastery and in traditional forms of piety. Christianity, the Bible, the contents and forms of ecclesiastical piety and the theological tradition were so broad and rich that a soul who *wanted* inner peace could have found enough points of reference and ways to attain inner tranquility. Luther felt compelled to focus one-sidedly on the wrathful God, on God’s absolute holiness, on the notion of judgment and of one’s having to attain justification before God. Furthermore, he even drew God’s judgment, which traditionally takes place only at the end of time, into the present by thinking that, standing alone before God in His eternal judgment, it is an absolute necessity to get *already now* absolute certainty about his relation to God, that is to say about his being justified or damned. The question is why.

All this is due to his emphasizing individual aspects, systematically selecting particular ones from the whole range of the doctrinal contents of the Christian message. God the loving Father, Christ the Redeemer—to name just these two of many quite different Christian motifs—are of course not unknown to Luther, but they remain without effect for him at this time. Why? Because the opus of the soul that reigns here, the special project that the soul realizes in and through Luther, has no use for them.

In summary, we can say that it is not simply a particular gloomy experience of God, an archetypal experience, which becomes effective here and at the mercy of which Luther happened to find himself. Rather, the experience of God, to which he is in this case certainly at the mercy of, is an experience already purposefully *shaped* by "the soul" itself on the basis of a certain conception. It is a fabricated experience. God, in his unapproachable holiness, is *sozusagen eingesetzt* ("*put up to it*, so to speak", to say it in the words of Jung's report about his own childhood neurosis, *MDR* p. 32), i.e., used for a certain "psychological *arrangement*", one, however, of which Luther, who is smitten with it, remains ignorant and unsuspecting. "God" is made use of. He has a function, a purpose.

The process which lived itself out in Luther was heading unerringly towards a *katastrophê*. In this process, Luther was forced to perform for himself a tragedy, not a comedy. It was not his personal tragedy, but the tragedy of the medieval form of human existence in general, or of man contained in the bosom of nature. This is what now needs to be shown, and for this we must, to begin with, clarify what is to be understood here by "medieval man's containment in the bosom of nature".

What does "nature" mean? Since we are in a psychological discussion here, nature must not be confused with physical or biological nature. Nature here does not mean the totality of plants, animals, stones, landscapes. Containment in the bosom of nature is rather that constitution of human existence in which man knows himself to be contained and embedded in a great comprehensive and "objectively given" meaning, in a divine, cosmic or metaphysical order, and in which he lives out of this containment, receives from it his "identity", his self-understanding and the concept of his essence. Conversely, we can say negatively that it is the constitution of human existence, in which he is, in ultimate regards, not thrown back on himself, does not experiences himself to be all on his own. The individual was relieved of the *essential* decisions and the *ultimate* responsibility. He was "metaphysically" sustained.

That does not mean that he would have been allowed to lie back and be inactive. He certainly had to make his active contribution. But this contribution consisted in the conscientious implementation of measures antecedently given and sanctified by tradition or authority or by the beck of the deity (oracles, dreams). Man was thus *essentially* obedient, essentially receptive; he was regardful, imitating established models, and "cor-responding" to the voice of heaven or earth. "*Essentially* obedient", that means, firstly: the obedience of which we are speaking here was not dependent on the contingencies of his personal peculiarity and his actual individual behavior, but lay in the essence, the logical constitution, of his humanness. And secondly it means that this obedience did not exclude the possibility that on the empirical surface level of practical *behavior* he could not be quite energetic, resourceful, and decisive. It only means that the ultimate responsibility did not lie with man; it lay elsewhere, in the customs and collective wisdom inherited from the ancients, in the authorities appointed to their office, or in the revelation of the deity. Everything truly important was always already decided or came (as in oracles) *as* decided to him. The only problem for man was in all cases whether he correctly recognized, understood and responded to what came to him as already determined.

Psychologically man was therefore (and only in this sense) a *child*. As a medieval person he was psychologically, for example, not for nothing contained in the *bosom* of the Mother Church. In still earlier times he had psychologically lived in the bosom of the Great Mother, Mother Earth (who for medieval man was, so to speak, his "grandmother", the "mother" of the already spiritualized Mother Church). He was (psycho-) logically still unborn (although empirical-factually he was as a matter of course born). Notwithstanding all empirical vicissitudes and hardships, he lived (psycho-) logically in the "childhood paradise". This is true even if, in empirical regards, he might in many cases have shown a higher degree of alert intellect, mature strength of character and personal decisiveness than the man of today often shows, who has become a subjective "individual" and is equipped with his personal "inner".

"Nature" in the psychological sense cannot be positivized. It is therefore also possible that the border between the containment in the womb of nature and having stepped out of or having being expelled from this containment (keyword: alienation) shifts in the course of history or from culture to culture, and thus that the particular form of what "nature" means changes in each case. The medieval form of containment in nature would presumably have been experienced by Stone Age man as an intolerable abstractness of life and as alienation, measured against what *for him* was containment in nature. Conversely, in later times an already largely technologized world, which would have seemed radically alienated to medieval man, can still afford the status of embeddedness in nature or at least intimate it, such as when for example steam locomotives and oldtimers arouse nostalgic feelings or when we modern city dwellers experience grain fields as nature, which were originally bold and highly controversial innovations at the forefront of culture ("agriculture"). What is and what is not nature in a psychological sense is not determined by fixed "objective" characteristics, but by the *place-value* assigned to something by and within the respective logical soul constitution of human existence and the world. What counts is the place and function within the psychological system. "Nature" and therefore also "alienation" are relative to the respective historical situation, to the historical locus. Just as the "now" is always a gliding border between the past and the future, so the difference between nature and alienation is an always gliding border accompanying cultural development and thus always newly set. From this border, wherever it happens to be at a given age, that which is on one side and that which is on the other side receives its determination and definition.

The form of nature characteristic of the Middle Ages can be designated above all by two formulations: the bosom of the Church and the world as divine creation and *ordo* (similarly to how we usually describe what was nature in archaic times with the words myth and cosmos: the world as animated by gods and spirits, a world directly *speaking* to man, immediately expressive of meaning).

The logical constitution of consciousness in the Middle Ages. Medieval man could not yet be divided from himself, dissociated. In the same way that he lived socially in fixed superordinate corporations, guilds, fraternities, feudal bonds, etc., he also lived psychologically in fixed predetermined states of being, in objective forms or types of life (Greek *bíoi*). For the devout there was the *bíos* of the monk, the penitent, the hermit, the Christian knight, the pilgrim, etc. In Japan there are similarly specific "paths" or "ways" (*dō*, Chinese *tao*): the path of Zen, of archery, of the sword, of tea ... Much like into a house or a train, the individual had only to enter into such an objective form of life, to tune into it and let it carry him. It was not he as an individual who was called upon to pave his way to salvation for himself. His task was at most to personally make use of a given, already paved path, such as that of monastic life. This form of life had its own intrinsic logic, its objectively given form together with its inner fulfilment and perfection. In it, everything essential—the salvation of the soul, the forgiveness of sins—was always already real. What was still open was only whether and to what degree the individual indeed participated in this always already provided and readily available salvation. This is remotely comparable to the situation of how knowledge imparted to children in school always already exists, ready-made, collectively and objectively known, but subjectively, to the individual pupil, still unknown, and how it therefore has to be personally acquired by him and how in reality it is acquired by different children to very different degrees of comprehension. The Pythagorean theorem does not have to be reinvented by every single pupil, it only has to be individually re-enacted in his mind. In much the same way, it is true for the Middle Ages in all essential things that the individual only had the task of re-enacting what was provided as a given option, an established model. The decision to become a monk or a hermit was, to be sure, a personal one in the Middle Ages (although not always!). But the status of monkhood itself, that a person had individually chosen, was an objective, universally valid, "finished" (accomplished) form of life, into which one could enter and into which one could also *abandon* oneself, that is, in which one could be released as a person. The individual was therefore fundamentally relieved. He did not have to bear the burden of finding meaning on his own, of solving by himself what we moderns experience as the *riddle* of life. He was not responsible for the authentic life and for the "answers". The answers were always already there. There were no puzzles. No need to search for meaning. Meaning was a matter of course, it was all around like the air we breathe. Just as with the decision to become a monk one externally entered the monastery in the sense of an existing building and institution, so one ipso facto got psychologically (i.e. logically) everything essential handed to oneself on a plate when one assumed the given *bíos* of the monk. Or with another image: he could lay down in a made-up bed. The Church and the religious forms of life offered by it relieved one of the fundamental responsibility for salvation of the soul. Certainly, the individual had to try to worthily carry out the (so I might say) "public office" of monk, once he had decided for it; that was his responsibility, his individual part. But the actual responsibility—the one for beatitude, indeed for all fundamental questions—was not his. The "office" of monk that he held and merely carried out through his personal behavior guaranteed beatitude, provided that he indeed carried it out conscientiously.

There had been many medieval people who, like Luther, were absolutely serious about the Christian religion, who became aware of their own sinfulness, who thoroughly searched their conscience and got into severe *vexationes* or *tentationes* (crises of faith, doubts, troubles of conscience). But all these crises and hardships, however radical and agonizing they may have been in individual cases, nevertheless remained fundamentally contained in or embraced by the Church. This Church, in its understanding of Christian piety, had room even for such conflicts, conflicts which, after all, contradicted the Christian piety, faith, and certainty of salvation. In other words, the Church had room even for what contradicted the Church's own actual demands. The lively sense of sin, the anguish of conscience, and doubt did not pose a threat to the Church. Rather, the Church had always already constructively integrated them into and for the Church faith. They were understood as *moments that belonged* to real life of faith and therefore were exactly that: a priori *sublated* troubles, so to speak institutionalized components of the monastic way.

The traditional medieval Church had very differentiated answers and aids to offer for such plights, with which these plights could be integrated as helpful elements in the inner religious life, indeed they were comprehended as promoting, intensifying and deepening it. There were various exercises of devotion, penance, as well as intellectual solutions for certain doubts; in addition there were the sacraments, the pastoral assistance, the help of the saints, the knowledge of the Church's inexhaustible treasury of merit. To experience such crises was ultimately not a catastrophe at all, no, it was even a sign of a higher degree and a more subtle form of piety—and probably even a method of achieving such a higher degree. Thus they also always were a mark of distinction. Insofar as man knew himself to be safely contained in the bosom of the Church and in the divine world order, the crises, however shocking they might be subjectively, could objectively not *fundamentally* threaten him with the danger of total despair (or maybe even the breaking up of his personality). They remained empirical states, particular cases of empirical ontic suffering and thus events on the psychic or practical level of "behavior", but psychologically (with regard to his "soul": to the logical or ontological constitution of his essence) unproblematic.

The psyche of the medieval devout could not be rent by the religious qualms, his personality could not be broken, because the religious qualms were not *his subjective* plight in the true sense of the word. They were not truly psychological. Rather, we must understand them by analogy with somatic wounds, symptoms, or diseases. With regard to the core of personality, they somehow remained external, did not get into his inner—because man did not yet have any inner into which they could have penetrated. The Christian dogmas were spiritual, nonsensible, but nevertheless "objective truths"; in this sense they were almost like (admittedly invisible, spiritual) "things", that is, not human conceptions, opinions, subjective convictions, but *realities*, which required a certain active human response. In the same way the doubts and qualms of conscience were also objective realities that could befall humans, similarly to how we imagine that we can be infected by viruses and bacteria: namely the said "*Anfechtungen*" (in the case of which demons were supposed to be the tempters). Viral diseases have their origin primarily not in myself as subjectivity, at least according to today's experience; they are objective natural phenomena, which, to be sure, take place in me and affect me, but which nevertheless always remain *vis-à-vis* to the core of my personality, my subjectivity, and in this respect are "objectual" (*gegenständlich*).[20] For medieval man the religious qualms were likewise objectual and not psychological. They were real attacks of the devil or of demons; visitations, trials coming from God, which as such came "from outside" and remained vis-à-vis. They were still ontologized ("reified"), i.e. mythologized. Doubts, torments of the soul, temptations, and the qualms of conscience did indeed play themselves out in the individual human being, but they were objective, factual nature events, only in nonsensible, spiritual nature, not in visible and tangible physical nature. Because of their objective nature event character, one had to deal with them only technically and expertly *lege artis*, according to the state of the art of religious technology. Subjectivity as such had no part of it.

In this respect, the psychology of medieval piety occupies an intermediate position between the psychology of ritual cultures and the psychology of the man who has become psychological. At the ritualistic level of culture, both the stuff and the form of spiritual contents as well as plights were material and sensual (and thus mythologized). There were cases of contamination that could be removed by literally washing. The highest values, the holy of holies, one's own self or the soul of both the tribe and the individual were externally located in things, in the statue of a god, in a holy tree or stone, in a staff or scepter, in holy masks and the

20 From here the question could maybe be raised whether the helplessness we experience in the face of such viral diseases as AIDS does not represent a call for consciousness to "demythologize" the viruses too, and that means, to "integrate" them: to learn to understand them no longer solely as external facts to be researched scientifically, but to comprehend them as forms of life *belonging to us*, in just the same way as modern man learned to understand the objective "*Anfechtungen*", still sent by demons in the Middle Ages, as his own soul states, which he therefore also has to answer for.

bridal or royal crown, in holy fire, in the flag, in a man's spear and a woman's basket. The soul was outside.[21] The will of the gods was recognized in the flight of birds, in the lightning strike, in the guts of animals, in the accidental fall of runic beech sticks or yarrow stalks used for divination. The relationship to the gods was mainly put (and kept) in order through the extremely sensual, even physical sacrificial slaughter of animals or humans, and also by libations, masked dances and similar ceremonies. For the medieval monk and his religious qualms, by contrast, the *material substance* of religious experience was already largely desensualized, decarnalized. Religious qualms, doubts, feelings of 'being a sinner', that is, of worthlessness, all these are *in themselves* purely psychic states. However, psychologically or logically they were not yet experienced at this stage of consciousness as psychological, as subjective and purely inner, as in each respective case really only *my* state, but still as objective-natural (albeit nonsensual) *entia* (natural entities, objective realities), which can attack me as well as any other person. (But even the spiritualization of the *contents* was not carried through consistently; for example, something thoroughly sensual like "illicit relations with the Devil", taken as literal, real behavior, was an integral part of the conceptual and experiential world of the Middle Ages.)

With all the differences that exist between masked dancers in ritual dances in archaic cultures on the one hand and the monastic execution of life in the Middle Ages on the other hand, one can nevertheless say that the monk, too, is in a sense only a player in a sacred performance. One can adduce a passage of C.G. Jung, *CW* 18 § 628, for the sake of comparison, where he speaks of a "symbolic existence", "... in which I am fulfilling my role, my role as one of the actors in the divine drama of life". The monk, too, wears a "mask" (not only literally: tonsure and cowl, but above all also spiritually: the role or the *bíos* of the monk)—with the only difference that for the ritual dancer the masked dance was re-

21 "... the soul is not always and everywhere on the inside. There are peoples and epochs where it is outside, peoples and epochs that are unpsychological, as, for example, all ancient cultures, and among them especially Egypt with its magnificent objectivity and its just as magnificent, naïve, negative confession of sins. ..." (*CW* 10 § 158, transl. modif.).

served for limited holidays or particular situations, after which he returned to his so to speak "bourgeois" life, while the monk is a player in a holy drama which is meant to last his whole life, that is, for which, apart from his death, no end is intended. In both cases, however, we must not confuse the player with the mask or role he has to play. One must not take the played role personally, not see it as *his* personal drama. *He* is not the subject of his actions. He is not living out *his* life. It is an objective, impersonal role play *into which* he has just released and relinquished himself together with his personal, so to speak "bourgeois" or "civilian" individuality for the duration of the play, in order to be engrossed in it to the utmost and, as far as possible, to *go through the motions* prescribed by the role. From this point of view, the crises of faith and the tormenting emotions of the monk are only something like the paroxysms of the dancer gone into trance: objective phenomena that can occur during and within the given role play. That which is demanded of the Christian consists analogously of *particular* given laws or recommendations and the corresponding good works and merits, and sins are *in the Middle Ages* likewise *essentially particular* objective events and facts, whereby the sins have similarly to be responded to with certain particular *behaviors* and are "settled" once this response has been given.

Psychologically, it was *as* "merely natural man" that medieval man could (and was meant to) be a Christian. When he became a monk, he certainly broke with "nature" on the literal, in its turn still naturalistic level. He broke with certain aspects of his (in the empirical sense) natural existence by vowing to renounce certain actions and thoughts which were considered sinful or at least distracting from God. These referred in particular to everything that had to do with bodily well-being and sensual pleasure. No doubt a radical break with nature. But now we also need to take note of the following other side: the in fact ascetically living man, who deadened his natural drives ("the flesh"), nevertheless was and remained psychologically or logically within-himself-unbroken, merely-natural man. The difference to before is only an empirical one, like a change of profession from farmer to miner. In practice the living conditions of farmer and miner are radically different, one works in the open air on and with the earth, the other in the narrowness below it, in the dark; one depends on the seasons, the other is largely independent of them. But these were only "semantic or content differences", not "syntactic-logical" differences. The logical constitution of human existence remains the same for both. By the same token, whoever became a monk chose only one other *bíos* among all the different *bíoi* that were open to man. He became a specialist for piety, just as others, the knight, the minstrel, the baker, the housewife, the prostitute, the executioner, each specialized in other aspects of life. They all exercised their profession within the total framework of the social fabric, and even if one profession may have had more prestige than another, these were only gradual, not essential differences.

Just like the man who lived out his sensuality, the monk, too, sought only his happiness; the difference is merely that he understood something else by happiness, namely "higher" or "supersensible" (spiritual) happiness, the salvation of the soul, eternal beatitude, in contrast to the "ordinary" this-worldly and temporary happiness of sensual existence. Again, the difference is only one in content, only "semantic": how happiness is defined. Since Augustine it was taken for granted in theology that man should seek in religion his beatitude and thus his *true* happiness (Holl). But no matter whether I understand my happiness as the quick gratification of carnal lust and earthly needs here and now or rather as a long term goal, namely my beatitude in God in afterlife, it is earthly, natural striving just the same. It is the expression of natural eudaemonism.

Medieval theology also ensured that the naturalistic level of thinking and experiencing was preserved and not overcome by experiences that would explode it. On the one hand it made use of *separations* and on the other hand, in combination with them, of *hierarchical gradations* in order to defuse whatever might impair it and thus to preserve an undisrupted logical continuity. Or, to put it the other way around, to prevent a logical rupture. Thus it divided human desires into those for baser goods (out of which, through a *privatio boni*, evil arises) and those for the highest good, the eternal, and by scaling them it preserved the non-contradictory *unity* of desire and the unity of everything desirable as *goods*: the *one* scale guaranteed natural unity. To love God was the highest, the true form of self-love, and ordinary selfish love and self-love were only deficient, perverted forms of actual love.

Man was divided into two segregated, self-contained quantities: the old Adam and the new man[22], the flesh and the spirit—very much like Jung, as late as in the last century, divided man into two segregated quantities, his ego-consciousness and his "shadow". Sin was then always the work of a subjectivity other than that which was truly his own, that is, the work of the baser, "old" (i.e. in principle already overcome) man or "the flesh"; all pious will, on the other hand, came from his actual self, his higher, nobler part, from the spirit. With this division, which of course was completely in accordance with the quasi materialistic (thing-like) view of religious experience,[23] man did not have to *fundamentally* contradict himself: everything that contradicted his highest striving for God was merely due to that other and non-authentic side, to the flesh, today we could say: to his "shadow", not due to his true being. Man himself was thus conceived as a natural object composed of different components. The logical, psychological consistent unity of man with himself as in principle good and as *natural child of God* was preserved by this division of man into various components on the one hand, and the disposal of sin (by placing it with the other part) on the other hand.

Similarly, theology divided sins into venial and mortal sins and distinguished between various ethical rules, those which only had the status of "advice" (a recommendation), and those which had the status of a "commandment", a distinction which mediated the moral or religious requirement with the actual capacity of the natural man, and thus relativized them. The duty to love God through the love of one's neighbor (charity) was graded according to natural social ties. Towards parents and brothers and sisters, for example, one was more obliged to practice charity than towards distant relatives, towards relatives more than towards friends and acquaintances, towards the feudal lord more than towards a stranger, etc.

---

22 Ephesians 4:24: "And that ye put on the new man, which after God is created in righteousness and true holiness."

23 If the phenomena of the religious experience are seen and experienced in analogy to naturally existing things, one can of course also categorize and arrange them as on a shelf according to whatever organizing principles.

The more painful it was and the more self-overcoming it required, the higher religious merit was regarded: it was esteemed and calculated according to one's empirical achievement. Being a monk, for example, was the highest, most meritorious form of life in religious regards. With a daring figure of speech I spoke above of the fact that someone who entered a monastery, so to speak, lay down in a made-up bed. Here it must be added that this bed was *only empirically* a very hard, uncomfortable, even painful bed, insofar as entering the monastic life was accompanied by the mortification of the flesh and the overcoming of literal nature. *Psychologically*, on the other hand, it was the highest delight: the knowledge that through the natural(istic), literal overcoming of literal human nature one was living the form of life that was most pleasing to God and that therefore one would one day be in the state of eternal beatitude, *ex officio*, so to speak, simply on account of one's "office" as a monk—and this is precisely what one's staying stuck on the natural(istic) plane consists in.

Thanks to the psychological difference between the empirical-factual (or the pragmatic level of factual behavior/suffering) and the psychological (or the level of the logical), the most terrible human suffering (e.g. the agony of a martyr) could be in itself the greatest pleasure, the triumph of being in the state of supreme salvation. This triumph is achieved through the glorification of and celebration of that which for a person is his own highest principle and absolute value (in the case of Luther: God). It is a glorification precisely because it is for the sake of *his* supreme principle (as it were *ad maiorem dei gloriam*) that the person suffers the martyrdom of absolute self-abasement, self-castigation, self-destruction. This absolute suffering *is* the victory of that which is most precious to him, and thus he experiences his highest satisfaction, even lust.[24]

24 One could also illustrate the ultimately unbroken preservation *of the natural level itself* with a literal reading of the biblical parable of the pearl merchant. The pearl merchant surrenders all the other objects he possesses to the one object most precious for him: the change is an exchange within the same sphere of objective possessions. It is, so to speak, a matter of taste whether one prefers the One Outstanding Object to a multitude of somewhat inferior but also valuable possessions.

The tragedy of the "Middle Ages", of man's natural sonship to God. Now it becomes understandable to what extent the terrible process which Luther went through with his religious qualms was the tragedy of the Middle Ages and of the natural sonship to God, a tragedy which Luther had to perform to himself, where he was stage, actor and spectator in one. In this process, Luther gradually had to conscientiously and with ultimate persistence try out and apply all the remedies and consolations of the medieval Church, not, as was his subjective, still medieval intention, for the purpose of finally attaining the certainty of salvation, but the other way around, for the purpose that the soul objectively pursued of step by step furnishing proof of the failure of each and every traditional religious aid for attaining salvation and thus ending the medieval *mediation* between the demands of religion and the nature of man and social life through the relentless experience of the indissolubility of the contradiction between the two. Contrary to his conscious intention, Luther was forced to systematically work off ("deconstruct") the medieval constitution of human existence as a whole. Of course, this could only succeed if he subjected himself *bona fide*, in all innocence, and thus precisely with full seriousness and ruthlessness towards himself, in detail to all those spiritual operations whose absolute ineffectiveness was to be proven by "the soul". Luther had to make use of them with full conviction that these operations lead to salvation and with the genuine will to achieve salvation through them. Had he intended from the outset to expose them as ineffective, their ineffectiveness would have been open to the suspicion of being nothing but a self-fulfilling prophecy. But because Luther tried with all his strength and honest effort to achieve his peace of mind by traditional means and failed in this very endeavor even to the point of absolute desperation, the proof of the ineffectiveness of the old means of pious living had the character of an unquestionable because unintended self-representation of the reality of these means.

The painful experience of failure is indispensable. Real overcoming does not happen perfunctorily in a sweeping way nor in abstract intellectual understanding, so to speak at one's desk. Luther had existentially to suffer the failure of the principle of medieval piety by going through it all himself, and the suffering had to be almost exhaustive, that is, to cover both extensively almost completely the whole spectrum of medieval salvational methods and to be intensively pushed forward in each case to their last consequence, in order to be *real* overcoming of the medieval consciousness. The price for becoming free of something must always be paid in full. And the name for the psychological price is pain, suffering. But I do not want to emphasize the value of suffering for the soul for its own sake, as some forms of mysticism do. Rather, suffering is simply the form in which a *real* transformation takes place, much as the flame is simply the place where wood is transformed into heat, gases and ashes. In suffering, farewell and arrival are inscribed in the flesh, so to speak.

In Staupitz's sentence—"I don't understand it"—it is beautifully expressed that Luther had de facto evicted himself from the "Middle Ages" as such (or found himself expelled from it) and transferred himself to another logical place. Staupitz here is, so to speak, the voice of the medieval mind, and if this voice feels compelled to say: "I don't understand it," then this means that Luther has crossed the border of the medieval mind. With his experience and thinking he was simply de facto in another, new place, which had to be absolutely incomprehensible for the consciousness that remained rooted in the "Middle Ages". From the point of view of the "medieval" consciousness of a Staupitz, Luther therefore had to appear almost as something like an alien, an "E.T.". "Medieval" stands here, within a psychological investigation, especially also for "medieval Church", and this in turn for the medieval "House of Being", for the vessel and at the same time the figuration of the medieval spirit, the medieval "soul". Luther was psychologically already now (and not only, as in practical reality, with the Reformation years later) *extra ecclesiam*, because he no longer had his real place in this vessel. For Luther, the door to the "Middle Ages" was slammed shut without his having understood this himself as yet. He had been thrown onto a "new continent", into absolutely new territory, without knowing for himself what had happened to him, even without knowing that this displacement into a completely new spiritual territory had happened to him and that he was therefore no longer on the same ground with Staupitz. According to his consciousness he was still in the "Middle Ages". Only the consequences of his actions showed that he was not. The process of being expelled had indeed taken place in and on himself. He had even had to produce it himself, but he had not pursued it *as* the very process of the deconstruction of the "Middle Ages" and his own exile from the "Middle Ages". It was the opposite attempt, to fulfill the "Middle Ages" in the most precise way, to lead a holy life, and to find peace of mind in the forms of medieval piety. He himself had been totally unaware of the actual purpose of the work of the soul, to undertake which he saw himself driven and which he had not seen at all as the work which it was. His conscious purpose, on the one hand, and the objective purpose of the whole event (one and the same event), on the other hand, moved in opposite directions. Following Hegel's phrase of the "cunning of reason" one could speak of the cunning of "the soul".

From here one can ask in what exactly the seemingly neurotic dissociation of Luther consisted. It lay in the fact that he, like a medieval man, claimed to be God's obedient child and thus pleasing to God by virtue of his choice of a certain *empirical* profession (the "holy" state of the monkhood) and of conscientiously leading his life in accordance with it by virtue of natural measures, although he *was* no longer a medieval man and no longer *in a natural way* the child of God pleasing to God. Jung once characterized the neurotic problem by saying about the consciousness of the neurotic: "It does not understand how its world has altered and how its attitude would have to change in order to be adapted again" (*CW* 9i § 61, transl. modif.). This was exactly the case with Luther at that time. The *world* of consciousness had altered, but *consciousness itself* lagged behind. When Luther hoped to be able to obtain a gracious God through the choice of a certain status and certain kinds of behavior, the underlying idea was that the fundamental sonship to God had been preserved, that the natural bond between God and man had not been torn, which is why it would only depend on empirical behavior (the choice of the *bíos* of the monk and the conscientious fulfillment of this *bíos*) in order to bring the *on principle* given relationship of grace up to date for himself. He believed that he could still see himself *from* above, that he could still be identified with God's point of view (in which containment in God or inalienable unity with him would have laid), although this natural unity with God had de facto already been broken for him and he was completely thrown back on himself, into his earthly humanness and subjectivity, so that he now stood *opposite* God as irrevocably separated by an abyss. Therefore, and because, unlike in Jung's childhood neurosis, play and suffering could not be placed on different sides as totally separated, his attempt to play once again "Middle Ages", once again "monk" and "saint", had to have the form of his performing a tragedy for himself.

The objective purpose of the process that took place in (and through) Luther was, as I said, to prove the failure of all traditional medieval means of grace, sacraments and consolations. These had to be irrevocably presented as ineffective. One might be tempted here to understand the word "proof" according to our scientific understanding. In science, proof means that something is, and always has been and will be, necessarily the way it has been proved to be, and that therefore all earlier opinions to the contrary about the same subject are false. In such a case, it is therefore hypotheses, opinions, theories, i.e. human propositions *about* something, that are proved or refuted. Within the soul's logical life and the history of the soul, on the other hand, "to prove" has a completely different meaning. The "soul" furnishes a proof by first itself *producing* that which is to be proved in the process of furnishing proof. It thus proves through the act, through the setting into work, through the production of the respective phenomenon. This also means that the phenomenon to be proved *is* itself the proof and that it is not some *sentences about* a phenomenon that are proved to be correct.

This means in our context that the proof of the obsolescence of the Middle Ages, which came to Luther through his process of suffering, did not mean at all that "the Middle Ages" with its methods of religious life and its paths of piety had been in error and that Luther now finally recognized "the truth" about it, saw through the falseness of "the Middle Ages". Here one must not succumb to the thought pattern of the Enlightenment, which declares as false convictions and forms of life that no longer correspond to *its* way of thinking and its position in the world. What happened through Luther was that a new form of truth was *realized*; that he had been *evicted* from the "Middle Ages" and thrust into a new historical situation. All this has nothing to do with right or wrong. From an objective point of view, these are processes of a *form change* of truth, processes of departure and at the same time of an initiating. From a subjective point of view, on the other hand, they are processes of transportation in which a particular form of human existence is transplanted from one time into another, from one constitution of consciousness into another. Speaking in Kantian language, the psychological type of "furnishing proof" has the character of "intellectual intuition" or is the achievement of "intuitive understanding". Knowledge is here not taking note of what has all along been in existence in its "objective" being-so. Rather, what is to be cognized in cognition is first determined and formed into that as which it is then cognized.

Certainly, the proof which was accomplished by Luther was the proof of the ineffectiveness of the previous means of grace. But according to what has just been explained, this means that these means of grace had to be *made* ineffective in that process of furnishing the proof. Nothing at all is thereby established about whether they were also ineffective before, or not. The psychological proof of their failure has the character of an active change: a destruction, debilitation, emptying, decomposition. In this process of the decomposition of the effective force of what has been familiar so far, something new establishes itself, a new status of consciousness, a new form of being human and of being-in-the-world, which acquires its logical constitution by having its place in another historical locus. The "soul" has abandoned *one* figuration of itself and eo ipso left it behind as a soulless and lifeless, depleted, functionless shell. At the same time it has entered into a new form of itself and presents itself as a new constellation. The cards, if this unseemly image is permitted, were now shuffled anew. The whole relationship between man and God was redefined, and from this new constellation both also received a new nature. The New, the new constitution of consciousness, was first worked out in the process of working off ("deconstructing") the obsolete form and on the basis of it. It is one and the same process. If, nevertheless, one still wanted to stick to the distinction between "right" and "false", then one would have to say that in the process experienced by Luther it was not the medieval forms of piety that were wrong, but conversely that Luther and the new *age* (the new historical locus, the new constellation into which "the soul" has now clothed itself) were proved to be *the wrong ones for* those forms (although in themselves not proved to be wrong either). But to prove oneself wrong *for* a traditionally given logical reality is the same as the real working off of one's own belonging to it and one's systematically, piece by piece, working oneself out of it, evicting oneself from it, which, however, is only the other side of one's gradually working oneself into a new status of consciousness and conquering it for oneself—or being initiated into it.

The principle and tool for the eviction from containment in the unity with God. Luther could not find soul tranquility on the paths of traditional monastic piety because he took the *standpoint of totality* and judged and experienced from it. The principle that had taken hold of him was the idea of wholeness. He saw man and his will as an acting unity. It is the whole person who acts and thus either sins or serves God. That Luther has advanced to the idea of the wholeness of the person is revolutionary. It was no longer possible for Luther to divide man up into individual impulses or into two opposing parts, *spiritus et caro*, spirit and flesh, or rather to comprehend him as a sum total or composite, the sum of his actions, traits, personality parts, etc. Since for him man was already set up as a personality and thus as a center, it was no longer possible to separate the various good and bad actions from the center of the personality as if they were individual quasi entity-like events. So he could not set off good works and meritorious achievements on the one hand against individual sinful deeds and thoughts on the other, not free himself from the latter through repentance and certain acts of penance (especially the sacrament of penance), and thus all in all arrive at the feeling of being justified before God. The righteousness of the whole person, the personality as unitary totality, has always been of central concern for him. *Anima tota est in qualibet parte*, the soul is whole in each of its parts. There are not two separate people in us, one who sins and the other who does God's will. But *totus homo*, man as moral wholeness, one and the same man, is the real subject of all action. Thus the concept of the I has been achieved. The level on which life is experienced is no longer objectual, substantial (in terms of individual entities), but purely intelligible-logical, and no longer semantic, but syntactic.

It is the principle of wholeness that functions as the lever with which the medieval methods of achieving salvation were deposed and rendered ineffective. For if man was a moral unity, then it did not help him if he, e.g., as a monk, tried to stand completely on the side of the New Man and kill the Old Adam in himself by practices of chastisement and penance, nor if he played off his striving for the highest good, God, against his carnal desire for baser goods. He never really got rid of the old man. He was always this old Adam, *too*. From the point of view of the "whole man", even if 99.9% of him might have been filled with a pure, holy striving, it was nevertheless of no avail: if there was only 0.1% Old Adam in him, he was corrupted as a whole man. This is the problem with innocence, purity, sinlessness, with the *level of principle*. For this reason, that man who has become a personal wholeness must also assume responsibility for that side which he wanted to overcome, since that side reflects on and soils even his noblest striving. He cannot get rid of it. It was therefore also not possible for him to simply identify himself with his other "higher" side and rigorously renounce the sinful "baser" side, as if he had nothing at all to do with it, as if it did not really concern him. Notwithstanding all his pious striving, he had to include inescapable, ultimately indelible sinfulness in his very self-definition.

This is exacerbated by the fact that even the distinction between a good, higher and an evil, baser will could no longer be made once the standpoint of unity had truly been adopted. Even man's most pious willing, to the extent that it was his own human, natural willing, was still the Old Adam's willing. It was not at all the willing of the New Man. Even *it* was ultimately selfishness, egoism, "willing *himself*". It was not really the free selfless love towards God from one's whole, cheerful heart, it *could not* be that at all. In everything he willed he *could*, as natural man, *only* want himself, his own happiness. Everything he aspired to *on his own*, even if it was the noblest and most pious aim, would ultimately revolve only around himself. Selfishness is inescapable. Man is completely and through and through selfishness. This is his nature.

This does not at all mean that Luther would deny the difference between obviously selfish and obviously altruistic actions in practical reality or would deny the existence of pious aspirations. Of course, in the reality of human life there are, on the one hand, clearly selfish behaviors such as robbery, exploitation, debauchery, and on the other, sacrifice for others and sincere efforts to lead a life well-pleasing to God. But, insofar as they are actions and aspirations that emanate from man himself, both belong to the side of the ego's striving. For then it is important for *me* to act altruistically, it is *my* desire to go to heaven, *my* need to find a gracious God and to attain eternal bliss. Egoicness.

From this it follows, however, that I have no chance at all to reach God of my own accord. A not only de facto, but structurally insurmountable abyss opens up between me and God. I can strive as I please, with ever so pious intentions—that which is actually to be achieved can on principle not be achieved by me, because all my own efforts systematically fall short. It remains on this side of the abyss. Now it is no longer simply a question of *what* is good, i.e. pleasing to God, and *what* is sin, as it was in the Middle Ages, no longer a question of the goodness or sinfulness of individual deeds and thoughts. With a catalogue of sins or vices here and another catalogue of what is demanded of a Christian there, one cannot get any further. It is no longer a matter of choosing between different behaviors and ways of life, between higher and baser striving. Why not? Because it no longer depends on the particular contents and aims of one's effort, but on the nature of the effort as such, which in any case is inevitably ego-willing, self-seeking, no matter what it may concretely be directed at in the individual case. Not whether one has chosen the right or the wrong is the problem. The problem is natural-human willing itself. Hence the hopelessness: no exit.

This is so because I can't get out of my willing. Even the mortification of my will, quite apart from the fact that it always only partially succeeds, is itself only a manifestation of my will, a will that is only *in terms of content* determined differently. In the ascetic deadening of my will I must even make use of a tremendously strong, unbending will; I am ego-willing to a much greater extent than if I only wanted to lead a normal, natural human life.

Luther's despair, which could even escalate almost to hatred of God, becomes understandable against this background. He is really caught in a trap: he cannot be how God demands him to be. There is a "should", a law, which he a priori cannot satisfy, because it is impossible for man to satisfy it. He sees eternal damnation before him and, despite his best will, has in principle no possibility to change anything. He is checkmated. For even if I do *not* pursue my interests, this not-pursuing is still *my* goal. Whether I strive for this or that, whether I assert myself or deny myself, is merely a semantic difference. But it is the syntactic difference that matters now.

You can see that a fundamentally new level has been reached, that of the I, of logical form, of the level of principle, of logical negativity.

The effect of the principle of wholeness. The idea of wholeness had implicitly been at work in Luther from the beginning as the guiding principle. It had been the means by which "the soul" could attain its new locus of being. At the moment when Luther found himself placed on the standpoint of totality (without of course already knowing this himself), he was in principle already evicted from the "Middle Ages", catapulted out (again without already knowing this himself!). This standing on the ground of this principle had specific inherent consequences or implications. These will have to be made clear now.

What we have already seen is the shift of the level of reflection from the particular *contents* of willing to *willing* itself. It is a shift from the semantic to the logical-syntactic level. The idea of totality obviously forces us to take a step back. The "soul", which had previously self-forgetfully been quasi spread out, released, into the individual goals and objects which might be desirable, withdraws from these and contracts into One, into a point. It focuses on itself, on its willing or desire as such, and gives itself a particular existence of its own. But this its own existence is not the existence in or as something sensually given. Out of the whole range of what is sensually-positively given, willing has precisely pulled itself out in order to come to itself. But it only comes home to itself as the *pure concept* of willing. One cannot see a will and identify it with anything visible or tangible. It does not exist like an object. It is not biologically something like an existing instinct or impulse. The will is absolute-negative. It hovers, so to speak, in empty space, is only an idea, an idea that only has an existence if a person is seized by this idea and is, obedient to it, determined in his thinking and acting by it. To be more precise: if he *comprehends* himself as willing, has posited himself as will.

That is the result of a psychological doing or achievement. The will is not simply an always already empirically given part of man's psychic inventory. Animals and babies do not will. The will receives its existence by the fact that man, in the logical constitution of his being, has himself become will and that is to say, become willing-all-of-his-own-accord, become *I* that *is* willing, *subject*.

Man has become "he who wills all on his own" when he no longer primarily feels drawn by desirable goals (be they gold, power, honor and sensual pleasure, or eternal beatitude), so that these are what pulls, i.e. the subject of pulling or of the attraction, whereas man is the object of their pulling or the one who is pulled.[25] Rather, he has become I or subject when for the first time he becomes reflectively aware *of himself as* the desiring, willing one, and of willing as *his own* willing. The withdrawal from the contents is thus a reflection-into-himself. In this (not abstract-intellectual, but psychically real) reflection on oneself as the one who wills, man has become the I, subjectivity, personality. He has snatched from desirable objects *their* being subjects and in their stead has swung himself up to being the subject of willing or desiring by having *in fact* grasped the *concept* of himself and relentlessly gone through with it, having placed himself entirely on its ground. In this sense, medieval man was not I. He understood and experienced himself fundamentally from superordinate frameworks, from God, from the divine world order, from the Church, from the social associations to which he belonged (tribal, feudal, clan, family ties, guilds and other corporations, for example). *He*

25 The same applies *mutatis mutandis* to one's being *driven* by something.

was contained in them and had in them his center, around which he revolved. He did not have his center in himself. Accordingly, the things and contents that might be desirable to medieval man were not mere objects in the modern sense (especially not those of the throwaway society), but they were *res*, realities, substances in the highest sense of medieval realism (realism regarding universals). They were, as it were, "personalities": endowed with divine dignity of being and meaning. In them lay soul. Especially also the nonsensual things of religion were substantial, quasi thing-like realities, perhaps more real than some things. Heaven and hell, eternal beatitude, Christ and the saints, the devil, sin and the Last Judgment were not only ideas, figments of the imagination, but "objective" hard realities. Using as a model how the priest, when he dealt with bread and wine in the Mass, in truth dealt quite concretely and really with the body and blood of Christ, one can recognize how real spiritual things were and how one could deal with them in a material, "hands-on" way. Religion was *dealt with "outside"*, in the sensual world, just as, politically and socially, relations between people and states were and still are dealt with "outside" through negotiations, treaties, violence, oppression, wars. Religion was essentially objective, not simply inner attitude, feeling, mental ideas in man.

The reflection upon oneself as the one who wills is a reflection on something that does not always already exist, but that is first *generated* in this very reflection. The I is not this demonstrable body of mine, nor is it some organ in my body. It is nowhere. It is just a concept, an idea—an air bubble; if you will: a pure "fiction", even a nothing. Absolute-negative. But if one unreservedly relies on this nothing—or rather more correctly: if one finds oneself based on it (because such a thing is never our own doing, but the "soul's")—then it is a psychic reality and one has become an ego-personality. The retraction of the willing from the objective goals and things in which it was previously invested (namely as their attractiveness or power of fascination), *is* only as the becoming aware of the non-existent "I myself" and as in this way *asserting* it, this non-existent "factor" (just as the other way around this asserting-the-I is only *as* the retraction from one's being spread out and released into the individual things, in other words, as reflection-in-itself or *as* the logical, not physical, sublation of the level of things). The I is only as an assertion, a thesis: the logical act of asserting it. It is not a something, not anything positive. It is nothing but this very *positing*, its positing itself as unity and wholeness, as dimensionless (= supersensible) "point", against all appearances.

Conversely, one must always keep in mind that it is not I who can "make" this assertion arbitrarily. It is "made", "done" to me if and when it is made, and I find myself in it—or maybe not in it. But if this assertion is present to its full extent, then I have been forged into "I". Becoming "I" is for its part not an egoic act, my own doing.

This also describes the difference between the physical and the psychological. Things of physical reality are characterized by a separation of existence and nature, character, or idea. With the mere idea of a chair its existence is not yet given. The representation has the reality of what it imagines outside itself. This is the trademark of positivity. The things of psychological reality, however, have their reality only in and by virtue of their idea. The idea has no external substrate. It gives itself a real existence, but only within itself, only as a psychic idea. (It gives itself this existence by taking root in a person, seizing his consciousness.) The logical negativity of psychological reality is based on this.[26]

The shift from the plane of entities is thus analogous to the shift from the "ontic" to the "ontological" (in Heidegger's sense). Expressed in another terminology: It is a shift from the "ontological" (now in another than Heidegger's sense of the word) to the "logical" (and psychological, which is the logical *as* real); from the substantial to the immaterial and nonsensible; to the level of principle; from the positive to the logically negative (e.g., to something as "fictitious" as "I"). With Luther it was no longer a question of individual, real, good or sinful deeds, but about man's no longer visible, objectifiable sinful nature as such. The level of the natural had been abandoned, and a purely intelligible, logically negative

26 In *CW* 6 § 66 Jung attacks Hegel's criticism of Kant's rejection of the ontological proof of God. Against Hegel's statement that God cannot be compared with Kant's 100 thalers, Jung says "But as Kant rightly pointed out, logic abstracts from all content" (transl. modif.). In this passage Jung himself misjudges the nature of psychological reality.

level had been adopted. When I speak of "level", it is to indicate that the intelligible now affected *not only the essential content*, as it naturally did also in the religion of the Middle Ages, but also the *logical form* of the content, or the syntax.

In the concept of the will, to which the essence of man has now elevated itself, the insight that we had already previously presented as Luther's, is already inherent, namely the insight that man's innermost being is ego-willing, selfishness. This will is not free to be either selfish or not, because willing "I" (i.e., *me*) constitutes its essence. Now that the plane of entities has been abandoned, "selfishness" is no longer a *special* quality of positive behavior (of particular individual actions in contrast to other altruistic actions), but it is the general determination of the essence of the will itself. Not semantically, but syntactically. Individual behavior itself is no longer decisive. The situation is no longer so simple, so natural, that it would still be about individual empirical acts and omissions. The level of religious experience and reflection is already the impalpable, namely *logical*, level of man's *being*, the *principled* level of his unity and wholeness.

The principle of wholeness causes a logical revolution also with regard to the direction of the essential demarcation, namely a rotation from a "horizontal" to a "vertical" division. In the Middle Ages there was a relationship of correspondence between the heavenly, divine sphere and the earthly world. The Scholastic central concept of *analogia entis*, whose ultimate background was the neo-Platonic doctrine of emanation, was not only a construct of lonely thinkers, but also expressed, in one concept, the real psychological-logical constitution of Being as a whole and thus also people's actual way of thinking and experiencing. No fundamental abyss separated the upper from the lower, the world of ideas from reality, God from his creation. Rather, both extremes (and what was between them) were connected in a graded yet ipso facto continuous way. Everything real, from the spirit via the soul, animal and vegetative life down to matter, participated in varying degrees in Being, which was ultimately the Being of God or God as Being itself. Even evil was only a *privatio boni*, not an independent absolute opposite of good. In a vertical sense (above – below) unbroken unity reigned. In *empirical* experience the impression of the complete incompatibility of what was demanded by God and of the real earthly being might very easily arise. But the idea of correspondence and participation made it possible to mediate this impression with the soul's basic experience of unity, and thus to relativize and neutralize the apparent rupture. The idea of gradation on principle took care and disposed of any possible experience of a "vertical" irreconcilable discrepancy by incorporating it within the thought of a continuous nexus, a uniform scale of the whole.

That is, in alchemical terms, the state of *unio naturalis*, the state of (in the psychological sense of the word) *natural* man. By virtue of this unbroken unity, man is irreversibly positioned into the whole of creation. It is not yet possible for him to fall out of the whole, and therefore he cannot be torn apart in himself, become dissociated: neurotic. He lives in the bosom of the divine *ordo* and, *despite* all distance from God, he is psychologically still directly connected with God by virtue of the prevailing correspondence and participation, as if with a very long, but nevertheless still attached umbilical cord. The nature (logical constitution) of the world guarantees this connectedness. This also means that there could as yet be no psychology in the true sense of the word.[27] One's being-in-the-world was essentially *cosmologically* (or ontologically) determined; man was *released* into the world, the things and events out there (into the existent as a whole or into the individual entities). His being was invested in *them*. There was no inner (in man). He could as yet not view and understand himself in terms of himself, but only in terms of God (as well as the Devil and demons, or angels), the creation, the whole that encompassed him. The natural condition is that man is outside of himself and with or in things, and accordingly sees his own being only from outside, only in terms of the things and spiritual powers in which he has his self. The state of the world can only become psychologi-

27 "It was therefore logical that the discovery of psychology was completely left to the last decades, ... It needed the *psychological plight* of our time in order to induce us to the discovery of psychology" (*GW* 10 § 159, my transl.). "As long as man still lives in the herd, he has no soul and does not need one either, with the exception of the belief in an immortal soul" (*ibid.* § 160, my transl.). To "live in the herd" is equivalent to living in the *ordo*, in the state of *unio naturalis*, etc..

cal when—as a first minimum condition—man looks at the world and the things in it intrinsically *from out of himself*, as subject, as his own center. A severing is indispensable.[28]

In contrast to its connectedness along its vertical axis, the essential *demarcation* in the Middle Ages (such a thing as a fundamental separation existed in the Middle Ages, too) separates the whole Being "horizontally" with a "vertical" cut into two opposites, which stand, so to speak, "left" and "right" of the demarcation line. In fact, the umbilical cord connecting vertically is, at the same time as it is that, the knife that separates horizontally. Just as in the hereafter, at the end of time, the Judge of the World separates the dead into the "sheep" on his right and the "goats" on his left, just as in transcendence God and the devil stand in opposition to each other, so here on earth, too, there is, analogously, a definite distinction between demonic and holy influences, sinners and the righteous, sinful and pious actions and, in us, between evil and good impulses and thoughts, Old Adam and the New Man. This has to do with the fact that in the natural situation all essential decisions and distinctions are made "outside" on the level of entities, better: the semantic level.

At the moment when man is no longer released into the whole, but is himself placed by the "soul" on the standpoint of wholeness, and is consequently himself established as wholeness and unity, the possibility of drawing the boundary "*outside*" between individual objective actions, forms of life, impulses, etc. has disappeared along with the whole withdrawal from the plane of things. Now that man has in himself and for himself become a center of his own, and there are thus *two centers*, two totalities, these two centers, God and man, (in a logical sense, not empirically) inevitably face each other directly, so to speak on one and the same "horizontal" level (for insofar as they are both *centers*, they are somehow on a par despite all other differences). However, an abyss between them now inevitably separates them "vertically" (because man as a center of his own no longer simply integrates into the original center, God). Man is now *unmittelbar zu Gott* ("in a direct relation to God"), of course directly *confronted* with Him. The world and its inner gradations in ontological regard and the Church in religious

28 Jung's "*psychological plight*".

regard no longer play a mediating role. Man must show his true colors before God without a mediating third. Luther, as we have seen, stood all alone and "naked" before God and was already *in the present* at the Last Judgment. All the responsibility which the Church, as an encompassing whole into which the individual was *integrated*, had previously borne for the salvation of the individual now falls to the individual himself.

Man is now no longer *released* into creation (away from himself) and no longer has his self in *it*, but has comprehended himself as a person, has become conscious of himself as a person. Because he has logically retracted from the world into himself, the consequence was that, as the other side of the coin, he must also *as himself* be on the spot and take a stand. This, in turn, means that the "Judgement" moves from the distance of the Last Days and the Hereafter into the here and now, into what can be personally experienced in this life. The "Judgement" becomes an insistent reality, because it has already been internalized, taken into the person. And this "Judgement" inexorably separates man, as irrevocably natural man, from God, the absolutely holy, and from his commandments.

This unbridgeable separation can be made understandable in two ways as an inevitable consequence of what Luther experienced: on the one hand contentwise, on the other hand with respect to form, or logically.

The first way (regarding content) refers to the already elaborated nature of the will as ego-will. The separation between the existing human being posited as *antecedently given* on the one hand and his good or evil will and action on the one hand, that is, of substance or substrate here and attribute there, has been abolished. The psychological experience has returned to man's "*being will*" itself. The commandment of God (which now, after the empirical level of things has been left and the level of principles has been reached, can no longer be split up into many different laws) is only this single one: To love God. But that is precisely what natural man is not able to do, because (notwithstanding all ontically-empirically undoubtedly occurring altruistic behavior and all selfless impulses) he can *essentially* only love himself. To love God would mean to hate oneself (whereby it must always be kept in mind that it is no longer a question of empirical emotions and behavior, but rather that we are already moving on the logical level of the *constitution* or *being* of man). But man *cannot* hate himself, it is impossible. It would mean extinguishing himself as his own being self, as center. As post-natural man, who has retracted himself out of his being spread out into the world and who reflected himself into himself, he *is* will and must therefore want. No matter to which concrete goal his wanting may be directed in particular cases, wanting as such, qua wanting, always also means wanting oneself, wanting one's own will. Sin is not only when one wants something specifically evil. Sin is already the will itself as one's own willing, one's ego-nature. The abyss between man and God consists in the fact that man, as inevitably ego-willing, is absolutely unholy, because before God he is always a sinner through and through, whereas God alone is the Just and Holy One. This is the compelling consequence of the principle of wholeness. For this principle demands that man always conceives himself as a whole person and not only focuses empirically and abstractly on individual, particular good works and experiences or pious intentions. It also requires that he does not *reductively* comprehend himself as nothing but an entity, a living being, an existing thing among a thousand other (living or non-living) things of creation.

Now I come to the second way, that of form, in which the unbridgeable separation of human will and God's will necessarily results from what Luther experienced. His realization that man's nature is self-will or willing himself, is, so to speak, tautological. This discovery is simply a different formulation for one's retracting oneself from being spread out into the divine order of nature and, instead, the reflection into oneself, in which man becomes the center for himself. To become the center for oneself or posit oneself as the center means to separate oneself from the One Center of divine creation and to posit oneself as something in its own right. That is by definition sin, a will counter to divine will, to the divine commandment to love only Him, God, and to recognize only Him as the true center. Thus Luther does not recognize, as he thinks he is doing, the general (universal) *nature* of man, but only the nature or constitution, *brought about* by himself, of man reflected into himself—the already sublated nature, the post-natural nature of man after his retracting himself from being embedded in and released into God's creation. Luther thus speaks only about himself, about the new early-modern situation of man. What he says is self-expression. For man in the state of *unio naturalis* was not yet self-will, because he was not yet at all constituted as will and center, not as I.

The mirror image that exists between the medieval situation and Luther's situation must also be taken into account. The medieval unity with God goes hand in hand with man's releasement out of himself, his *relinquishing* himself and his nature or his self into the world, into the hereafter (Last Judgement) as well as into individual empirical acts ("works"). Exactly the other way around, Luther's brusque vis-à-vis of God and man goes hand in hand with the retraction from the releasement of his nature into the world and man's contraction into himself, into the wholeness of person, as his own center.

If man has become his own center and now stands on his own feet, then this also means that he has to continuously *maintain* himself, his own identity, in the face of all events. Man is no longer primarily released into the flow of events. He is no longer logically *symbolic for himself*, no longer only a role-*bearer*. He is now something in his own right, all by himself, because he carries his selfhood or his identity as his property within himself. He lives on his own account.

So now we have the situation that good and evil are radically cut off from each other and distributed on two different sides, according to the well-known motto given here in Luther's version: we have to *tribuere deo omnia bona, nobis autem mala* (attribute to God everything good, but everything evil to ourselves).[29] In addition it follows that God is, to begin with, experienced by Luther as an angry God and a punishing judge who condemns sin and the sinner with absolute severity. This inescapable consequence was, as we know, the cause of Luther's despair. One is used to seeing in such one-sidedness and *splitting* something unnecessarily pointed and exaggerated, and in such an exclusive positioning oneself on the side of evil and damnation something morbid, perverse and above all also something that violates the spirit of psychology.

29 *Psalmenkommentar*, WA IV, p. 241, cited from Holl, p. 31, note 2.

Was it not a morbid desire that drove Luther to drive himself, in such an extremist way, ever deeper into the hopelessness of a dead end? But for a psychological understanding (though not for a theological one), the question of "right" or "wrong" does not arise, so here too with such valuations we must not obstruct for ourselves the insight into what the sense and rank of the described experience is. This radical, one-sided split is first of all not Luther's work, that is, it does not originate from his personal complexes or his needs (be they legitimate or misguided). He *finds himself* in this experience. It is the *opus* of the soul that is realized in Luther. The power of the soul to split is just as important as its tendency to unite. Without radical separation there is no *mysterium coniunctionis*. Secondly, separation is logically justified, a compelling necessity. One must not react here in an emotional judgmental way, but instead consider its logic and meaning.

Conversely it is psychologically also not acceptable to regard the one-sided idea of the wrath of God and the damnation of man as an experience of God that simply happened to be so constituted and that therefore had to be accepted as such, i.e., to regard it in a thing-like and naturalistic way as a factual event. Psychologically it must be understood as posited, as the work of "the soul", as part of *its* self-representation.

The "soul" *needs* (and uses) the relentless wrath of the judging God as a means to an end in order to be able to perform the reflection-into-self. One must be aware of how improbable it was to abandon the natural point of view. One must take into account the enormous forces of perseverance, of the "psychic law of inertia", so to speak, against which the revolution taking place in Luther had to prevail. The wrathful God is the psychological means by which the tremendous work could be accomplished (at least in one single person, here Luther), namely the work of pulling the soul that had previously been dispersed and invested in the world out of its releasement into this world of things and to throw it completely back on itself, for the first time to contemplate itself, become irrevocably reflectively aware of itself. The wrath of the absolute judge constellates eo ipso the feeling of absolute guilt, and the absolute feeling of guilt is the *eye of the needle* through which alone the idea of the I could *in fact* gain entrance into the real psychological being of man. The feeling of guilt is not a natural fact that simply comes upon man like an external storm. Nor is it an anthropological constant. It is an invention, an achievement of the soul, produced and used for the certain purposes that it has in each respective case. In the history of its logical life as "formation, transformation, the eternal Mind's eternal recreation", in order for the soul to give itself the unheard-of, completely new form of subjectivity or personality, it needed the staging, arranged by itself, of the radical, mutually exclusive opposition of man and God. The feeling of being a sinner and thus of being condemned, and of the absolute, total Divine Judgement, was the burning fire, ignited by "the soul" itself, in which *omnes superfluitates igne consumuntur* (everything superfluous is burnt away), as alchemy puts it. It was in this feeling that the *mundificatio* (purification) of the pure I could take place, its *mundificatio* from the previous stance of its naturalistic (i.e. mythical-symbolical) self-understanding and its detaching itself from all entanglements and investment in the world of things. This process was the edification of the I as a *psychically-real* PRINCIPLE. What Luther experienced in his crisis does not speak for his morbidity, but is a component and characteristic of that one, particular "archetypal" moment in the soul's play with itself that lived itself out at this time of history, and in him, Luther, of all people.

The realization of the principle. The transformation from a world situation in which people are *logically* given over to the world and its One Center, to the situation in which there is the ego-personality, which is ego-personality because it is its own center, is not simply based on a new insight, a change of perspective, an understanding of the new principle. It is not just something intellectual. It is a real and gradual and painful process, a process that cuts into the flesh. It needed strong, perhaps even brutal spiritual means, namely absolute feelings of guilt and worthlessness over against God, feelings that went to the point of complete despair, to make the transformation real. It will now be necessary to take a closer look at how the principle that Luther was seized by became reality and how it, if I may put it that way, "worked" internally.

That aspect of Luther's crisis, which from an external point of view is analogous to neurosis, was, in addition to and apart from pathological exaggeratedness, the fact that he had already been seized by the principle of wholeness and, already committed to it, had all along been expelled from the "Middle Ages", but that he nevertheless wanted to live once again the medieval form of existence of a monk, of holy life. The new principle was alive in him from the beginning of his crisis, perhaps it even was already the driving force behind his decision to enter the monastery. Where else than there could the eye of a needle have been found, the obstacle that is indispensable for the realization of this principle? One could therefore quite well view the abandonment of his law studies and his entry into a monastery as a manifestation of the fact that Luther had long since been gripped by the new principle. Implicitly he was already "I". Implicitly he had long since left the naturalistic and thing-based level of thinking and experiencing, that level on which it was a question of individual religious remedies and the goodness or sinfulness of individual actions and psychic impulses. Where he had been placed, it had already become absolutely impossible to get rid of the status of the lost and damned by any pious efforts on his part. But he was nonetheless driven to exhaust with desperate effort all the individual possibilities of the devotional exercises, mortifications, rituals of the Church in search of "a gracious God". And he could only see himself driven to do so because he himself had no idea as yet where he had long been and where the journey he was on inevitably was heading.

The aim of the journey was to make the principle real. The new principle existed ready-made from the outset, but it still had to be realized. At first the (already "finished") principle is only an idea, a standard and measure, something airy, unreal. For Luther, being already committed to his new principle from the beginning, it was at first only hovering high above him like his sun or his polar star (and on top of it all as an unconscious, tacitly existing celestial body). Although he saw himself forced *a tergo* to orientate himself (instinctively, so to speak) to it, the principle was not yet realized. It only became real when it came down from the state of floating high above and became the ground on which he stands, i.e., on which his whole existence is founded and of which his thinking and feeling now makes use also consciously and explicitly. Only when the principle, as indispensably binding principle, is also known and acknowledged, only when it is integrated into the form of consciousness, has man, has a figuration of human existence, truly positioned himself/itself on it as his ground.

Luther's problem was, therefore, that he subjectively remained in his consciousness entirely bound to the medieval way of thinking, while objectively his real experience was already determined by what was yet to become. Thus there is a dissociation between consciousness, on the one hand, and the soul driving Luther forward, on the other. This dissociation is the instrument, I would almost like to say: the (psychological) *machine*, with which the "soul" gets the psychically-real translation or transportation of itself from *one* status into a new status. It is the machine with which, in other words, the principle of the new status of consciousness is first merely posited, in order that this principle thereafter realizes itself, gradually brings out its realization, forces this realization all by itself, and at the same time presses on with the real expulsion from the old status (the decomposition of the principle of the latter). This machine works by means of contradiction (or *as* a contradiction), as self-contradiction, and therefore it leads the person in whom it is at work into a hell of a mess, which then, from the outside perspective, gives the impression of something abnormal, like an illness. The machine simultaneously works in opposite directions, of course in such a way that the internal contradictoriness of its goals does not thwart the true purpose of the course of events, but is precisely the way, the only way, that it can be realized. The no longer natural principle of the "whole man" edified and established itself in reality exactly by Luther's striving *with* this principle *against* this principle. His ostentatious aim was to achieve justice before God through individual efforts in the spirit of the Middle Ages; he did not want to be "post-medieval", as some people today want to be "post-modern". Luther's consciousness was turned back, away from the destination of his journey. This destination was completely unknown to him. But only by striving away from this goal did he in truth move toward it.[30]

30 As Greg Mogenson kindly reminded me, one might compare here John Donne's

This is because Luther, with his devotional efforts committed to the Middle Ages, gave the new principle—that is a first point—a concrete *real substance* for the first time, on the basis of which it could become operative in practice, applied again and again, exercised, and in this way gradually be realized. It was not allowed to be, as they say, a "merely theoretical" exercise in a dry dock, or like an armchair decision. It had to come into play *in that arena* where it was taken deadly seriously. To the extent that Luther was striving to return to the Middle Ages, the new principle inscribed itself more and more into him.

A second point is that the realization of the new principle was not allowed to simply push the old constitution of being aside, leave it behind and *replace* it (in which case the old form would still continue to exist as an alternative with which one could toy), but it had to systematically destroy it, work it off. Not the substitution of certain forms of life by others, but the transformation of the whole constitution of being-in-the-world was intended. Not an extension of the existing building, but a complete new constitution. Only if the new principle prevails without competition and alternative and there is no possibility whatsoever to switch to another principle or to switch back and forth between different standpoints or possibilities of life, does it really prevail and has consciousness placed itself unreservedly on its ground, or more correctly: *has it been* placed on its ground and *is* it now indeed standing there. Only then is the transition from one status to a new one indeed accomplished. This is another reason why Luther had to play the tragedy of the Middle Ages for himself in his painful process.

Now I would like to recapitulate by way of summary a little more schematically the various logical moments of the movement in which the realization of the principle takes place.

- The first moment: Luther, i.e. the soul in him, has already been seized by the new principle or, conversely, been expelled from the Middle Ages. He is already placed on the ground of the I, the personality as its own center. He already lives in the "future".

poem, "Good Friday, 1613. Riding Westward."

- The second moment: But the principle keeps him, i.e. his consciousness, completely in the dark about the fact that it has settled in him. It makes him almost blind to his having been expelled from the "Middle Ages". So the new does not approach him openly and directly from the front, in the form of an epiphany, a revelation that would demand acknowledgment or faith, nor even simply in the form of an inspiration, a sudden idea, a discovery. It asserts itself from behind and secretly. It has, as it were, subverted him covertly and from within.
- The third moment: Luther had been a law student. The study of law was a pioneering study. Jurisprudence was exactly in line with the development of the modern I, just as it was also of great importance for the formation of the modern State. It would therefore have been in the interest of the principle to encourage Luther to continue along this path. But no, the way of the soul is contradictory. The principle compelled him to abandon the study of law contrary to the actual direction of this principle and to move *back* to the monastery, to the "Middle Ages".
- The fourth moment: The move back to the "Middle Ages" is, however, the way into the future. By honestly struggling to achieve his spiritual tranquility on the paths of medieval piety, Luther necessarily exposes himself to absolute failure on account of his being already expelled from the "Middle Ages" by the soul. *Failure*, however, is the soul's way to realize the new principle of consciousness. The psychological realization is not an ego performance, not the egoic "implementation" or "application" of an idea into practice (only technical realization proceeds in this way). For the soul there simply is nothing that could be implemented or applied, and everything that has been implemented or applied is ipso facto external and irrelevant for the soul, merely "ego". It remains on the old level. The soul does not aim at empirical results, not at other semantic possibilities, but at the transformation of the logical constitution of consciousness. *Its* realization therefore has the form of sending man deeper and deeper into failure and exposing him to it, so that failure can come upon him and work on him, im-

> part itself to him. The realization of the new principle consists in letting *the failure* realize *itself* and letting it gradually take hold of and permeate everything. The soul is negative and realizes itself through negation. Just as a long bar of metal is gradually introduced into a melting furnace in order to be melted down, so consciousness is led deeper and deeper into failure, so that failure, which is after all the failure of the obsolete, now false expectations of consciousness, allows the illusionary nature of those expectations to be experienced *psychically-really* at first hand and as beyond all doubt. It is not theoretical, argumentative refutation, but experience in the flesh, an experience that befalls man. The new "has to be learned the hard way". The experience of the untenability of the old attitude must inscribe itself in the flesh. And insofar as the untenability of the old attitude is not based on *its* internal falsehood, but is solely due to the fact that the *new principle* has secretly already long since been actively at work and become implicitly real, insofar is the accomplished failure also the true, explicit realization of this new principle.

This is in general, it seems to me, the way "the soul" rises to a new level of itself: via failure and dis-appointment. It is a highly complex logical process. It takes place by means of self-contradiction, enantiodromy: moving (consciously) in one direction in order to arrive objectively and factually (but unconsciously) at the goal lying in the opposite direction. The progress of the soul is recursive progression, retrograde advance.

Differential diagnosis. Previous psychologists have tried on various occasions to understand the crisis Luther experienced from his biography, e.g. from his highly problematic relationship with his father. Provided that the interpretations and reflections presented here capture something and are not unfounded, they make it understandable why such a recourse to childhood and the family constellation (i.e. to the empirical, to positive facts) fundamentally misses the *dimension* at issue here. Luther's struggle is about *psychological*,[31] logical conflicts. He had his true life in spirit and soul.

Moreover, the view presented here makes it clear why *Luther's* crisis was by no means *neurotic*, although the absolutely exaggerated sense of guilt into which he maneuvered himself was in itself clearly "pathological" and, if I may say so, "highly eccentric", though "pathological"[32] only in the psychological, not in the clinical sense. Nevertheless, what happens with *Luther* is the exact opposite of a neurosis. The antagonism becomes visible in the symptoms: With Luther, "the symptoms", his, realistically-pragmatically seen, absolutely unnecessary and homemade despair, are *pointing the way forward*; they are in the service of the future, of further development. The soul *productively* develops through its own labor something unprecedentedly new, something also culturally new. His crisis has, so to speak, the character of a *rite de passage*.—In neurosis, on the other hand, the symptoms are based on a refusal, a defiance, against the very development that has already taken place. Contrary to the *already experienced* (!) obsoleteness of the previous attitude or constitution of consciousness, the *neurotic* soul stubbornly insists, precisely against its better knowledge, on the *regressive* simulation of the old attitude.[33] In contrast to Jung's view, neurosis proper is by no means a "failed attempt at solution or adaptation" (cf. *CW* 7 § 438 and § 18) and even less a *morbus sacer*. It has no redeeming value; it is simply sick.

The situation in neurosis in the 2nd and 3rd moments is therefore exactly the opposite to that in Luther. As far as the 2nd moment is concerned, in the beginning Luther knows nothing of a rupture between the Middle Ages and modern times. But the neurotic soul *has* experienced its rupture. This is why it is neurotic. And with regard to the 3rd moment we have to say that with Luther the driving force was the New that wanted to become,[34] while

31 "Psychological" in its rigorous sense of a psychology with soul, not in the nowadays ordinary personalistic sense.

32 Etymologically "pathological" goes back to the Greek word for suffering, pain, mishap.

33 "Regressive simulation or simulated restoration" versus "recursive progression, retrograde advance"!

34 This is what makes the psychological situation of young Luther analogous to

the neurotic soul tries to push itself off from the New that has already become real and return to the old and dig itself into it. That is one difference.

A second difference is that with *Luther* the symptoms are negative, in that they are the *path of failure*, of systematically working off of the obsolete, whereas in neurosis the symptoms are the positive *celebration* of the obsolete, a celebration that is successful. In compulsions, in phobic symptoms, in hysterical stagings, in neurotic depression, in anorexia, the respectively celebrated neurotic idea *triumphs* and is constantly reaffirmed anew.

A third and crucial difference is that neurotic symptoms are irrational. Their meaning and the reason for them remain mysterious; not even the neurotic himself understands why he has to wash his hands innumerable times in a row, or why a perfectly harmless plaza makes him panic or why he suffers from hysterical blindness. Neurotic symptoms belong essentially to the *unconscious*. By contrast, Luther's "symptoms", his religious qualms, exclusively take place in the full light of consciousness. They are decidedly rational, immediately comprehensible as perfectly logical consequences following from certain religious ideas, theological dogmas and presuppositions, provided that they are taken absolutely seriously and are rigorously thought through. They have their home in *theology*, on the *intellectual level*, not in the *person*.

Even though many neurotics are not obviously persons of the mind and the soul the way Luther was, the drama that takes place deep down in their neurosis is one in which also purely *psychological-noetic* concerns are at stake. But they are those of the *neurotic* soul, which is entangled in the petty and shameful, thanks to the fact that it defiantly passes off an already known untruth as the truth. What makes neurosis neurotic is precisely that the psychological/logical concerns are relegated and pushed down into the positivity of empirical realities and held down

---

the psychology of the artist. Cf. C.G. Jung: "That which in the last analysis is the subject that wills in him [the artist] is not the man as person, but the work of art." (*GW* 15 § 157, my translation. The wording in the English *CW* is too unspecific.) The work produced by the artist does not belong to him as private individual. It belongs, *if* it is a great work, to the culture as a whole or even to mankind. The same is *mutatis mutandis* true for the "I" that was produced in Luther's psychic anguish.

there, in such a way that, thus constricted, they are pressed into the narrowness of the private "interior" of the personality or, another possibility, into personal relationships (with dad, mum, partner, boss, colleague, etc.) or into irrelevant things (the spider of a spider phobia, the elevator or tunnel of claustrophobia). Furthermore, the neurotic soul keeps the personality itself out of intellectual, psychological life [the true life of the soul] by letting the personality keep *itself* above it, because this true life is depressed beneath the personality and locked within it.

Part Two of the Case History: The Solution

The breakthrough through the "sound barrier". Just as a tragedy strives from within itself towards its lysis, so does the rite of passage, *provided that* it is lived through unreservedly, with full commitment. This is a further difference to neurosis, whose inherent goal is to preserve itself forever. Luther's whole striving was to work his way out of being a sinner in order to reach the state of the just or righteous, but it was precisely this striving to get out of being a sinner that *was* his systematically digging himself deeper and deeper into the cul-de-sac of being a sinner. Through his exhaustive struggle, Luther demonstrated to himself beyond any doubt the hopelessness of his struggle and its goal. That was the result of our previous reflections. The picture of the dead end and the concept of hopelessness imply an end point at which we absolutely cannot go any further, we could also say: where one bumps into a "wall". What kind of wall is it, what does it consist of? It is not a physically existing wall against which Luther collides. Rather, it is a wall he himself *established*, by his attitude. It is the result of his own doing and thinking and thus his own work (or rather the work of "the soul" in him). He himself (i.e. "the soul" in him) builds up the hopelessness against which he desperately runs, builds it up always anew and always further. It is one and the same act that runs against the wall and ipso facto builds it up.

The wall is nothing other than his insistence on his attainment of righteousness before God. He *absolutely* wants to overcome his sinfulness, which, however, is *posited* anew and anew equiprimordially through this very willing. "Sin" is not a fact of nature (like the height of one's body), but an idea, a truth, of the soul. It is Luther who experiences himself as a sinner and absolutely concretely *experiences* himself as such! The concrete-like hardness of the wall results from the relentlessness of the contradiction: from his running against that very thing that is *his* very own experience and truth. Luther does not want to allow *his* truth to be true and fights doggedly against it.

The wall would disappear the moment he would stop running against his experience and truth. Something would open up as soon as his consciousness, dominated by "medieval" expectations, dropped these expectations and surrendered to the dead end. The cul-de-sac—that very thing that only a moment ago appeared to be a cul-de-sac—would suddenly turn into a passageway, into the eye of a needle of which we have spoken, into the gateway to a new *dimension*.

The concept of a "new dimension" is essential. What lies behind the former wall is not simply, as with empirical walls, some more of basically the same as what lies before it. It is not on the same level with it. Rather, it is something like a break through the sound barrier, more correctly: through the time wall, into a completely different dimension. Therefore one must also take the picture of the dead end at face value. At its end it is really over. *Non plus ultra.* It is the inexorable end of this "world", of this dimension, and with the breakthrough through the wall, the path is not continued into a previously only factually, only on account of the wall, *inaccessible* area, but "the world" *as a whole* is newly created, i.e. the previous world has disappeared and been replaced by a new one.

Normally the wall at the end of a dead end is experienced as an obstacle and the idea of a "dead end" or "hopelessness" awakens the desire either to somehow get through after all, or to turn back and try one's luck elsewhere. The former was what we see also in the case of Luther. He desperately tried to get out of the cul-de-sac of being a sinner. But *this* dead end is not an obstacle, but rather the goal itself, it *is* (to say it with Hölderlin) "*das Rettende*" ("that which saves"). The wall *is* the opening. The opening is not a door *in* the wall through which one could step out into an open area beyond its boundaries, nor is it the disappearance of the wall, the overcoming of it. No, the wall *is in itself* the breakthrough into the open, the only breakthrough there is. This is how contradictory things are in the sphere of "the soul". So it needed more of a dead end, not a way out, because here dead end and way out are strictly identical. It was necessary to go deeper and deeper into the cul-de-sac, not simply externally-literally, deeper in the spatial sense, but so deep that one would arrive at its *concept*, i.e. be able to comprehend its hopelessness as the goal, or the opening itself. The concept, as the dead end's soul or inwardness, is the "new dimension", and that is why entering into its concept is the breakthrough into the open, a breakthrough which nevertheless remains *in* the "dead end", indeed which is nothing other than the breakthrough into the "in". The movement can only continue through the *self-application* of the "dead end" to itself.

The cul-de-sac is and remains a cul-de-sac in the everyday sense of the word, as long as one either wants to get out of it again or, conversely, over it, to the other side of that wall through which it becomes a cul-de-sac. For then one remains in the same old dimension, on the old level of spatial thinking, and this remaining in the spatial dimension *is* the very impasse. What is at stake in our context is not a movement from here to there across a spatial boundary, but a breakthrough from a first, familiar dimension into a completely different one.

The knowledge of such a breakthrough into a completely new, different dimension by the entering into the interior of a dead-end street or a wall is ancient. It precedes all conceptual thinking for a long time. We find it expressed in numerous fairy tales and legends, for example through the idea of the open and light[35] stone. One record can be found, for example, in Snorri's *Heimskringla*: a Swedish king named Sveigðir goes into a massive rock the size of a house on the evening of a feast day without ever returning; all his life he had longed to meet the god Odin; he had already made an unsuccessful five-year trip to get to Odin; now, back home again, a dwarf beckons him, standing below the door of the stone:

35 "Light" in the sense of flooded with light.

there he will meet Odin. Sveigðir, we hear, jumps into the stone and the stone closes behind him.[36] "In Central European mountains there are countless stone walls that open at the right hour or for the miracle key."[37] This is the pre-conceptual, visual image for the breakthrough into a completely different dimension (Sveigðir jumps from the ordinary world into the dimension of the gods) and at the same time the sign for the clear knowledge that the other dimension is not given positively, but has its place in logical negativity (expressed figuratively in the ἀδύνατον, the "impossibility", of a (despite its massiveness) light, within-itself-bright and open, stone, as well as an entering only with the help of a miracle key or at the "right" time). God is not to be found in the distance. The five-year journey to the East did not lead him to his goal and would not have led to his goal even as a ten- or twenty-year journey: the path to God does not run in sensual space, in positivity. The impenetrable stone (just like the cul-de-sac) is the image of the *closedness* of the sensual space, the image for one's winding up with it, for one's *having* finished with it. In this respect, the five-year trip to the East was not in vain, just as little as were Luther's protracted struggles: it was necessary to exhaust the idea that in sensual space or in the space of imagination there was a natural way to God. This journey had been Sveigðir's way of failure.

The idea of a cul-de-sac must itself be comprehended as a cul-de-sac. One must not fall for its everyday sense. If the notion dead end is applied to itself, then the dead end, the wall or the stone, will open up and it becomes possible to leap into it. The idea of the dead end only reveals that one wants to go *beyond* it. But in the soul it is a matter of fully and truly getting *into* it. One must not rest content with the banal sense of dead end or stone, one must not make one's peace with the dead end, for example, the way Kafka's man from the countryside, in "Before the Law", resigns himself to the prohibition of the doorkeeper.

The transition into a new dimension must therefore not be pre-

36 *Snorris Königsbuch* vol. I. In: *Thule*, vol. 14, Jena 1922, p. 38. Quoted from Heino Gehrts, "Vom Wesen der Steine", in: *GORGO 11* (1986), pp. 3–27, here p. 18. For a more detailed discussion of this whole topic see my "The Leap Into the Solid Stone", in: W.G., *The Soul Always Thinks* (= W.G., CEP 4) 2010, pp. 165–172.

37 Gehrts, *op. cit.*, p. 18, my translation.

sented, for example, as an ascent to a higher level, to a new "storey", because in this way one remains in spatial thinking, which in turn means: in the mode of imagination, and thus in the same old dimension. The leap into the solid, massive stone cannot and must not be imagined; it would be an absurd idea. In terms of the imagination, it is a miracle. But logically speaking, it is by no means a miracle. That the stone "opens up" is not a wonder or fluke, but results from the willingness, no matter at what cost and risk, to dare the impossible, to do what is absolutely feared: in other words, to go all the way through with the experienced *necessity*.

Now it also becomes clear why there must be a dead end and why the open lies not beyond the wall but *in* the "obstacle", *in* the impenetrable stone of the wall itself. If the wall were nothing more than an obstacle to be overcome, then consciousness would remain, even after its overcoming, in the dimension whose crossing was the very issue. Psychologically, it would have been a waste of time and energy. Consciousness must really experience hopelessness, suffer it through to the bitter end, it must collide with the impenetrability of the stone, because only in this impenetrability is the "sound barrier" or "time wall" really there for it, which (in contrast to positive walls) *is* nothing other than the clash of two dimensions. In the relentless end of the cul-de-sac and in the impenetrable hardness of the stone, the real and absolute end of the hitherto ordinary dimension is indeed experienced and does this dimension really *end*. And only when this *real end* is experienced and the price that it demands paid, which also means: when the experience has been made that it is really over (only then is it a real end at all), is the breakthrough into the new dimension accomplished. The old dimension must not simply be bypassed and ignored and thus remain, because then it would continue to exist; that is, it would not be finished.

The end of the old dimension is therefore not simply an end that as a new fact would be inflicted on it. Rather, the end only happens because man as subject is *exposed* to the end of the old dimension and *himself* has to die *its* death. Otherwise the "wall" of the cul-de-sac would remain external, physical, a soulless fact, a senseless obstacle. It would not have become psychological at all.

A merely positive-factual overcoming of the old dimension would be tantamount to avoiding its end and would rob this end of its soul. The process is animated only by the fact that *we* lend it our soul. It needs us as we need it. *We* must take the "impossible" leap, *we* must get into the stone, so that the constitution of our consciousness can experience its transformation and suffer it through. The new dimension is not simply an existing reality. It is not a place in the world. It first arises and only becomes real when and because a consciousness has *entered* into it.

Continuation of the "case history": The resolution of Luther's crisis. Luther's process drove him into the despair in which he had *his* crash against the sound barrier. *His* impenetrable stone was the thought of being a sinner, of eternal damnation. And so also the solution of his "crisis", his breaking through the "sound barrier", lay solely in leaping into the concept of sin without reservation. Exactly what he had wanted to prevent *at all costs*, what he had struggled to overcome, was his salvation. In the soul the illness itself is the cure. The healing does not lie outside, beyond the illness. The illness is the initiation into the illness itself. It *is* illness as long as the initiation into it is not yet complete. The liberation in this sense for Luther lay in the unconditional surrender to the worst, most extreme eventuality, and his formula for it was: *se resignare ad infernum*, to resign oneself to the possibility of exile to hell. That was the step that gave Luther inner peace. He had to lay down his arms, no longer allow himself to kick against the pricks (Acts 9:5 and 26:14). After all, he had had to learn that there was no freedom from ego-willing, *that* ego-willing which was the heart or principle of all sin.

But now a single needle's eye appeared: at one single point the will could free itself from the ego, namely in the act of voluntary submission to God's judgment, even if it meant eternal damnation. For that is no longer the eudemonic ego-willing. In this unique act, the unity of man's and God's will that had previously been striven for in vain, was established. If God so pleases to reject me, and I agree with the possibility of belonging to those rejected by God, then I no longer want what I want, but what God wants.

A kind of union of opposites takes place: The acceptance of the absolute separation from God ("eternal damnation") is the restoration of oneness of his and of God's will, along with the simultaneous undiminished recognition of the modern discontinuity in the relationship between man and God. The complexity inherent in this contradictoriness is the sign of the new stage of consciousness.

Previously, Luther had always radically separated Salvation from judgement and damnation. Salvation and damnation were mutually exclusive opposites. Now he had to realize that the gate to salvation is the Judgement itself. Salvation lies in the stone of stumbling and the rock of offence, if I may combine two different images here, the literal image of the stone of offence and the image of myths and legends of the impenetrable stone, which as solid is nevertheless in itself bright and hollow. And he can only pass through this gate into the open, namely into the impenetrable stone as into the logical negativity of a completely new dimension, if he adopts the verdict of rejection at the Last Judgement as his own, if he carries it out himself as a judgement of rejection of himself, a judgement which extends to his whole person (not to individual offences). He had to go all the way down, to the zero point of self-abasement (mind you: *logical*, not emotional nor devout, pious, self-abasement). That was the κένωσις (*kénosis*, Phil. 2:7), absolute emptying, which of course is to be understood here primarily as being emptied of ego-willing. In some ways, Luther has *psychologically*, though not empirically, or literally, performed a descent to hell. To put it more realistically, he has found his way into his status as Prodigal Son.

This is expressed most clearly in such extreme formulations as: *esto peccator et pecca fortiter*, "*Be* a sinner and sin heartily". This, in the context in which it is spoken, is not a call for a debauched, immoral way of life. That would be the sentence semantically understood. But it refers to the logic or *concept* of being human, not to behavior. This thought has nothing at all to do with the way of life and behavior. As we have already seen, Luther had long since left behind him the whole level of the empirical-practical, and we too find ourselves on a psychological level, not the level of behavior. What is at stake here is, as the first word of that Latin sentence indicates, alone man's logical *status of being*. He is to let himself fall completely into his real state of being as a natural, sinful man as into his *truth*,[38] to settle without reservation in it, to take up this state of being into his definition, into his self-understanding, and thus to take relentlessly seriously the insight that he *is* a sinner by nature (and that means inevitably), and therefore absolutely lost. He is to stop the whole contorted struggle of wanting to be better and more than he is. The hope that he might still be able to prove himself to be able to attain justice before God must be completely abandoned. No more games to fool himself into believing in a chance *known* not to exist. The full, even absolute price for one's being "natural man" is to be paid down to the last cent. One cannot *be* a natural (here = earthly, "fleshly") human being and still claim to achieve unity of one's will with God. Paying this price is the admission ticket for the transfer from the Middle Ages into the dimension of the modern I.

"The Birth". These insights are an expression of the fact that Luther has "metaphysically" fallen out of the containment in "Abraham's bosom" as well as of the fundamental embeddedness in "the bosom of the Church", and has received this loss of containment into his consciousness, even actively *renounced* the idea of containment. He is now standing outside, (in the psychological sense of the word) *extra ecclesiam*. He is no longer by nature, simply by being born into the Church, in (potentially) irrevocable connection with the heavenly Father, so that all that would still be needed for him to do would be, through special efforts in his real behavior, through a particularly pious way of life, to prove that this logically unbroken, "metaphysically" existing relationship of unity with the Father is also empirically and practically actual. With the *se resignare ad infernum*, the break of unity, the fundamental separation from the Father, is irrevocably accomplished and acknowledged.

The state of being inalienably contained in God's grace or of having an unshaken harmony between God and man as the background of his existence means *psychologically* living high up in

38 That is his psychological, not a positive truth.

"heaven", so to speak in "Cloud-Cuckoo-Land". As much as in the Middle Ages, too, empirically real existence was naturally an earthly existence and as such was exposed to all the hardships, plights, and sufferings of life on earth, the *logical* place of human life was nevertheless in the Pleroma or in paradise and not on this earth. Wherever there is an intact, living mythology and an equally living ritual life, existence is, psychologically or logically seen, pleromatic, and man is ipso facto psychologically still unborn because he is completely contained in and embraced by mythical meaning. Just as with his biological birth man, as individual person, is not yet psychologically born, but his birth as a *human* being has yet to take place in several mostly painful stages, so also does the simple fact of the existence of the species homo sapiens not mean that the human being would already be born psychologically. The psychologically natural man is in the state of being unborn. In the Middle Ages we of course no longer find myth in the original sense, but we still find something like its equivalent: the fundamental embeddedness of human existence in the grace of the heavenly Father. (Because "bosom" and "birth" here are psychological concepts, there is no need for a mother.)

Luther, however, has descended from the original height, from heaven as man's a priori place of existence, to the *empirical* earth. He has irrevocably stepped out of the Pleroma as natural man's essential home. The *empirical* earth is no longer a priori embedded in the divine meaning and thus at the same time also a logically sublated one. He expressly renounced his a priori connection with God by accepting the idea that—seen from a purely earthly-human point of view—*man's essential homeland is hell* and not heaven. This is his psychological birth, his psychological incarnation.

"Hell" is here no longer a mythological place. It must not be imagined and ontologized, for example, as a literal place where souls are tormented by little devils in eternal fire. The experience of hell in the case of Luther must already be understood as a real *thought*, albeit a thought in the still traditional form of an image. *Hell is simply the name for the absolute distance from God*, the fundamental having fallen out of His grace. To have logically established oneself as one's own center (opposite God as the other center) is in itself already hell. There are not three places: Heaven, earth and hell, but only two: heaven (the place of God) and earth (the place of man). But in order to in fact come down to earth from the original existence in heaven, the thought of hell as the thought of the abstract negation of heaven, the absolute separation from God, is required. Otherwise it would not be possible to cut through all the bonds that logically tied back the existence of natural man to or into the Pleroma.[39] Here one also sees how misguided are Jung's ideas about evil as "the Fourth".

Luther lets himself fall into his earthly, "carnal" being and once and for all puts an end to the wish to patch up a relationship that was already broken. Luther no longer *has* a gracious God and cannot win him either. The loss of a priori containment in grace by virtue of his natural humanness has been suffered through and *abgetrauert*, grieved to a finish (as we say today). Luther is completely thrown back on himself, on his empirical humanness. He has given up the higher blessed status of God-childhood that came

"Man's Position in the Cosmos"

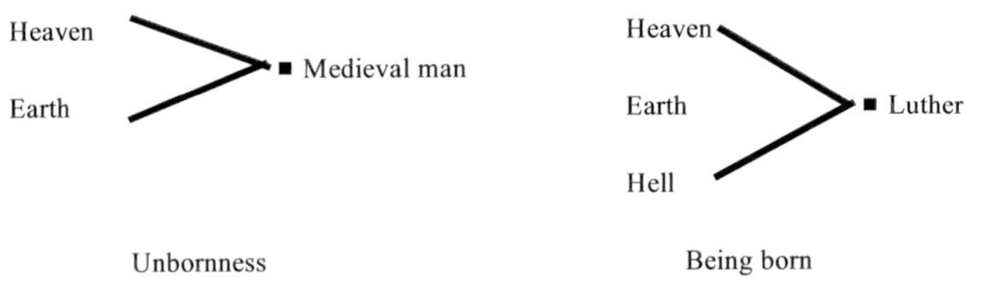

with his natural being. He has divested himself of the still "mythical" garment of a child of God; having accepted his position as an earthly man, he has distinguished himself from the archetypal role which he had previously still claimed for himself. At that time, to be sure, he still wore the monk's robe and lived a monk's way of life. But logically this mythical garment and the status of potential saint it claimed had already been discarded. The whole

39 Concerning the necessary two-steps move (double pace) cf. W.G., "Der Doppelschritt: Vom Buchstäblichen über das Imaginale zum Konkret-Wirklichen. Eine Antwort an Frau Vetter-Lüscher", in: *GORGO* 16/1989, pp. 60–67.

mode of the imitation (re-enactment) of the *exemplary* life of the saints and the *constant practice* of a prescribed attitude of humility (as, for example, in mysticism), which was characteristic for the medieval form of being-in-the-world, had been abandoned in favor of a life completely to be lived on one's own account.

The nature or essence of man is now *demythologized.*[40] And that is the birth of man as "I" and as a *psychologically* adult. It is the explicit stepping out of the "Middle Ages", out of "immaturity" (no matter whether self-incurred or not), out of "nature",[41] and entry into having to stand up *for oneself.* Man now stands on principle *extra ecclesiam*, as an individual and therefore naked and destitute before God. Luther confesses to his nothing but empirical humanness, his being nothing but human, all-too-human. He lets himself fall completely into this status. The "umbilical cord" which directly connected him psychologically with the divine meaning (a meaning that could be immediately extracted from the natural world as creation and *ordo*) is cut. The embeddedness in something encompassing, supporting and relieving is over. It has been replaced by the essential *being vis-à-vis* (vis-à-vis God and the world, Being as a whole). (Medieval man did not only *not* stand opposite the world, but also not opposite God. No doubt, God was indeed infinitely high above him, but at the same time by virtue of the *analogia entis* not *absolutely* distant.) Insofar as (the psychologically understood) nature = containment in myth, insofar is the demythologization of the human being at the same time also the "sacrifice of the merely natural man" (in the sense of C.G. Jung, *CW* 8 § 751). This sacrifice has been made by one's on principle

40 It goes without saying that along with this, also nature in general (here as much as: the world as physis) is demythologized.

41 Through this stepping out of nature, two meanings of "nature" now fall apart, because stepping out of nature in the sense of being contained in something comprehensive and meaningful is in itself stepping into nature as the creaturely "sinful" constitution of man. So there are several ambiguities of the word nature: besides the difference between nature as essence or constitution (the nature of man or the nature of the thing) and nature as physis or geological-biological environment we have the contrast of "merely-natural man" as unconsciously encompassed by divine meaning and "merely-natural man" as earthly, human-all-too-human man, empirical homo sapiens. The appropriate sense of "nature" and "natural" must be inferred from each respective context.

agreeing with the eventuality of being condemned a priori by God.

As the logical birth of man means having broken once and for all with being embedded in nature, it also means that man has now become *conscious* of being himself a piece nature. Becoming conscious is always accompanied by the parting from or loss of what one has become aware of. The reception of the idea of "being a sinner" (= of being a natural ["fleshy"] human being) into conscious self-understanding is man's birth (*zur Welt Kommen*), his coming down to earth, and casting off of the mythical garment of a child of heaven. Or it is at least the *first immediacy* of this casting off. Luther has overcome the (psychological) natural state because he has his naturalness *as a reflected one* in his consciousness.

But the *se resignare ad infernum* does not mean that Luther has now deliberately *committed* himself to hell, especially not with morbid lust; it means nothing more than his *de-identification* from the original claim to be able to stand, (fundamentally) by nature and (*actualiter*) by himself (through his own behavior), in the grace of God. The "marriage" between God and man is (to begin with) divorced. The pleromatic background of being and the empirical foreground have split apart; the connection between the two, by virtue of which the empirical foreground has always already been *contained* in and *sublated* by the divine background, has broken. This renunciation and loss is the κένωσις. But at the same time it is also the release and letting go of God: God is no longer with might and main to be coerced to still be a God gracious to me. It is entirely up to him to judge me as he wants or must. But with this "letting God be completely free to pass his judgement on me", that judgement that He wants or must pass, I too become truly free. I am no longer dependent on a favorable judgement. I have paid the price that freedom requires.

It is true that Luther did all this. But it is crucial to see that this achievement does not simply belong to his personal psychology, to his individual development. Luther did not simply overcome his crisis and win a solution for himself. Rather, what happened in and through him is the fundamental historical birth of man as such (of course not civilian man, man as empirical fact, but man *in his "metaphysical" essence*—the Self of man, as Jung might have said), albeit only at the *one* point of *his* person. From now on the "sound barrier" is broken in principle, the human being is ejected from the Pleroma, potentially for all human beings. The *concept* of personality, of subjectivity, of the I, has become psychologically real and is from now on available, so to speak. This concept now exists and unfolds its own dynamics—admittedly in long periods spanning centuries; its logic works (above all also underground, unconsciously), it is infectious. The people who come *after* Luther do not all have to go the same way of suffering on their own in order to become a personality, just as the Pythagorean theorem does not have to be invented anew by every schoolchild. Just as the crisis had been created in Luther by "the soul" for its own purposes, so has "the soul" in Luther also evicted itself from itself, from its original Pleroma, *for its own sake*, not for him and not for us, in order to transport *itself* into another status of its own.

A poignant image of this fundamentally new life situation of man is expressed in the words that Luther is said to have spoken at the Imperial Diet in Worms (the tradition concerning the exact wording of his dictum varies): "Here I stand, I cannot do otherwise, may God help me. Amen!" Just imagine: Luther, an insignificant monk from Wittenberg (and we must also take into account that monastic status was at that time generally very little respected), stands all alone—in the truest sense of the word: *mutterseelenallein*—before the assembled imperial princes, archbishops, cardinals and the emperor of the Holy Roman Empire and presents his convictions, which had been condemned by the Church as heretical. And he ends his remarks with the dictum quoted. This statement contains multiple aspects:

1. I am all alone, all on my own, isolated, lost, abandoned. I cannot invoke any higher authority, any protective power that would back up my claims and thus give credit to them, or whose mere speaker I would be. I have to shoulder the responsibility for what I say all by myself. I have to rely exclusively on my own poor human insight. I am speaking only as the subjectivity that I am and claim no more than that for myself. I do not claim to be in possession of the truth or to speak, as it were, *ex cathedra*. The fact that in principle I could also be in

error is conceded from the outset; but if that should actually be the case, it would have to be demonstrated to me in detail.

2. But speaking in this way only for myself and in my admitted weakness and mere subjectivity, I nevertheless *stand*. I stand firm, hold my ground. I really stand up for what I have to say before the whole world and with all the possible consequences.
3. And I do this because I cannot do otherwise, that is to say, because I unreservedly let myself fall into the necessity of my being-so, my actual insight, which *is* what it is, and I let it bind me.
4. Because I only stand up for myself and my human-all-too-human insight, I completely surrender myself and what I have to say to the judgment of God as the last and actual authority.

By subordinating himself to God as the ultimate authority, Luther at the same time implicitly says that he does not recognize the judgement of human beings or authorities as *ultimately* authoritative. This implies that the individual, as subjectivity, is now primarily thrown back on himself, on his own mind, *his* real insight, *his* experience. Not the Church, not tradition, not society are, in ultimate matters, binding. By contrast, the Church could still invoke the idea that God has spoken and continues to speak through her, that the Church administers God's revelation. But the God to whom Luther submits here no longer speaks *directly* in revelations, be it through dreams, through signs of nature, holy institutions, the mouth of prophets, etc. The umbilical cord is cut. There are no longer any direct and positive (positivizable) messages from God. God—as the ultimate authority—is now out of reach, logically negative. No one can now claim that *God* has spoken to him and that He speaks through him: "I am the voice of God". It might of course be the case that God indeed speaks through an individual, also through this Luther before the Imperial Diet of Worms, but the point here is that whether this is the case or not must be left to God. There is no human, empirical proof of this. The risk of going astray is always given. Thus the invocation of God as the ultimate authority is nothing other than Luther's confession that he has unreservedly and as honestly as possible and with as much critical intellect as he possesses, surrendered himself to what *appears* to *him* to be the truth. Because Luther now speaks only on his own responsibility, his awareness of his absolute dependence on God's help is indispensable.

No matter whether or not Luther actually said that sentence exactly in that way—it is certain that the sentence excellently expresses the new state of being he had reached in a single concise formula. The break with the natural state of shelteredness and embeddedness is obvious. He no longer believes that he can see and understand himself primarily from God, from a given eternal truth, but knows that he must stand before God from the standpoint of his subjectivity and thus on his own account.

So far I have described the soul's construction of the early-modern I as a process that took place in Martin Luther. This exclusive focus in my representation might give rise to the wrong impression of a solitary significance of Luther for the emergence of this new mode of being-in-the-world. But the principle of the early-modern I emerged, and has been expressed, in different ways, in different places, on completely different levels and in different regards in the centuries around, before, and after Luther's lifetime. I will mention some major instances and regards.

- For Luther it was the real process of *personal existential experience* in which the birth of man was realized and painfully inscribed into the soul. Here we have the psychological transformation, the *psychically real* transport of the soul from one logical locus to another through the experience of a personal crisis. Luther's experience could be seen as the modern psychologized and personalized equivalent of what would have been an initiation ritual in archaic times.[42]
- Already earlier, the principle of the early-modern I had presented itself in painting in the invention of central perspective as a principle of aesthetic intuition. Here it was not an existentially experienced principle, but a formal one, a construction principle for pictorial representations. It presents itself externally as a visible image, but not as the content of the image, but as the general schematic form into which any content

42 Conversely, the initiation ritual in archaic times served only to bring the individual to the level of adulthood and "metaphysical" knowledge *reached by the tribe*, by the collective, while in the individual person Luther a *further development* of the *whole culture* or of the status of consciousness as such, of the general psychological being, took place.

is fitted. The scientific description of the inner logic of the central perspective required a new mathematics, the infinitesimal calculus, which was only developed later, in the 17th century.

- The development of the monetary economy and early capitalism on the real, "materialistic" ground of economic activity is a "symptom" of the emergence of the early-modern I.
- *After* Luther it is, in the sphere of *thought*, especially the philosophy of Descartes, in which it is not only theoretically formulated as a principle of philosophy (*ego cogito*) and rationally argumentatively justified, but *ipso facto* inevitably makes itself also *de facto* felt by the fact that Descartes can no longer orientate himself on authorities, but must exclusively and systematically rely on the insight of reason itself, that is, on the *inherent* principles of *reason*. Although this is a completely different sphere of the mind, the parallelism with Luther is obvious. I do not want to go into these facts, which are largely known. Rather, I would like here to present
- a fifth form in which the same thing articulated itself: that form of articulation in which it has coagulated into the *primal image* of a human being who has become the I, the first immediacy of the psychologically truly born man. Instead of "primal image" I could also use the word "archetypal image", but that evokes the idea of timelessness. The image to be discussed here, however, is not valid at all times. It is essentially historical, fundamentally new, characteristic of a new epoch in the life of the soul. The primal image has found its realization or representation in the figure and fate of Robinson Crusoe, and it appears in narrative form, as a novel. It is the equivalent of what would have been a myth in primitive times. The modern I cannot appear in a myth, because myth is the form for the soul when it is not I, when it is still contained in a world of meaning shining forth from nature. The religious stage of the soul is also already beyond myth.

Excursus: The primal image of born man, man having come down to earth: Robinson Crusoe. This figure was invented by Daniel Defoe (1660? – 1731) and is the protagonist of his novel *The Life and Strange Surprizing Adventures of Robinson*

Crusoe ..., which appeared in 1719. So with this novel we are a full two hundred years after Luther. But what we found in Luther as a personal experience is, in the fate of this figure, captured in an image, coagulated into a picture. The extent to which this quasi-archetypical image has hit the psychological form of existence of early-modern man at its core and expresses it, the extent to which it responded to a need of people to have their own existence vividly and objectively in front of them in an image and thus to be able to reflect on it, can be seen from the fact that the book became a worldwide success within a short time and was not only disseminated in countless translations, but also prompted numerous imitations. As the future would show, Defoe had with this book founded a whole genre of novels, the Robinsonades.

I said the character in the novel was invented by Defoe, but that is not quite true. Defoe made use of the real story of a shipwrecked sailor who lived on an island in the Pacific for four and a half years before (in 1709, ten years before Defoe's novel) being rescued by a ship's captain, a story that had caused a sensation at the time. But in the context of our psychological question this real, factual background of the novel's content interests us as little as does *the way* in which Defoe, as an empirical author, *processed* and *shaped* this story in his novel with all its details. We cannot be concerned here with the literal novel as a literary work and work of art, with the actual text and its individual episodes, with its embellishment with special features and with many reflections that the specific *consciousness* of the author and his time, the English Enlightenment, and the pragmatic-utilitarian ethos of the merchant class are reflected. What the author wanted to say with his novel and how he saw things is irrelevant to us. It is the image, hidden in the *core* of the plot and behind the temporal embellishments motivated by ideological ideas and moral goals, the *image of man as having been cast away on a deserted island*, that we must peel out from its incidental rootedness in a specific mental world and in the personal idiosyncrasies of the author. And we must also sometimes protect the immanent, "autonomous" *logic* of this nuclear image from the explicit intentions of the narrator and the literal text of the novel. For only that approach gives us the primal image.

The two central moments of the image are the shipwreck and the existence alone on an island. They form a unity. First, I turn to the logic of the idea of shipwreck. This shipwreck is neither one on the high seas, where the ship with man and mouse disappear into the depths of the sea, nor a shipwreck in sight of inhabited land, where through a possible rescue the impact of the shipwreck would be cushioned and reduced to a painful material loss. Robinson Crusoe is suffering shipwreck in *such a way* that he can neither drown nor continue to live in the human world. Rescue to an island deprives the shipwreck of the literalness of 'catastrophe', of 'doom'. The loneliness of the deserted island deprives the 'rescue' of its literalness, insofar as *this* rescue is in itself a catastrophe (absolute isolation, solitary confinement, total expulsion from the human world and civilization and becoming suddenly and directly exposed to the wilderness). It is, in other words, the shipwreck itself! Precisely for this reason, what presents itself as an adventure novel opens up to other dimensions. While an ordinary adventure is something that happens to a certain individual in reality, without affecting the ontological or logical constitution of the world and being-in-the-world or man's self-definition, the shipwreck in our novel, together with the hero's being cast away on a deserted island, is the image of or *exemplum* for a revolutionary change in the constitution of human existence in general. The shipwreck and the abandonment not only happen to this one individual, but also to the image of man in general, to the logical state of consciousness, which this one individual merely represents and displays for us. So, for our psychological standpoint, the novel is not about the *life* of a person, it is not a fictitious biography, indeed it is not about a *person* at all, but about the logic of human existence, of course in such a way that this theme is presented pictorially using the example of a person's life.

Even if Robinson Crusoe does not die physically, there is an experience of death inherent in "being shipwrecked". It is an image for the rupture of continuity: for the radical break with the world from which he comes, with tradition and with the human community. With the sinking of the ship it is over with his containment in an a priori existing security, with his embeddedness in a larger comprehensive meaning-providing order, with his reliably being supported by solid ground. Certainly, the ship's floor is not the floor of dry land. But it is the "sublated" ground of the mainland, taken with him to the sea as a sublated moment or symbolic representation. Figuratively speaking, it is the *internalized* ground which man can take along with him wherever he goes, even when he leaves the mainland. The ship is, so to speak, the portable memory of the homeland in the form of a concrete shape, the memory especially of solid ground. The ship is the symbol which guarantees one's staying *essentially* (even if not in practical reality) connected with one's origin. When the ship sinks, the parting from one's own origin is irrevocably accomplished.

The sailor is the image of that man or that way of existence where *literal* dependence on the solid ground was abandoned but internalized as the *idea* of the solid ground, which in turn was projected out of the interior and objectified as the ship's floor. This means, however, that *psychologically* dependence on the solid land remains intact. Even while at sea, the sailor is in this sense still a "landlubber", the floor of his ship being still being a kind of ersatz ground beneath his feet.

The two logical operations of the soul that have been presented here in a sketchy way, are so important and of such general importance that I would like to describe each of them briefly again.

- The first operation that the soul can perform is to internalize a given external reality, that is, to transform it into a memory image, a concept, an idea, a principle. This is a process of sublation (or, alchemically speaking, of distillation, evaporation). Through this process, the original object is deprived of its ultimate and full meaning, which at the same time means that man logically—albeit not completely factually—frees himself from his dependence on this object. In its transformed form as concept or principle or category, the latter is now a property of consciousness. In this respect, the operation described is also a process of integration: what was previously an external object and as such the *content* of consciousness, has now—in the form of concept, principle, category—become a part of the logical *form* of consciousness, *the way* consciousness thinks and experiences.

- The second operation that the soul can perform is that it can set up outside of itself that external reality that has been internalized as a concept or principle and give it *as sublated moment* or *as symbolic representation* a sensual, thing-like form in reality. This is not a relapse into the initial situation, but a further step forward that is carried out on the sublated content and now again sublates it (by depriving it of its pure inwardness). In our example, it is the planks of the ship's deck in which the *mental* image or principle of the solid ground takes on a sensual-material form.

Because the soul is capable of performing these two logical operations, humanity has been able to rise above the (biological) nature state, in contrast to animals, which remain largely attached to their instinctual patterns of behavior and their direct relation to their environment. Human civilization is largely based on these two possibilities of the soul.

To the extent that the ship is the symbol in or through which (not the literal, but) the psychological connection with the mainland and home is still guaranteed to the seafarer who has overcome his literal dependence on solid ground, the breaking and sinking of the ship is now also a brutal attack on the still remaining *psychological dependence* on solid ground.

In the novel, Robinson Crusoe is the son of a merchant who expressly warns his son against risking the blessings of the golden middle state. My father, he writes,

> told me it was for Men of desperate Fortunes on one Hand, or of aspiring, superior Fortune on the other, who went abroad upon Adventures, to rise by Enterprize, and make themselves famous in Undertakings of a Nature out of the common Road; that these things were all either too far above me, or too far below me; that mine was the middle State, or what might be called the upper Station of *Low Life,* which he had found by long Experience was the best State in the World, the most suited to human Happiness, not exposed to the Miseries and Hardships, the Labour and Sufferings of the mechanick Part of Mankind, and not embarass'd with the Pride, Luxury, Ambition and Envy of the upper Part of Mankind. He told me, I might judge of the Happiness of this State, by this one thing, *viz.* That this was the State of Life which all other People envied, that Kings have frequently lamented the miserable Consequences of being born to great things, and wish'd they had been placed in the Middle of the two

Extremes, between the Mean and the Great....

But an irresistible thirst for adventure drives Robinson Crusoe to sea. One can think in this connection of the words from Goethe's *Faust* written more than one hundred and fifty years later, which Faust, animated by his idea of the "Earth Spirit", exclaims:

> Ich fühle Mut, mich in die Welt zu wagen,
> Der Erde Weh, der Erde Glück zu tragen,
> Mit Stürmen mich herumzuschlagen
> Und in des Schiffbruchs Knirschen nicht zu zagen.
>
> "I feel courage to venture out into the world,
> To bear earth's woe, earth's happiness,
> To grapple with storms
> And not lose heart in the crunching noise of shipwreck" (lines 464–7).

In both cases, albeit in quite different contexts, we have the image of a person who strives to get out of the given containment and shelteredness within a community, who is willing to *expose* himself to life entirely on his own account and risk, thus consciously taking the risk of shipwreck and destruction. "To bear earth's woe, earth's happiness": this is the overcoming (negation) of the narcissistic urge to avoid pain under all circumstances and to attain well-being, and it is the readiness, if necessary, to allow life to wound oneself—all for the sake of the full intensity of an unreservedly lived, exhausted life. Indeed, in the sacrifice of his narcissistic dependence on the topic of pain and well-being, man has already *logically* performed the cut into his own flesh. The notion of a possibly threatening disaster no longer has the power of an argument for this person. It cannot shake his decision.

One's risking oneself as long as one is still on the mainland and hopes to get through unharmed remains in the status of a mere *possibility* and thus a noncommittal idea. The real test comes, of course, only when what was an idea turns into reality. The merely imagined shipwreck is harmless. The enticement by the world and its exotic charms are strong enough to allow one to lightly disregard the possible disaster. However, the enticement that a man like Robinson Crusoe feels does not, psychologically, at all have distant miracles as its intended goal. These serve "the soul" only as a lure for ego-consciousness. What is in truth *intended* is real shipwreck as the veritable initiation into exactly that which had previously only nonchalantly been imagined as a mere eventuality. To remain within the imagery of the Robinson Crusoe story: it is not enough to *de facto* leave one's home and the mainland, to board a ship and sail to foreign parts of the world. For as long as that is all, one always takes along with the ship and its floor one's psychological connection with solid land and the land of origin. What is necessary is the shipwreck itself, being cast away on a deserted island, and thus the absolute negation of psychological attachment to the homeland. This is the telos "of the soul" here.

Now I turn to the second aspect, exposure to a deserted island. What does this feature of our image contain and imply? By being cast away on a deserted island, Robinson Crusoe is (in modern existentialist terms) "thrown into existence". He had not been *thrown* into existence before. He had previously not only been metaphysically a child of God, but also contained on earth in the bosom of the human community, the bosom of a Church. Being thrown onto the island is his psychological birth. Only now did he really come into the world, has he arrived in the earthly reality stripped of all mythical garments. Now he has been completely thrown back on himself, is completely on his own. He no longer lives primarily as part of an encompassing whole, such as the Church, which assumes ultimate responsibility for him and provides the ultimate answers in all essential things. In this way, however, he has also completely fallen out of the meaning it had given him.

He is now solely responsible for himself. He now stands in direct relation to God. Ultimately, if one disregards his obligation to God and thinks only of human and pragmatic realities, it is also entirely up to him whether he assumes any responsibility at all, or not. He could, for example, simply remain lying on the beach if he were too lazy to take action in order to find shelter and food. But if he remains idle, he has nothing to eat then or the next day, and has no protection at night from cold, rain and wild animals. He *can* behave like that, nobody cares two hoots about it. There is nobody who could tell him what to do or wag his finger at him. It is all entirely up to him. But, of course, he will not remain lying there, because his *own reason* tells him that he must take into his own hands care for the security of his life and for his comfort, not because he *is supposed to* for reasons of social morality, but because he *wants to* out of self-interest, quite pragmatically according to an "if – then" logic.

He also does not have to prove anything to anyone, nor try to impress anybody. He cannot lose face. He simply lives in his truth, as good or bad, smart or stupid as he really is. Things are now just the way they are and must be. No dressing up through ideologies. The only reason for acting and forbearance is his own, albeit rational, will and being-so. Life is demythologized, enlightened, freed for soberly pragmatic viewpoints and freed to focus on empirical causal connections. Under these circumstances there can be no feelings of guilt, no feelings of worthlessness, nor any self-aggrandizement (ideas of grandiosity), because reality step by step mercilessly abrades all silly ideas and illusions.

There is no one on whose shoulders he could cry, whom he could ask for consolation when he feels miserable, whom he could ask for advice when he is faced with pressing questions and decisions, but also no one with whom he could share his joy. He must settle everything with himself. There is also no Other from whom he could expect anything and hope for anything, to whom he could have claims and from whom he could feel narcissistically offended if his expectations were not fulfilled. No one with whom he would have to get somewhere, by whom he would absolutely want to be "meant", wanted, loved.

He also has to mobilize himself to whatever is to be done, because there simply is no one who could take the initiative for him and from whom he could hope to get the impetus for his own actions, and above all hope to be taken by his hand and told where to go. He is freed from all this. Freed to what? To simply being-himself. The shipwreck forced him completely into himself, settled him in himself.

He who has become so logically lonely (truly "*mutterseelenallein*") is psychologically adult. He is I, a subject, because he is completely thrown back on himself.

It goes without saying that this primal image does not depict the *empirical* situation of the adult human being who has become an ego-personality, an I, but only his *quintessence* or the *logic* of his situation. In the practical reality of one's way of life, this logical loneliness by no means excludes living in a human community, in modern society, and in close relationships; indeed, the fully appropriated logical loneliness is even the precondition for a happy interpersonal relationship under the conditions of the consciousness's constitution as the consciousness of man having become a modern individual. This is so because the desire for an a priori existing, not empirically laboriously *to-be-established* bond, when it occurs in a relationship today, necessarily destroys it. (Incidentally, this is a decisive difference between an interpersonal, intra-empirical relationship and the relationship between *man and God* that we find in Luther's case, which is not an empirical, natural relationship, but the relationship between the empirical-natural as a whole and the "metaphysical" or transcendental. Here, too, the naturally existing bond is of course cut, so the relationship must for a start be restored secondarily (be laboriously established, as it were). However, in this case, as Luther experienced quite clearly, the restoration can only take place from the other side of the human persons in the relationship, namely from God. All efforts of the natural man would not only be in vain, but downright counterproductive. Man is absolutely powerless in this respect. He can only *receive* reconciliation.)

At this point it becomes very well possible to show the difference between the psychological situation of *early-modern* man, that is, the situation into which Luther also belongs, and the explicitly *modern* situation in which *we* have our place, and thus also to understand why a neurosis could not yet occur in the premodern *Neuzeit* (early-modern age) and why, on the other hand, it was possible in the *modern age*, that is, since the 19th century. Neurosis is a *historical* phenomenon and not a timeless possibility of being human, an anthropological constant. I have said about modern man that he is the logically lonely man who is thrown completely back on himself and therefore I, subject. But I also pointed out that his *own reason* tells him what to do.[43] So his free-

43 This must of course not be understood as if his reason were a subject behind subjectivity! The I, as the sublated result of what is on the subject side and the object side of consciousness, is reasonable. Reason is the I via its producing itself by pulling itself up by its own bootstraps.

dom is not arbitrariness, not "anything goes". He is only free from heteronomous authority, from external determination, but not from any determination at all. In his reason he has his own inner authority. Still much later, shortly before the beginning of modernity, this shows itself most clearly with Kant when, for example, he defines the Enlightenment as the maxim of *thinking for oneself* at all times, that is to say "seeking the supreme touchstone of truth in oneself (i.e. in one's own reason) ...". And it is through reason that in modern times man is connected with God and the divine world order, insofar as the natural light of reason in man has its origin in God, just as the *ego cogito* does not exist without God as the infinite substance encompassing both the *res cogitans* and the *res extensa*. This means, however, that the solitude of early-modern man is not yet absolute, it is not *metaphysical* solitude.[44] He has not yet been forsaken by God; just as lonely Robinson Crusoe, cast away on his island, still often and extensively lingers with God in pious thoughts and prayers. Even the world is not an alienated *vis-à-vis* for him for the simple reason that, as Spinoza teaches, "the order and connection of ideas is the same as the order and connection of things" (Eth. II, p. vii). Thus man is born out of his embeddedness only in relation to the bosom of the Church and all institutions and customs.

In modern times, this has changed. Now solitude is total, namely *metaphysical*. For now man is abandoned by God and reason. He has only an intellect (in contrast to reason), only what Heidegger called "*rechnendes Denken*" (calculating or operational thinking), Horkheimer "instrumental reason". Unlike man at the time of metaphysics, he stands as a subject isolated and alienated, i.e. without mediation, *vis-à-vis* the object, especially the world, a world which is only a raw material for human utilization (whereby "utilization" also includes sentimental tourist consumption in the romantic experience of nature). Now everything he does and wants becomes arbitrary and all events merely empirical-factual, and that means *psychologically*: it becomes banal.

In this situation neurosis can occur, the neurotic soul can take

44 Which is why I had to stress that in early-modern times it was only *the first immediacy of* the birth of man.

possession of certain individuals. Because there is no relativizing Absolute any more, in neurosis personal suffering as well as the desire of the neurotic human being become, just like that, absolutized, endowed with unconditional meaning. Under the conditions of modernity, the place of the Absolute that God once occupied falls to certain, often trivial, empirical concerns the moment that neurosis sets in. Certain things, situations or experiences, one's own person or other persons are not only artificially attributed a higher importance by the neurotic soul than is empirically inherent in them, but an *unconditional* importance is attached to them. A normal disappointment or offence thus suddenly becomes *absolutely* unbearable; a rather harmless dog appears as an *absolutely* terrible danger; staying in a completely normal elevator becomes *absolutely* unbearable; neurosis also often posits and celebrates the idea of one's own *absolute* worthlessness or one's own *absolute* guilt, etc. All this serves the purpose of once again, just as at the time of metaphysics, simulating the reality of an Absolute, of an unconditionally valid truth and thus of one's being embedded in a higher meaning, which has long since been irrevocably lost and deep down is also *known* to be lost, and which can therefore only appear *negatively* in the undignified form of a neurotic symptom.

Neurosis can in each case only seize individual parts of reality (these or those persons, things, situations) and produce absolute significance in these parts of reality by inflating and exaggerating them. That is to say, it can always only in very small, completely private things or aspects provide neurotic proof of the existence of the Absolute. But psychologically, unconsciously, this undertaking actually aims pars pro toto at the logical character of the world as such and as a whole, which, however, itself remains inaccessible. The work (*opus*) of establishing a recognized untruth as the truth can only succeed selectively, in tiny instances.

After these side remarks about neurosis let's go back to our main line of thought. The new constitution of consciousness that becomes visible in the image of Robinson Crusoe brings with it the liberation from a superior authority. Thus the possibility of absolute arbitrariness and immorality is theoretically also given. But just as Luther had not completely lost God with his resigning himself to the extreme distance from God, so it is also true here that man, insofar as he still understands himself as a being of reason, can comprehend his liberation *from* that morality which comes from outside as a liberation *to* morality in the high Kantian sense, that is, to self-legislation. Only he who has the freedom to be a "bum" or live a "dissolute life" can give himself the moral law that forbids him to do so. Then authority is sublated: not eliminated, but integrated, pushed down in me to a mere moment.

The image of Robinson Crusoe can be seen as an answer to the place of the soul that was expressed in a text by John Donne (1572–1631), a *negating* answer or one that reverses into the opposite what it is the answer to. Donne's statement, written down a century earlier in 1623 in an often quoted sentence from "Meditation XVII", reads: "No man is an island, entire of itself; every man is a piece of the continent, a part of the main." It is not only by chance that Robinson Crusoe finds himself on an island, he is not only forced to lead an insular life. His insular existence is not a circumstantial condition of life. For a psychological or logical interpretation, Robinson Crusoe is much rather the image of man *as* "an island, entire of itself". That's what it is all about. He is the image of the man who has become his own center, man as atomic subjectivity. Insular existence is not the *empirical state* of modern man, but his logical destiny.

And vice versa, Donne's image of man as part of the continent, part of the main (= mainland), is once again a wonderful image for the "medieval" mode of being-in-the-world: the logic of the individual embedded in a larger whole. In the same meditation we read a little earlier: "The church is catholic, universal, so are all her actions; all that she does belongs to all. When she baptizes a child, that action concerns me; for that child is thereby connected to that body which is my head too, and ingrafted into that body whereof I am a member."[45] Here again the essence of man is described as released and fitted into a greater, comprehensive reality, as whose member he must therefore experience and understand himself. I as an individual have *my* head in that body, the Church; I do not have it in myself as my own reason. This image is directly analo-

45 John DONNE, *Devotions upon Emergent Occasions*, Meditation XVII.

gous to the physical image of the embryo contained in the womb of the mother, the embryo who does not have to do his own breathing and eating, his own thinking and protecting himself, because the organism of the mother provides him directly with everything necessary because of the containment of the embryo in the womb of the mother. This is a containment by which the embryo is almost something like one of her own body organs and not an independent individual. The born baby, on the other hand, is already "thrown into existence" and has to breathe and eat by himself, and if he is hungry or in pain, he has to shout selfishly to force others to attend to his needs. The embryo knows no needs. It cannot therefore be selfish. These literal biological realities may once again underline what is meant by *psychological* birth in a metaphorical sense.

The fact that Donne can formulate the deeper conditions of the "medieval" form of existence in such clarity, suggests, of course, that what he formulates, and formulates as the valid truth, is in truth for him, albeit unacknowledgedly and unconsciously, already a past that in itself no longer applies to him. Reflected knowledge is always the sign that one has left that of which it is the knowledge, so that one can have a view of it from the outside and therefore see it with clarity.

The true explosion of the "natural". The descent from the height of the heavenly, pleromatic place of being down to earth has taken place. This descent or crash, which we have also called the (first immediacy of the) psychological birth of man (in his metaphysical essence), demanded the payment of a high price, namely the unreserved willingness to expose oneself to the worst possibility, the possibility to be condemned to hell by God in His unfathomable decree. The formula for this, *se resignare ad infernum*, could of course now be read as if man had simply "resigned": he suffered a loss by having to give up an illusion; he has to be content with his human all-too-humanness; he may no longer have any high aspirations since his wings are clipped once and for all. He can only struggle along in the dust of the earth. He is no longer allowed to raise his gaze upwards. The topics of "Heaven", the "grace" of God, being righteous before God, are over once and for all.

But, as we have already seen, this is not the situation of the early-modern I. Rather, we must recognize that such persistence in mere disappointment would not at all be the real birth of man *as* human. Luther, too, did not stop at the depressing insight, or more correctly, the *se resignare ad infernum* in itself did not have only this abstract-negative meaning for him. Abstract or simple negation is only one half of the experience which was formulated for him in this phrase, and it is also only one half of man's birth or one half of the blasting of one's containment in the natural Pleroma (or put differently: the Pleroma *of the* "natural"). As a simple negation of the original expectation, pure renunciation still remains related to what it renounces. It sees only that the *fulfillment* of what is expected remains denied. It does not become free of the expectation itself. The desire or the ideal remains untouched, only its attainability or realization has been renounced.

Resignation in the nowadays usual sense of the word is therefore not a *re-signatio* at all (not a being placed under a new sign, not being transported to a higher or deeper level of knowledge). It is not dis-illusionment (being un-deceived). The domination of the old "sign" and the previous "illusion" does not change, although one admits their impossibility and unreality as far as their *content* is concerned. In empirical-practical behavior and "semantically" one has then, in order to return to Luther, given up the demand for a gracious God, but *logically* (structurally, "syntactically") it still remains, despite the negation of its content, as the central point of orientation. So what, then, is the other half of the simple negation? What brings the real breakthrough into the open?

What the answer to this question has to be can be demonstrated using Luther's understanding of true humility. Humility is unreserved submission to the judgement of God. It is not one's own self-degradation, one's ducking (for the purpose of avoiding possible condemnation from the outset). It is not, in the sense of the defense mechanism of "identification with the aggressor" worked out by psychoanalysis, the self-damnation executed by oneself, i.e. an anticipation of a possible condemnation under *one's own charge*, in order not to be *exposed* to the much more terrible experience of a condemnation *actually pronounced by the other*, by

God. Empirically and factually, there is of course no difference between the pain caused by an external wound and the pain caused by a self-inflicted wound. But psychologically the external factual (empirical) pain is not that which is at stake at all. People are usually quite willing to take a fair bit of physical pain and real plight. As a rule, this is not the real problem for them at all. Rather, what really matters is the logical or metaphysical pain (which can, of course, also be projected onto an external pain, so that the difference is not conscious and the external pain is considered to be the actual pain). This logical pain consists precisely only in the "it befalls me" character, in *being exposed to* an attack or judgement from outside, and not in the literal content of the judgement or in the empirical-real effect of the attack itself. The pain is that one's own majesty and sovereignty is offended; it is the experience that there is something else besides oneself that is beyond one's control. (In Kafka's "Judgement" we read: "So now you know what else there was besides you, until now you only knew about yourself!" The second half of this saying applied to medieval man or the constitution of medieval humanity. He knew of himself only because he was not yet I and did not yet have the world and God vis-à-vis himself. He was still retained in the whole, and God as the center of this whole was the only real subject.)

As psychological, the pain of being exposed is either the pain of the experience that one is at the mercy of a trespassing on the part of the other, which is not legitimized by one's own consent, and that one's own integrity and self-assertion is thus impaired. Or, what is more important in our context, it is the pain of the loss of the inalienable unity with the other, the pain of a sudden condition of standing alien and possibly hostile vis-à-vis one another. This loss is unbearable and must be prevented under all circumstances. I can (seemingly) prevent the breaking apart of the original unity by antecedently performing the literal act of attack (condemnation) on myself. I then gladly accept the literal or empirical pain, because I am psychologically or metaphysically reestablishing and securing my identity with the aggressor by taking over under my own control the act of attack.[46] This procedure is rightly

46 In an analogous way, I protect myself against another's trespassing (e.g. by my

regarded as a defense mechanism, because what should *actually* be suffered through is not the physical or literal pain, the psychic pain caused by the attack, but the much more fundamental (psycho-) logical pain of the loss of profound oneness, the loss of "grace", of sympathetic unity. What is horrible, unthinkable, is the *logical* rupture, the banishment from harmony; it is metaphysical loneliness: being alone with oneself, being thrown back on oneself alone.

Very much in this sense, there is an attitude of humility in which man practices humility as empirical behavior, in order to escape the possibility of being exposed to the Last Judgement and its verdict. That would again be just another example of the ego-willing that Luther recognized as the core of his conflict. True humility, therefore, is not an attitude to be adopted by man and more and more acquired or deepened through constant practice. That would still remain his own action, guided by his *will*. Submission to God's judgement, a submission which I have described above as "voluntary" (*freiwillig*), is with Luther, by contrast, to be thought as really *frei-willig*, that is to say, logically free *of the will*, the simple *realization* that we *are* subject to God's judgement. The self-rejection judgement which Luther demands and which is supposed to extend to the whole person (the person *as such*) is a judgement (verdict) about one's own being and in this sense an insight, *cognition*. It is not the kind of "humble" self-condemnation in which I, as the self-condemning one, would rise high above myself as the condemned one 'down there' and thereby precisely prove to myself my moral or pious attitude. Letting oneself fall unreservedly into one's own sinfulness can only happen as an act of knowledge, as *cognitio sui* (self-knowledge), as the *intellectual* act of taking this cognition as decisive, inevitable, and binding. Humility, says Luther, humility—*id est agnoscere et credere,*

---

father who wants to chastise me), against an intrusion into the integrity of my person, if I anticipate his judgment, or carry out his punishment on myself. The empirical content of the judgement or punishment remains the same, but by anticipating and executing it myself I escape the *attack* character that the judgement or punishment would otherwise have for me. I take them into myself and thus make them *ego-syntonic*. The character of being exposed to an exterior other, to a vis-à-vis that has a free hand to do with me what *it* wants, without respecting my sovereignty, is (seemingly) eliminated.

nos esse gloria dei vacuos, plenos nostra ignominia et omnibus malis, et sic timere in hac paupertate: "That is to recognize and believe that we are empty of the glory of God, but full of our unworthiness and all evil, and so to be afraid in this poverty". Accordingly, Luther in his early days called the cognitive organ of faith "intellectus".[47] It goes without saying, however, that "intellectual" here cannot refer, as it nowadays so frequently does, to a split off, abstract intellectuality, but the cognitive act of the whole man, the person as a whole.

The judgement consists in the insight that I am exposed to God's judgement and that it is impossible for me to comply with God's commandment, that I therefore *deserve* damnation. It is simply a question of recognizing the absolute discrepancy between what God demands of me and what I can achieve.

Psychologically, Luther's step from a humility that man acts out as his feeling and as his humility-pose to a cognitive or *logical* (intelligible) humility is of utmost importance. At bottom, it is already the blueprint, on the basis of a special theme, for the step necessary today away from a personalistic, egoic, subjectivistic stance of psychology to actual psychology. As long as humility is still emotionalized, it remains bound to the ego and its interests. Only logical humility is liberated to itself, is free, *released* into simply being true.[48]

But with what has been said so far, true humility has only been determined halfway. The unquestionable submission to God's judgement as a simple act of knowledge is only one side. For true humility must also place itself under God's completely free mercy,

---

47 Walther VON LOEWENICH, *Luthers Theologia crucis*, München (Chr. Kaiser Verlag) 1954 (first 1929), p. 17.

48 With respect to *intellectus* as the cognitive organ of faith and logical humility we can compare, as Mogenson kindly reminded me, Hegel's description of thinking: "... thinking is only genuine with respect to its content insofar as it is immersed in the *matter*, and with respect to its form insofar as it is not a *particular* being or doing of the subject [as subjectively biased me], but consists precisely in this, that consciousness conducts itself as an abstract 'I,' as *freed* from *all* particularity of features, states, etc., and does only what is universal, in which it is identical with all individuals. ... the worthiness that consciousness ascribes to itself consists precisely in the giving up of our *particular* opinions and beliefs and in allowing the *matter* to hold sway over us." (Encyclopedic Logic, § 23)

that is, allow itself to be bound by God's promise of grace. Full submission to God, which even openly consents to eternal damnation, if this should be God's will, also demands submission to God's grace (promised *just as much* as His judgement). Therefore Luther says: *Necessarium est* ***sub periculo aeternae damnationis et peccati infidelitatis*** *credere his verbis Christi* ("it is necessary *risking eternal damnation and the sin of unbelief* to believe these words of Christ").[49] Just at the low point of the feeling of unworthiness before God the heart must "turn from such feeling, and grasp and hold the deep, secret yes that is under and above the no, with firm faith in God's word ... and to bear God out in His judgement against us; then we have won."[50] The *cognitio sui* (self-knowledge) needs to be supplemented by the *cognitio dei* (knowledge of God). Man owes it to God to *contra spem sperare*, to hope against all hope, to consider himself to be in a state of grace, in possession of the Holy Spirit.[51] With such an action man would carry out his *Hic Rhodus, hic salta*, to perform which is refused if he settles down in his original resignation and disappointment.[52] Conversely, if man were to reject the promise of grace because of his clear insight into his irrevocably being a sinner and to insist one-sidedly on his being a sinner and on his unworthiness, then he would only be wanting to *anticipate* God's decision again and decide for *himself*, have *himself* the control over himself.

---

49 WA II 13, 31, quoted from Holl, p. 112, note 2. The reference is to Matth. 16:19.

50 E.A. 11, 125, quoted from Holl, p. 75, note 5.

51 "Against all hope" means against all human-all-too-human hope, empirical or *psychic* hoping of finite man, which is easily realized as being fundamentally unrealistic, or more than that, totally in vain, illusionary. One's hoping against this hope is the psychological or transcendental hope. It is not illusionary because it is based on the real presence of the *soul* and thus of *infinity* in finite man. In this sense, *contra spem sperare* expresses the actual performance of the psychological difference.

52 Cf. W.G., "The Rejection of the *Hic*. Reflections on C.G. Jung's Communion Fiasco", in: *The Flight Into The Unconscious. An Analysis of C.G. Jung's Psychology Project* (= W.G., *Collected English Papers*, vol. 5) New Orleans, LA (Spring Journal Books) 2013, pp. 91–136.—As the performance of one's *Hic Rhodus, hic salta*, the phrase *contra spem sperare* is *psychologically* the call, to express it in Jung's words, to go through with our psychological reality, namely with the fact that we are "more than autochthonous *animalia* sprung from the earth, but as twice-born ones ha[ve our] roots in the divinity itself" (*MDR* p. 333, transl. modif.).

True humility is therefore open to God's will, and it can only be that because it is the ego-will's full-fledged exposure to the judgement of God. The openness of which I have spoken, however, is not one's leaving everything open, indeterminate. On the contrary, it is certainty.[53] The very fact that it is certainty *is* the real turning point, the real reversal that humility brings about or experiences. The openness does not remain stuck in indeterminacy because it allows itself to *be* reached and *be* told, *be* given something, by the Word of God: namely, both the judgement or wrath of God, and the grace of God. Leaving open would be readiness for the Either/Or of condemnation or justification. Both would be understood as alternatives. But judgement and grace, anger and justification are the Same, though not alike. They are not at all, as the ordinary mind sees it, opposites, but two sides of the same coin: in that man seriously holds his ground against the inexorable wrath of God, allows himself to be struck by it, this judgement completely crushes man's self-willing (and with it the core of sin) and ipso facto *makes* man "just" (i.e. ready for communion with God) and partake of grace.

To see that is true humility. This, as realized κένωσις, as one's really being emptied of the ego-will, does not stop at the view of God's wrath motivated by the fear of punishment, i.e. by the human will for self-preservation. Consequently, it does not, from the purely earthly-fleshly point of view, see in the wrath of God anything other than just this wrath. Rather, it looks through the (admittedly fully admitted) outside of the unrelenting wrath and recognizes in the cruel image of the judging God, God the most gracious Father, and in the wrath, love. It recognizes that God is the author of the *Anfechtung* and its overcomer. Man is not capable of this seeing-through on his own. It is possible only as the gift of God, as the result of *His* work, precisely of God's wrathful work on man.

This work of anger will have to be discussed in more detail later. Here we stay for the time being with the idea of seeing through the front that offers itself to the gaze from the human-

53 It is certainty because it is based on our *being* "more than autochthonous *animalia* sprung from the earth", our *essential* nature as soul and because one's *Hic Rhodus, hic salta* has become an accomplished fact.

natural point of view, seeing through to a deep view, which sees *the same thing* with spiritual eyes, so to speak from the perspective of God. Both visions are equally valid, both are true, although they directly contradict each other. The front or outside, which is directly visible to the human gaze, is not simply removed, as having been overcome by the second view, it is preserved, even if it is at the same time invalidated by the opposite truth. The full or actual truth is the contradiction itself, the contradiction of both truths. Faith is the state in which man thinks both opposing judgements of God about himself as a single one, namely the intransigent judgement that he, this man (he who is "I" in each case), *is* utterly a sinner and thus falls victim to rejection, *and* the judgement that he is nevertheless absolutely justified before God. Man is, as Luther's formula reads, *simul iustus et peccator* ("*simultaneously* just and sinner"). He is *at the same time* "flesh" (*caro*) and "spirit" (*spiritus*), *at the same time* "healthy" and "sick". He must acknowledge his real forlornness and yet necessarily believe himself not lost.

The "simultaneously" (*simul*) is to be taken quite strictly. It is not softened by "a partly so, partly so" or "sometimes so, sometimes so", not even by the introduction of different respects. "At the same time" does not mean that man is composed of both, *has* a "flesh" side and a "spirit" side, to which the two opposing judgements would apply respectively. No, the *simul* expresses the *contradiction* as which man *exists*. We have already spoken of the principle of wholeness (unity) of the person, which is Luther's guiding principle, and accordingly Luther also insists that man is as whole person just *and* as whole person sinner. This necessarily leads him to the contradictory statement: *sunt duo toti homines*, there are two "whole men". The *whole* man exists twice, once as "sick" through and through and once as "healthy" through and through, and both at the same time. This doubling of wholeness shows that the contradiction is indeed endured and sustained without attenuations and excuses.

This is a revolution, and with it the true break through the stance of the nature standpoint of consciousness to an entirely different dimension, to the *Geist (Mind) level* of consciousness, to the status of the *logical*, has happened. For the natural view, man as a whole person can always only be either healthy or sick. Or he can be partly ill and partly healthy. Healthy in the head, sick in the body, with pneumonia, but a healthy heart—this is how it looks for the natural consciousness, which primarily orients itself by means of visual intuition/perception and imagination. But the simultaneity of one and the same *whole* person of being both healthy and sick can no longer be imagined. This contradiction goes beyond the whole level of imagination or representation, because it can only *be thought*, can only be *for* thought. Now, with Luther, healthy and sick, *iustus* and *peccator*, are no longer names for positive, empirical states or qualities. They are logical determinations, opposites, which *both* permeate me *totally* and, as logically negative, are also able to *permeate* me totally, whereas contradictory empirical states are inevitably alternatives.

"Thinking" here must not be understood as specific empirical behavior, one's practicing the "thinking function", since it designates something completely different, namely the form (the logical status, the general constitution) of consciousness, a level or stage for *whatever* perception, experiencing, feeling, thinking, etc. Likewise, "breaking through the natural" or "overcoming nature" by no means expresses hostility to nature the way one often likes to portray it today. That revolution consists precisely in the fact that the level on which one might, for example, be concerned with being hostile to the body, has been overcome. The Middle Ages had been the time of asceticism and the killing of the flesh. The breakthrough leads to a higher (or deeper), more subtle, level, where such things as the literal body, empirical, positive health or sickness, the practical behavior of sinful doings or doing good deeds, etc., are no longer the topic, because its topic is, for example, the whole person, who is not an empirical, observable reality at all, or the topic is this whole person's *being* a sinner or *being* just, or the state of grace, the new life in faith, all of which are not positive objects of experience, but have their place in logical negativity. *Nemo scit se vivere aut experitur se esse iustificatum, sed credit et sperat*: "Nobody knows whether he lives as justified or experiences himself as justified, but he believes and hopes it". It is not *nature* as positively existing reality and not the *body* as positive object that is disregarded. Rather, the *positivity* of whatever reality (no matter if it is bodily or spiritual) is overcome, that positivity which is the very point of view of the natural consciousness.

Therefore, for Luther the believer stands in freedom vis-à-vis nature and the whole of material reality, also vis-à-vis the "law" (the commandments), as he will later explain in his essay "On the freedom of a Christian". The world of things, of the empirical, of positivity, is logically *sublated.* They are no longer the bearers, or the scene, of *true* life. In a certain sense they have become indifferent, which does not mean that they may be arbitrarily maltreated and degraded. From freedom with regard to them also arises a responsibility, even a higher one.

One might perhaps think that Luther's overcoming of the "Middle Ages" and the explosion of the "natural" in favor of the modern ego-personality could only be a loss: something is cut off. Embeddedness in nature and in the bosom of the Church, the a priori harmony with God are lost. What remains is demythologized nature and a man who is likewise stripped of his mythical garments. But that would miss Luther's full insight, as it has just been presented in this section. It is not the amputation of essential aspects of being-in-the-world and the retreat to the miserable rest. What really happens with Luther is rather that the *whole* logic of being-in-the-world is transformed, translocated, namely sublated: negated, but also preserved in such a way that the whole situation is raised to a completely new level, on which all questions about human existence, about meaning and about the relationship between God and man must be answered and determined anew. In alchemical language one can say that the constitution of being-in-the-world has been distilled, sublimated, evaporated.

If it has emerged that true humility is both one's placing oneself under God's judgement and under God's love; if concerning man it has emerged that he is both just and sinner and both simultaneously; and if, therefore, it has emerged that there are two totalities, then this is simply the consequence of the dissolution of the "natural" unity (*One* Center) and its bifurcation into the vis-à-vis of *Two* Centers. Luther thinks the difference, the separation of the unity, the newly emerged vis-à-vis. He does not amputate (God is not simply cut off and eliminated); nor does he replace

One Center (God) by another (the ego-personality as subjectivity), which would inevitably be accompanied by inflation (the unconscious identification of man with God)[54] because in the "soul" what has been cut off as a psychological reality is not simply "gone", but only disappears from consciousness. He takes the process of "cutting the umbilical cord" fully seriously and thinks it all the way through in his existential experience: so that the dialectic is brought to light.

The duality of judgement and mercy, wrath of God and love, *iustus* and *peccator,* simply corresponds to the fact that the original unity (with the One Center, God) was not destroyed just like that, but was stretched, bifurcated, differentiated into the much more complicated contradictory relationship of two centers (God and man as I). God's judgement and anger, inescapable sin and eternal damnation, as the essence of man: this is the view from the perspective of the one center (man) to the other center. Conversely, God's mercy and justification are what shows itself from the perspective of the other center. Both the fact that for Luther there are both perspectives (self-knowledge on the one hand and God-knowledge on the other hand) and therefore the *simul* that unites them, and the other fact that in each of the two perspectives the gaze always goes from one center to the other, shows that, unlike in modernity, unity is not given up abstractly, but continues to exist in a new form.

Also, the thought that no way leads to God from natural man, but that man can only *receive* reconciliation from God, inevitably results from the separation of unity. I cannot step out of unity to establish myself as my own center and then claim to be able to establish unity. Because then I would not have taken the separation seriously at all. But the separation has really taken place, the vis-à-vis, the separation *has been* established. The fact, however, that separation does not mean absolute discord and hatred or even total indifference, but that on the contrary reconciliation can indeed be *received*, or to put it another way, that in addition to God's work of wrath there is also God's *love* for man, this fact is

54 At least this was Jung's repeatedly expressed view, which I, however, disagree with. See, for example, CEP IV, p. 226, and, more extensively, the "Excursus on inflation", in Chapter II below, pp. 159 ff.

due to the other fact, that separation is not physical-literal, but takes place in *spirit* and in "*soul*", where separation, even relentless separation, always remains as an *internal* differentiation within the bond, that is, remains syzygic, dialectical. The bifurcation is not a falling apart. In concrete terms, the fact that man has become the center for himself does not mean that the previously only center, God, is not still *the* center for him. What ultimately has separated are not man and God (taken as entities), but positivity and negativity, finiteness and infinity. Man has become aware of himself as center, because he has become conscious of his naturalness and finiteness (= has *settled* there). To be more precise one would have to say the other way around, that he has become aware of true infinity and can more precisely appreciate his finiteness from it. He is center in the sphere of finiteness, and only there. Early-modern man (other than modern man), who had become the center for himself, still has in God his true, his infinite center, just as before.

The words for the level of the logically no longer positive and finitely apprehendable that Luther uses are above all the traditional Christian words faith and hope (see above: *sed credit et sperat*, "believes and hopes"). *Peccator* is the whole man *in re*, in reality, thus as positively existing, but he is *iustus in spe*, in "hope". Of course, "hope" here does not mean an uncertain state, a vague "maybe" only based on pious wishful thinking. It is not an empirical emotion that is referred to. Rather, it merely states that "*iustus*" is not an object of empirical experience, not to be pinned down to any positively existing characteristic, not of a quasi thing-like nature. Hope is the real presence of the infinite in the finite human being (as, correspondingly, also "faith"): the presence of the soul in empirical man. It is already the designation of a logical status in which a content can stand, and not a psychic event or behavior. Because of his insight into the non-positivizability of salvation (redemption, "justice" before God), Luther explicitly opposes the scholastic doctrine of the "signs of existing grace". To fall back on the sentence quoted in the previous paragraph, he holds out his *nemo scit...*, "nobody knows", to it. There are no visible signs. Grace cannot be pinned down to anything empirical. The formula *simul iustus et peccator*, regarded as the definition of man, thus presents the essence of man as spanned between positivity and negativity. Man *is* the contradiction insofar as he as a whole belongs to positivity and yet at the same time also belongs as a whole to negativity and infinity. In a sense, *peccator* and *iustus* are even synonymous with logical positivity and negativity.

Since for Luther the difference between these two dimensions of being explicitly opens up in its dialectic, i.e. in the unity *of* its unity *and* its opposition, and the essential place or scene of the essential now lies, and is to be discussed, on the level of this logical difference (a difference that has become logical, intelligible, and can no longer be adequately formulated in natural images), the "Middle Ages" have been abandoned and consciousness has been catapulted to the logical or noetic level of itself. Bernhard Lakebrink has coined the phrase "Thomistic analectic" as a counter term to the dialectic (of Hegel). The analectic, if it is understood beyond Thomas as the analogous thinking that characterizes the entire Middle Ages, is philosophical, and in part already pre-philosophical, thinking at the natural level of consciousness, insofar as the analogy involves proportions and participatory relationships between *existing things* (persons, powers, at any rate substantial entities) and between levels of being, that is to say between what is (according to its form) *imagined* or *represented*, rather than thought. With dialectic, e.g. with the formula *simul iustus et peccator*, however, the level of reflection is no longer directly the "semantic" or "ontological" one of Being, of the existent and what is imaginable according to the model of things. Rather, the reflection is directed only "syntactically" towards the strictly noetic, logical, intelligible of the *statūs* in which standing the existing can then be seen. Man is no longer taken at the corner of his empirical givenness and from there viewed as a natural being, a creature. He is (grasped as "wholeness" and "unity") a *noumenon* and is apperceived as the tremendous tension or *movement* between opposites.

With Luther the New Testament insight that God is spirit has been caught up with, brought home into consciousness inasmuch as now the whole *question* with which God, man and the relationship between man and God is approached is a thoroughly spiritual or noetic one. Before, spirit, *Geist*, had still quite concretistically (semantically) been something like an existing quality of only one *content* of consciousness, "God". Spirit, *Geist*, was still pictorially imagined. Now it is—integrated into consciousness—the form of consciousness itself for the contemplation of all that is, and only then can the special content "spirit", *Geist*, be adequately thought.

For Luther, totality has not been lost. Therefore there is no loss of meaning, unity, embeddedness, but instead **the transformation and translocation of the whole question from the level of "nature" to the level of *Logos*.** Luther's *simul* is the successor of the post-mythic-Christian (medieval) form of the whole, the harmony between heaven and earth, the human and the divine, the empirical and the archetypal, which in turn was already a successor of the mythical form of the whole. Luther did not bring a reduction to only one side of the whole. What Luther lost on the natural level of human consciousness he regained on the level of logical negativity, where now one evidently can no longer speak "naturalistically" of heaven and earth, but must talk of logical *statūs* ("sinner" – "just").

The path of absolute negative interiorization. When man exposes himself unreservedly to the *religious qualms* and lies entirely under the wrath of God, then a reversal of perspective takes place. In being struck by the wrath of God, man is not at all separated from God. The wrath of God is recognized as His work on man, through which He works redemption (justification). God needs the wrath in order to *work off the obstacles in man* that stand in the way of faith or of the unity of willing with God. But, as we have seen, this wrath work has not only the negative purpose of clearing away disturbing things in order to make room for something new. Rather, the anger is in itself the way that leads to justification. So there is no splitting: the negative work of abrasion of the old, the positive work of construction of the new. Rather, the whole work is that negative work of anger, because it is *in itself already* God's positive work of love. The direction of the way, as the path of true humility, is the way of negative interiorization, recursive progression, not that of ascension to something higher, of refinement, of sanctification, of expansion, of supplementation. The believer never becomes a "saint" in the sense of approximate perfection. Throughout his life he remains the sinful (natural) man he is, because this is simply man's nature. No *positive* (externally verifiable) result is achieved. Man is merely *absolute-negatively inwardized* by God's wrath work into God's love, into another status or "style" of his being.

In this one point there are certain similarities to the form of the work of alchemy, which is also a negative work, an *opus contra naturam*. In alchemical terms, the work of God's wrath is an etching away, burning away, a *logical mundificatio* (purification), a *mortificatio* (killing), also a *putrefactio* (rotting) of the "prime matter" man, as well as of the *unio naturalis*. As in alchemy the path of work is the negative one of inner refinement and spiritualization (*distillatio*, *sublimatio*, *evaporatio*, etc.) and should lead to an end product that is likewise not of a positive but of a spiritual or noetic nature (*aurum nostrum non est aurum vulgi*, λίθος οὐ λίθος), so the path that Luther describes does not lead positively to gain, to new acquisitions, to new possessions, but simply deeper and deeper into what always already is and was, i.e. into its essence, its noetic content, its truth. Perhaps one may say that it is a process of growth in cognition. The wrath work of God, which corrodes away all obstacles, causes the eyes to become a little more seeing, more subtly seeing.

From here it is understandable why Luther had to comprehend devotional exercises, mortifications, the acquisition of an attitude of humility through constant practice, all efforts to overcome oneself, as an evasion of what is actually necessary. Expressed in modern terms, they are an *acting-out* of what is actually required, an acting-out of what can only be "inwardized". By definition, acting-out belongs to the logic of positivity. It is a positivization of what is meant negatively. It is one's treating within the space of "semantics" something that belongs in the dimension of "syntax". By acting-out, consciousness withdraws itself from the corrosive effect of the operations that are to be carried out upon *it* (upon the logic or "syntax" of its consciousness), and thus consciousness withdraws itself also from its becoming absolute-negatively interiorized into its new truth. In order to save the old internal logical constitution of consciousness and to avoid the experience (suffering) of being interiorized, consciousness carries out these operations firstly by itself and secondly on its contents and objects.

The necessity of "God". The process which took place in Luther could be comprehended as his very personal, existential suffering-through of the transition from the "Middle Ages" to the early-modern status of consciousness as I, or personality. Although the process took place in him personally, it is not primarily and not only his personal initiation into subjectivity. Personal initiations belong to the shamanistic, the ritualistic, the mythological level of culture. The philosophical-religious level of consciousness, by contrast, has left the individual behind and always deals with consciousness at large, even if the changes first always take place in certain individual persons. It is much rather the initiation in which the soul, as the Occidental form of human existence, has translated itself as a whole, on the level of the whole culture, into the status of itself as subjectivity. The question arises why this process of *transporting* the soul from one status to another has taken place as a *theological* one. Why the reference to God, and why of all things the one-sided emphasis on a judging, angry God (which does not really suggests itself from the Christian gospel), indeed, why the whole focus on the question of justice and certainty of salvation? Was this necessary? Or could one have imagined that precisely because it was also a matter of the transposition of human existence into subjectivity, and thus ultimately also of creating certain *pre*conditions for the possibility of psychology, the same transport process could have been executed and carried through on a level of purely earthly-human themes?

An external necessity for the theological level of experience to prevail can be seen in the fact that the religious theme was simply dictated by the age in which it took place. Religion and theology at the time of Luther still quite naturally provided the material as well as the level of one's thinking about fundamental issues. But this is not an answer, but only a reformulation of the question. That religion was quite naturally "in charge" at the same time logical and thematic place and medium of change, is precisely what gives rise to our questions. The psychological answer seems to me to be the following.

"God" is used by the soul and for the soul as an "Archimedean point" by means of which it can lift itself out of the hinges of its previous being and bring itself into another form of being. Only by means of the experienced idea of God is man constellated as *totus homo*, because only in it can he reflect himself as a whole, as the living concept of himself, and distinguish himself from himself, so to speak encounter himself from outside. Only by means of the idea "God" is he addressed *absolutely*, in a depth that ensures that the transformation does not merely shift some surface aspects, but hits and grasps the real essence of man, i.e. him in his very concept. If his concept were not reached, all initiation would simply pass over the essence of man. There would only be cosmetic changes—figuratively speaking, a rearrangement of furniture, when what is actually demanded is a reconstruction and new design of the entire house. The transformation must take place on the absolute level of the logical, psycho-logical and must not remain in the realm of the merely empirical. Without "God" the radicality and the unconditionality indispensable for such a process would not have been achieved. The "soul" would not have ventured forth into its outermost possibility at all, would not have raised itself to the absolute. Wherever "the soul" aims to fundamentally expel itself from a previous constitution into a new constitution of itself, it posits its highest principle for itself and expressly reaches out for it. And that highest principle was at that time the Christian God.

With Luther it was a question of lifting human existence out of the natural level and into the noetic level. With regard to "God", "level of nature" means that man, as the natural, empirical man that he is, rises to God through certain concrete acts of piety and a certain pious way of life. *Psychologically* (though not empirically, factually) he lives in paradise, in unclouded unity with God. But with Luther, the task was extraction from man's immediate identification with God (that is, with the standpoint, the level, of God), the extraction from that direct oneness which had its concrete expression in the institution of the Church as the representative of God on earth.[55] This task was about a separation, about

55 *Immediate* oneness with God thus goes together with an only indirect relationship with God *mediated* by the Church, just as conversely, the falling

departure from man's natural being-a-child-of-God, about the breakout from the Pleroma and thus about being psychologically born as an individual. Man was to find *himself*, as an ego-personality and a center of his own, and to face God all alone and for his own account.

Why did it need such extreme ideas as hell and eternal damnation, the idea of God as an angry judge and, on the human side, the corresponding feelings of fundamental guilt and absolute unworthiness (worthlessness), not founded on individual real acts? Here one has to realize how improbable the detachment from the firm rootedness of existence in heaven (Pleroma, Paradise) was. Empirically, man had always lived on earth and thus had to experience all possible predicaments and sufferings. But that was the empirical foreground of existence, which did not reach and did not at all concern the (psycho-) logical or metaphysical background. Everything that happened in the empirical foreground was logically surrounded by and contained in the divine background of the world. No empirical misery, no real catastrophe was psychologically able to serve as an *objection* to the metaphysical embeddedness of existence in the divine meaning. On the contrary, even misfortune, pain, illness, epidemics, death, famine, earthquakes, etc. were manifestations of the gods or at least (in Christian terms) expressions of divine will, God's act of providence. All suffering was in this respect always already a priori (in the logical sense) *sublated*. Whatever happened thus confirmed and fortified only the metaphysical embeddedness of Being as a whole in the pleromatic background. The radical idea of eternal condemnation to hell as the fundamental opposite pole to being in Pleroma, as well as the terrible insight into one's own being a sinner or guilty, were (as the idea and the real feeling of absolute remoteness from God) the razors that could cut the umbilical cord that tied man and all Being back to the pleromatic background, cut it once and for all, turning the cut fully into a psychic reality. These specific ideas and feelings generated (posited) by "the soul" are its means to free itself—*in* a human being—from a primary unity and to throw itself back on itself.

By "the soul's" and thus also the individual person's being

out of immediate unity results in a direct vis-à-vis.

thrown completely back on himself, the communion, the congregation, is disempowered. Before that, *it*, not the individual, was the actual place where salvation was won. *It* administered the mystery, the myth or the "metaphysical". Now the individual stands directly before God; the place of the "metaphysical" has moved into him, and the community is released for other purposes.

This creates a *pre*condition for the possibility of a personal psychology and thus also of a personal neurosis. But historically it would still take centuries until the "condition of possibility" turned into a reality and "the struggle of light against darkness" fully "moved its battleground into the interior of [the human soul]" (*CW* 13 § 293, transl. modif.), and man has become the sole center. This has only really been the case since the middle of the nineteenth century. If today the struggle of Luther with an angry God and for his justification and for gaining the certainty of salvation, if his religious plights, which bring him to the brink of literal death, seem quite alien to us, indeed, are hardly comprehensible to us as a real problem any more, and are even rather boring for us, then this shows to what degree what Luther conquered for the first time under the greatest personal pains as a possibility for all future is today already integrated and has become a self-evident common possession. What was for the people of his time an exciting offer—an offer that in its entire extent and depth could only be accepted and appropriated in the course of several centuries—has long since become for us the ground on which we stand, indeed, which we are already about to leave again. The whole complex of ideas of being sinful and just, of the uncertainty of salvation, of the wrathful or gracious God has done its duty. It can go. It *has* already gone. ❦

Chapter Two

The Western Soul's Historical Project of the Development of the "I"
A few selected aspects

The topic of this paper is such a huge and complex one that all it can do is present a few highlights of the development of the I.

Preliminary clarifications

We need to remove popular misunderstandings of what I is.

Jung spoke of the I as a complex (the *Ichkomplex*) and as the center of consciousness. Both ideas are naturalistic. The notion of a complex makes us think of an entity, something thing-like, e.g., as if the I were an organ of the psyche similarly to how the heart or kidneys are organs of the body. The I as a complex would also imply that it is something separate from all other complexes, just like the heart is not the lung and not the kidneys. But my father complex or whatever complex I have is *my* complex, i.e., the I is "in" each complex. In psychology we must leave the thing-ontology behind. The I is not an existing organ or part of the psyche. The idea the I as the center of consciousness does, of course, not necessarily imply the idea of an existing object, but it tends to be naturalistic, too, because it invites a spatial fantasy. If the I is thought of as the center point, this is in analogy to the axle of a wheel. Erich Neumann even spoke of the ego-self-axis. The I is seen as the unmoving center, around which the experiences and contents of consciousness revolve. But the soul is nothing spatial. There is no spatial center-point and nothing around it. This is not how things are in psychological life.

Another problem of the I as complex and center is that it treats the I as the private possession of each individual. Just as we have to overcome thing-ontology and naturalistic thinking in psychology, so we also have to overcome people's psychology and personalistic thinking. Very often psychologists say: this patient has a weak ego. His ego needs to be developed. Or we speak of "my I". This is nonsense. I don't have an I. You don't have an I. Nobody has one. The I does not develop in us the way in small children all of a sudden teeth start to emerge or how in puberty the sexual organs develop. We must not look for it *in* people, individuals, if we want to study the I. It is not to be found in them. Nor must we look introspectively into ourselves.

But if it is not on organ in the personal psyche and if we have to leave thing-ontology behind in psychology, then what *is* the I? Here I give two preliminary answers, which at the same time refer to two fundamentally different senses of "I".

But before I come to my answers to this question, a further clarifying comment is necessary. In English "ego" has been used in psychology for Freud's and Jung's German word "Ich" ("I"). This is a great handicap. "Ego", as a Latin word in English, is inevitably a third-person word. It cannot be the first-person word "I". In many cases, for example when you read in English about the "ego-self-axis", what is actually meant is "I-self-axis". We have to be aware of this ambiguity. "I" and "ego" are clearly different. I is the existing concept as well as the cultural form of modern Western man's being-in-the-world. "Ego", by contrast, is a particular *style* of consciousness, one that psychologically borders on the pathological, because it is a literalization and straitjacketing of the fully developed psychic I and one's being personally inflated by it, one's having become identical with it or confusing oneself with the objective soul structure of "I".

A. Two senses of I: The *psychological* vs. the *psychic* I

The first sense of I is what we most commonly mean in psychology when we speak of the I and the ego-personality (*Ichpersönlichkeit*),[56] namely the modern Western I, and my first answer is:

56 In English the standard psychological terminology uses the Latin word "ego-",

The I in this sense is a *form* (and not, as indicated, a complex, an organ of the psyche, a part of the personality). A particular form of consciousness and of being-in-the-world, a particular logical constitution of man's identity *and* of the world at large. Just like government can take on different constitutional forms such as monarchy, oligarchy, democracy, dictatorship, etc., so man and the world can take on different forms, one of which is the form or logical constitution of I. The I in this sense is all around man and the world in modernity. We are in it. It is a form that produces a particular stance in those people or cultures in whose consciousness it prevails. It is a special type of self-relation and world-experience/world-relation characterized, for example, by a pronounced sense of 'autonomous subject' (vis-à-vis an 'object') and correspondingly of self-determination. It is the predominant form of consciousness of modern Western man. The I in this sense is, like all *psychological* reality, something cultural and general, not personal, not individual. As *psychological I* it cannot be understood in terms of personalistic psychology.

I criticized the phrase "my ego" or "my I". If the I is cultural, this does not mean that this excludes personal differences. When we study mathematics or biology, these fields are cultural realities, not "my" mathematics or biology. Mathematics or biology is the same for everybody. But individual persons may have a very different *grasp* of these fields, know more or less about them. Another example: We live in a democracy. But this does not mean that all individuals in this democracy are themselves 100% democratic. Democracy is *their* reality, too, but they may nevertheless personally be little dictators. The same with the I. It is the cultural reality of modern Western man and much of the modern world, but the I may be present and realized in individuals to very different degrees. So there is much opportunity for a discrepancy between the *cultural* psychology and *individual* psychology. The main two different types are:

- an individual's lagging behind the cultural development, as Jung explained (e.g., physically and objectively living in the

---

which is misleading as pointed out above.

21st century, but subjectively, psychologically still being in the 19th century),

- personal *pathology*, e.g., neurosis.

The second sense of I refers to the use that people universally, the world over, make of the first-person pronoun. This I is more than a logical constitution of consciousness. It is not merely a structure. The I is also, and above all, the psychic event or performance of a logical act, a doing and achievement. We see this best in individual psychology, when small children first acquire the capability of referring to themselves as "I". Before, they also spoke of themselves, but in the third person singular, namely by using their name: "Paul is hungry". This self-reference by *name* instead of the first-person pronoun means they saw themselves from outside, from an external point of view exactly the same way they (and we all) see everything in the world, all other people, animals, and objects. Paul was just one of all the existing beings among the other entities. *Psychologically*, Paul did not make a structural difference between "Paul is hungry" and "the cat is hungry". Paul was for himself "he" or "it" and saw himself as an object, not as *subject*. The moment the child can say "I am hungry", he has *established* himself as I. The VIEWPOINT from which he used to experience (avant la lettre) "himself" has now immigrated from outside into himself and thus come home to himself: he has turned into *himself* (*being* self). It is now in him, nay, he now *is* this VIEWPOINT from which he sees. I in this sense is nothing else but the absolute personal *identity* with the VIEWPOINT. Paul sees himself from within. The child now exists in the first-person status. In a revolutionary act he stepped out of the sphere of all the many beings and entities in the world and *dares* to single himself out, giving himself and claiming for himself the special, absolutely singular status of "I" in contrast to everything and everybody else in the world.

But here I need to add that "viewpoint" in this context does not mean an empirical, psychic point of view. Rather, it is one that we objectively find ourselves *in*. The said viewpoint (and whether it is outside him or in him) is our a priori, our logic, our psychological constitution. We have no choice, no say in the matter. It comes with our being consciousness, being mind or soul. As such it is completely different from the various viewpoints that we can take (and shift) at will in our actual thinking about things, and it is even different from those particular viewpoints that (qua complexes, prejudices, or "archetypal perspectives") "have *us*" without our being in the least aware of there being a special viewpoint involved in our experience or in our opinions. We take our experience for the simple truth.

Such unconscious viewpoints can be made conscious and, e.g., through analysis, perhaps be overcome. Not so the VIEWPOINT inherent in the word "I". By the same token, the "performance of a logical act, a doing and achieving" that I said constituted the I in the second sense of the word is not a literal behavior, not a psychic act, something *we* do, but a logical act that happens to us and forms us. Likewise, the *child's* "establishing himself" and "his daring" that I spoke of is not *his* conscious and willful act, not a psychic behavior, and therefore also not truly *his* establishing himself. It does not come about as the result of his doing. Rather, it is an event that *happens* to him spontaneously and unconsciously, without his own volition or personal involvement. How could a child have personally performed this act as his own deliberate doing, when, after all, the possibility of performing deliberate *acts* (instead of unconsciously *being* moved by impulses, feelings, desires) already presupposes that very I? The revolution is a logical one, it happens objectively, not subjectively, on a transcendental level. And when it happens, the child all of a sudden finds himself as an "I"-saying person—and irrevocably so.

The I achieved in this way is the "psychic I". It is a *psychic* fact, a real event in the person (and not just a logical form of consciousness) because as I-saying it appears in empirical reality, as the actual speaking of real people and is their real making use of this self-reference, of "first person". However, it is this psychic I only in its first immediacy. It is merely the *linguistic I*, as I call it (without wanting to trespass into the field of linguistics, I merely use this designation to describe a psychological phenomenon by its most obvious feature). While empirically clearly expressed, the psychic I qua linguistic I is nevertheless psychologically only a fundamentally *implicit* and *unconscious* I—just spoken, a mere word that is used, but not consciously made the speaker's (e.g., the child's) own lived truth and not comprehended as such. It is only the assertion of I, the abstract form or empty outline of it, not yet the fulfilled reality, inasmuch as the child is objectively not self-determined (and does not subjectively feel self-determined either). Therefore, this I must not be confused with what in psychology has usually been referred to as the "ego-personality". It is still in the custody of parents and teachers and, on its part also feels in need of them as its superiors, caretakers, and those that know what is necessary and right. This of course does not exclude the possibility of its being strong-willed, obstinate, egocentric, unruly, or even have ideas of grandiosity in some cases, inasmuch as this empirical, behavioral contrariness happens within the psychological structure of acknowledged authority and precisely confirms it.

I illustrated the second sense of I with the emergence of I-saying in childhood.[57] One might perhaps think that with growing up, with coming of age, the linguistic I would become an explicit or fulfilled I. But as the longest part of history shows, this is by no means the case. For thousands of years individuals *psychologically* (i.e., in their objective logical status and their own self-feeling, not only literally, factually) remained in the fold of their family, tribal traditions, and group spirit; they stayed determined by parents and social customs, socially dependent as bondsmen of feudal lords, as subjects of majesties, or as servants of wealthier people, not to mention their own psychologically extremely telling conscious feeling of being by definition in the hands of gods or God

57 As an aside let me, in the context of the topic of the first emergence of the I in childhood and for completeness's sake, refer to the related, but separate topic of the primordial origin of the I in the prehistoric process of man's (*homo sapiens's*) becoming *human* (not in the sense of biological hominization, but of his psychological-cultural development). I briefly advanced my hypothesis about this absolutely first appearance of the I in the world—on the collective level and as a cultural potential—in my book *What Is Soul?* pp. 258–260. With the idea in mind that the first form of hunting seems to have been that of persistence (or endurance) hunting, in which a human hunter pursues prey until it is exhausted and just stops, letting the hunter approach and kill it, I suggested that the dramatic *moment* of the face-to-face encounter between game and human at the very border between life and death, the moment of the hunter's seeing, and feeling penetrated by, the *knowing* gaze of the animal expecting his killing spear, was the first instance of I or (momentary) self-awareness.

[*children* of God(s)!] and their fundamental containment in nature or in the fold of the Church. My pointing to this dependence and containment does not imply that people in this status of consciousness were on the empirical-practical level childlike and immature. By no means. *Psychically* they could even be impressively imposing and resourceful personalities of moral strength and vigor, maybe even heroic personalities that would make many a modern, fully developed "ego-personality" look pale. Nevertheless, *psychologically* even these strong personalities remained on the level of the implicit, merely linguistic I.

B. The nature of the psychic or *linguistic* I

"I" in general is not a new, different material reality or substantial *content*. It has no particular concrete characteristics or descriptive attributes. This is why "I" can be said with equal right by any and every human person despite all their particularities and personal differences and is nevertheless always the same and always true. It is something strictly logical. Although "I" means specifically "me", it is paradoxically fundamentally *impersonal*, it is only the abstract general *concept* of a (one could almost say: *empty*) form of "first person", form not as static structure, but rather as logical act. The concept "I" *has no content* of its own. Rather, it is nothing but a demonstrative for the first person, much like "this" or "that" are demonstratives for the third person, that is to say, simply an act of pointing.

But what kind of a pointing is it? It follows from what I said before that "I" is not *my* (personal, intentional) pointing. Secondly, it is not a pointing to anything positive-factually existing (the way "Paul" in "Paul is hungry" is. Paul literally exists. He is conceived as visible, tangible being). Instead, I is the word or concept "I"'s uroborically pointing back to *itself* and thus establishing the sense of "self". What it points to is not visible, not tangible. It only points abstractly to "first person" or to "subject", which are not empirical facts, but only concepts that like fantasies and fictions belong to the ideal, purely mental sphere.

But that is still not the whole truth. "I" does not point to the abstract concept of "first person" as a free-floating concept in the generality of the mind. It points concretely to the invisible VIEW-

POINT *as which the speaker is speaking.* It points to the concept actually inherent in the act of here and now *thinking* or *saying* "I". It ipso facto turns Paul, the speaker *as speaker* (*not* as human animal), into a self. "I" is not pointing or crossing over from the realm of concepts to the wholly other realm of empirical reality and existence. Rather, it *begins* concretely down here in reality as the actual I-*saying*/I-*thinking*. Qua concept it is real from the outset. I is, as Hegel said, the *existing concept.* As such "I" *is* a contradiction in terms.

Because of the I's strictly logical reality as *concept*, we should not let ourselves be misled by Lacan's thesis of the "mirror stage", which explains the origin of I through the child's self-recognition in a mirror. In one's mirror image one does precisely not see "I", but "it" or "that" ("that's me"). I is not an object to be seen. To derive the sense of "I" from one's self-recognition in or self-identification with a mirror image would be a petitio principii. In a mirror image I do not *primordially* know myself. I at best *re*-cognize myself in it. In order to be able to recognize myself in a mirror image and to perform this identification, I must already know myself as I and thus possess the necessary criterion for any identification of myself with the mirror image. As Johann Gottlieb Fichte realized[58] "I" can only be understood as an *immediate* consciousness prior to any subject-object division (and therefore prior to any mirror image or the like, from which it could be derived). The act of self-recognition presupposes this immediate consciousness of I. It has been said that certain higher animals are able to realize that their mirror image is a reflection of themselves (Gordon Gallup's "recognition test" with chimpanzees). But even this amazing skill does not turn them into full-fledged I's or subjects, does not initiate them into "first person". What is completely mistaken is taking recourse to sensual reality in this discussion, to the visible mirror image and the picture of the empirical, physical body. As I said, "I" points exclusively to the invisible *logical subject* inherent in the I-*saying*, not to the visible human being. My body is

58 Johann Gottlieb Fichte, *Grundlage der gesamten Wissenschaftslehre* (1794). Cf. also Dieter Henrich, "Fichtes ursprüngliche Einsicht", in: *Subjektivität und Metaphysik*, Festschrift für W. Cramer, ed. by D. Henrich and H. Wagner, Frankfurt am Main (Klostermann) 1966, S. 188–232.

not "I", but "it" (third person), merely "my" *body*. As demonstrative, "I" has no specific empirical content, as I pointed out; it is not an image. If it were an image, if it were tied to my looks, nobody else but I could say "I".

But every human person can say "I". "I" is in this sense absolutely indiscriminate. And yet each speaker's in fact *saying* and *thinking* the thought of "I" gives that speaker his absolutely unique identity and selfhood, establishes him as I and makes his seeing and experiencing, feeling and thinking *his* in the first place. It removes him psychologically from the level of existence as human animal and transports and initiates him, together with his bodily being, into (the first immediacy of) his existence in language, concept, mind or soul, in which alone one's personal identity and selfhood, one's being "I", are possible. The sense of personal identity with oneself is retained across the changes of time because one's saying "I" is always *the same*, always points contentlessly to "self".

Ordinary concepts are abstract concepts, that is, concepts that have the existence of what they refer to outside of themselves. One can speak of one's body. But the *concept* "body" and an actually existing body belong to two different orders. Concepts as purely mental phenomena have in common with labels that it is always a question of whether we are applying the right label or concept to a given thing or, conversely, whether a concept (e.g., a "gryphon" or "Martians") has a referent in reality. A statement like "this is an oak tree" can be false, because maybe this is really a beech tree. But "I am I" can never be false, never be a lie or error. "I" is not an attribute of "me". It is my *being*, my *essential nature* as human being (where "nature" is not the empirical, naturalistic one that is accessible to biology, physiology, or any other science). I is, the moment that it is truly thought or said, already real, it is its own reality. Referring back to my notion of "the psychic I in its first immediacy" we can say: even as "linguistic I" it is already the *existing concept*.

When the child says, "Paul is hungry", Paul exists, too, but Paul is not a concept, but a person, a human being ("third person"), or, linguistically speaking, the name of a person. That beings exist is nothing special. But when he has learned to say "I am hungry", a *concept*, the concept of self-identity, has become an existing reality *in him or he in it*, and that is something incredible. "I" is not a name, not the name of a person (just as "this" is not the name of the thing pointed at). It is just a concept. And yet, through saying "*I* am hungry", "I" refers to the real Paul and allows him to live as explicit self-identity. This is the human distinction. No thing, no animal exists as this explicit identity with itself. And other concepts, e.g., "tree", stay on the ideal plane and remain separated from their real referents by a gulf. I, the existing concept, has its referent within itself.

I is on principle absolutely singular and solipsistic (notice that I say "I *is* ... solipsistic", because what I mean is not meant to suggest that people who can say I have to *be* solipsistic.). It is solipsistic because all other "I"s are inevitably not "I" but "you", not 1st (and not 3rd) but 2nd person singular or plural.

C. "Anthropological constants" versus the historical transformations of the soul's logical form

Now we need to distinguish the I as which the individual generally exists from the I that is of psychological concern and the particular topic of our discussions. The fact that healthy humans beyond the baby age all over the world can say "I", and as such inevitably exist as the existing concept, is an anthropological constant. It is rooted in the humanness of man, in the fact that man is the *zôion lógon échon*, the linguistic animal. As rooted in human nature it is something psychic (part of personal psychology) and not really psychological. I called it the linguistic I. But the I in the sense of this discussion is the *psychological* I, the *cultural form* called I, the I as "modern subject". This I is not an anthropological constant, but a particular logical form and late result of a special historical development. It is one of the logical forms or modes of being-in-the-world in which psychic Is in certain historical times can find themselves.—Psychic Is can also live in non-I modes of being-in-the-world. But it is inevitable that they have to live in some logical form, just like people in a community inevitably live in some form of government. Soul is logical form, logical constitution. The form of government defines the citizens in some way. It defines what is possible or not possible, right or wrong, necessary and desirable, or out of the question. The same applies to the modes of being-in-the-world, such as that of the I. The difference is that we can leave the states or forms of government (but usually only by entering another state), whereas we are always inevitably stuck in the prevailing form of soul. Psychology has the job of studying not people or societies, but the soul, that is, the different logical forms that people or societies are defined by and within which they inevitably live.

The soul is eminently historical.[59] This means that it is numerous different forms, or rather not a plurality of forms, but only one form that undergoes a process of change, the process of a metamorphosis. This form change creates the impression of a plurality of forms. Jung's first major book was entitled, *Transformations and Symbols of the Libido*. Applying the logic of Jung's title to our topic, we could describe the historical nature of the soul as the transformations of its logical form. The soul goes through different forms and stages or statuses of itself.

We cannot see these logical forms or modes of being-in-the-world. We can only see their "symptoms". I use this term deliberately. By symptoms we mean in medicine visible signs or indications or evidence of an illness that is on principle not visible. We can never see the illness itself. We can only see signs of it. But the illness itself is only a hypothesis, it is conjectural, inferred on the basis of the seen symptoms. I use the term symptom here in the same way, however without any of the pathological connotations that "symptom" has in medicine. We cannot see the logical forms of the soul, the different garments that the metamorphosizing soul wears at different epochs of its history, but we can turn to symptoms, signs, indications of them, to what sometimes has been called "documents of the soul". And we will have to do this if we want to see the emergence of the I in Western history.

59 This is what Hillman vehemently wanted to deny, whereas Jung was fully aware of it.

D. The soul's construction of the *psychological* I

I. Introduction: Jung's experience of the sympathetic world-relation

As my starting point I use by way of example a particular description of a pre-I world-relation that can serve as a contrasting foil for the discussion of the emergence of the I. It is a passage from Jung's *Memories Dreams Reflections* in which he describes how he feels in his private retreat at Bollingen. Jung tells us:

> At times I feel as if I am spread out over the landscape and inside things, and am myself living in every tree, in the plashing of the waves, in the clouds and the animals that come and go, in the procession of the seasons. ... (*MDR* p. 225 f.)

We see immediately that while Jung on the *psychic* level certainly speaks as a self-identical conscious modern I, the *psychological* form of being-in-the-world that he describes is not that of the I. It is rather the opposite. In the situation he describes there seems to be no border between him and the landscape or things around him. It is as if he seamlessly extended into his environment, as if invisible hyphae or threads connected him immediately with the inside of everything else around him, much like an embryo is immediately connected with the pregnant mother through the umbilical chord. He is in this situation not at all a modern individual who as *subject* is strictly vis-à-vis the world *as object* and who is completely dependant on his eyes and other sense organs for becoming aware of things outside of himself. The form of existence that Jung describes here makes him feel as if he was a priori and directly living *in* the things and processes of the world.

In other words, Jung's description is that of the sympathetic world-relation that in one way or another was also the mode of man's being-in-the-world during the ages of mythology and ritualistic cultures. There was at bottom a basic sympathy of all things and a fundamental *Inständigkeit* (in-ness) and containedness of man in the world. Logically, psychologically, man wittingly or unwittingly perceived himself objectively as an *essentially*, that is to say by definition, *integral element* of and within the fabric of the world, like a cell in the tissue of an organism. The whole is the true reality, the individuals are sublated components of this whole.

The modern I is, as I said, the very opposite of this stance. The modern I means, among other things, the mode of being-in-the-world as subject that has the world (and even the person's own human body) irrevocably vis-à-vis itself as object. "Vis-à-vis" versus "in-ness", "containment".

What I said here needs to be understood as ideal types in Max Weber's sense. In practical reality and in the course of history there can be many transitional positions or the co-existence in one person of what is closer to the one and what is closer to the other type at different times and in different situations of his life. Whether either type has ever existed in its pure form does not concern us here.

I spoke above of our need to turn to "symptoms" of the psychological modes of being-in-the-world. Now I have to state that the cited text from Jung is not a symptom of the *described* mode of being-in-the-world, is not a "document of the soul" attesting to this mode of being-in-the-world. Jung's being spread out in the landscape is not his truth, his being, but a *representation*, a representation in the form of a *feeling*. This feeling is already a *reflected* feeling and thus in itself the opposite of *what* it is the feeling of, namely the unreflected immediacy of the sympathetic world-relation. To be sure, *semantically* it is an adequate description of the pre-I mode of existence and a truthful description of what he subjectively experienced. I already pointed out that on the psychic level Jung is speaking here as self-identical conscious modern I and he only describes a feeling that he, as I, *has*. The important point here is that this feeling is a construct. It is made possible through much effort, through Jung's creation of his private retreat which had the purpose of producing *in modernity* a replica or simulation of a *historical* house and historical living conditions. To express it with Beaudelaire, Jung created his own *paradis artificiel*. Modern romanticism and historicism is unwittingly already at work in Jung's Bollingen project, and this ego-project of the imitation of what is definitely a thing of the past is the condition of the possibility of his having at Bollingen at times those feelings of a primordial oneness with nature. *Syntactically* Jung's feeling is the downright modern feeling of a modern I, but semantically it is the feeling of long bygone times. What historians and also Jung as scholar of the historical psyche try to do intellectually, theoretically, namely reconstruct the spirit of former ages, Jung did here on the emotional level of personal experience.

Jung can only describe his *feeling as if* spread out into the landscape because he is already irrevocably outside and vis-à-vis nature. Such a feeling is precisely evidence of the fact that it is felt from a distance, from outside. He who is really in it, does not feel it, because it is simply his truth, the actual form of his existence, not a content of consciousness, not an experience. At the times of myth and ritual nobody could have said what Jung said, nor could he have *felt* that he was living *in* every tree, etc., precisely because he *was* objectively *inständig* in, and sympathetically connected with, the world around him, in fact an integral part of it. The status of in-ness means that a subject that could *feel* to be in trees or whatever did not exist. Instead of feeling to be living inside the things of nature, the people whose real mode of being-in-the-world was that of in-ness objectively saw nature *from within*, that is to say, they saw the divine face or the manifestation of the nature spirit appearing from within the things of nature or they heard their divine voice speaking to them. The counterpart of man's in-ness in nature was nature's appearing as *presences*, that is, the individual natural phenomena's manifestly presenting themselves to him in the concrete eachness of their inner image and compelling demand.

Precisely because Jung's brief passage is in itself the contradiction between the semantically portrayed pre-I position and the actually, syntactically displayed modern-I position, it lets us clearly see the two poles between which that soul history that is the topic of our present reflections moves, and between which it moves exclusively in a one-way direction with no return.

II. Three moments in the history of the emergence of the I

This is a highly complex topic. Of all the many relevant events in and aspects of the history of the soul I will select only three of the major moments.

1. The emergence of reflection

The first moment is the *emergence of reflection*, above all in Greek pre-Socratic philosophy. This is in itself a highly complex history with many facets, but here I will only discuss it summarily and with respect to our topic.

The most essential aspect of "reflection" is the freeing of thought and truth from its attachment to real people and thus the rise to a fundamentally higher *impersonal* or better *supra-personal* standpoint above the natural one. It is the standpoint of thought that has come into its own. Prior to reflection, all thinking and mental processes aimed at gaining (or deepening) knowledge of truth were *person-centered*. Initiation and illumination always meant a particular person's initiation or illumination into higher wisdom or deeper mysteries and the refining and perfection of the person. It meant the person's immersion in and staying completely contained in the respective truth or wisdom. The sage, the wise man, the shaman, the "enlightened one" were the model figures. But the rise to reflection meant the abstraction from oneself as existing person and thus the soul's rise from the personal level to the strictly impersonal *conceptual* level[60] and at the same time gaining a critical distance *to* what is thought. Following Wilhelm von Humboldt we can say: The essence of thinking consists in reflecting, i.e. in distinguishing the thinker from the thought. The rise to reflection amounts to thought's having stepped out of

60 The fundamentally impersonal character can also be found prior to reflection, namely in mythology. But myth does not require any abstraction from the personal level inasmuch as it does not have its logical origin in individual persons the way philosophical thought has it in the thinker, philosopher. There is no need to acquire or deepen mythological knowledge because it comes as always already complete. And it is knowledge of truth that precedes all individual persons from the outset.

its containment or entranced envelopment in traditional mythical ideas or wisdom and its having become able to actively examine its contents.

It is the entrance into the generality of thought *as such*, liberated, independent thought as a *reality* in its own right, thought that stands on its own feet, inasmuch as it is *objectively* a general conception that has and follows *its own inner laws*, its logic and dynamic (just think of mathematics as an example familiar to most). It is autonomous thought,[61] thought thinking *itself* (ultimately Aristotle's *noêsis noêseôs*). It is thought that is no longer a person's initiation or illumination or wisdom, *not a personal more perfect state*. An initiation is neither needed nor results from it. What is needed for reflection is that the mind stands still for a moment in its continuous activity, gathers what it imagined into a unity, and in this way places it as an object vis-à-vis itself and with definite *criteria* of truth objects it to the "labor of the concept", rigorous thinking. This also means that comprehending the most sublime philosophical thought does not turn *you* into an "enlightened one", a sage, or holy man, nor does it mean your becoming "individuated" in Jung's high sense or your achieving (or approaching) "wholeness". It just means that you have conceptually comprehended something.

Reflection is working on an objective *opus*, contributing to a cultural work like science or like the building of a cathedral. Only the cathedral counts, not the generations of construction workers who built it. They and often even the major architects remained anonymous. The construction of a cathedral does not imply that it serves the personal self-development of the individual workers, *their* becoming better, more pious, wise, "whole", or "initiated". Their benefit was simply that they earned their living, plus, possibly, the personal satisfaction that any serious work and above all

61 Analysts may here be reminded of Jung's similar move of clearly separating what he called the "autonomous" or "objective" psyche from people's own thinking, wishes, and doings ("... that there are things in the psyche which I do not produce, but which produce themselves and have their own life", *MDR* p. 183). But Jung did not really go through with his own insight, since he nevertheless held on to the personalistic standpoint in psychology and the focus on *people*, declaring that the goal to be striven for by individuals was the "wholeness" of *personality*.

the participation in a highly esteemed project may bring. The "cathedral" that reflection qua philosophy is working on is the objective logical form of *consciousness-as-such*, its insight into the ultimate truth of the world and existence.[62]

In connection with reflection's abstraction from the personal level and its rise to a suprapersonal standpoint we may also remember the crucial episode from the Odyssey in which Odysseus, who needed to escape from the murderous giant Polyphemus, told him that his name was Nobody. This is probably the first evidence of the crucial possibility of one's complete abstraction from oneself, from "person" and the thereby gained freedom from and towards one's personal emotional needs and preferences.

This also means that reflection presupposes and amounts to the act of the soul's emigration from its primordial in-ness in nature, a rise above itself to a new status. All the invisible threads that tied consciousness like so many umbilical chords to the things of nature must have been cut in order for reflection to become possible. In the mythological and ritualistic mode of being-in-the-world man's connection to nature had been to the individual concrete phenomena that immediately and in actuality presented themselves to his experience, so to speak here and now. This is just as Jung had spoken of his feeling as if "living in every tree, in the plashing of the waves, in the clouds and the animals that come and go, in the procession of the seasons", that is, in their eachness. By contrast, reflection, in order to establish itself, leaves behind the individual phenomena and the presences shining forth from them and, for example in Parmenides, apperceives instead Being as such (in the singular), the world, the cosmos, as a whole. Cosmology takes the place of immediate *soul relation* to what is in fact before one's eyes. The two parts of the word "cosmology" are revealing: "cosmos" instead of this tree, this plashing of the waves, etc., and "-logy", i.e., *lógos*, concept in the mind, in-

62 To highlight what I said about reflection by a stark contrast let me mention that it is only during the 19th century and the emergence of the modern positivistic focus on factual existence that "the person" and the personal reentered philosophy, above all in Kierkegaard and Nietzsche, but also to some extent in 20th century existentialism. Paradigmatic for the personalistic turn to the philosopher *himself expressly as I* is Nietzsche's *Ecce homo*, especially with its last chapter, "Why I am a fate".

stead of what presents itself to immediate experience. In order to conceive of Being as a whole the soul must have pulled itself out of nature and gained a fundamental distance to it. Only once reflection has firmly established itself can it return its attention also to individual entities and later even study them scientifically in much greater detail than before, but now on the completely different level of logos and reflection. Being, as well as the cosmos, cannot be seen or experienced. They are inevitably *thoughts*. Reflection means that the soul is concerned with its own thoughts, not with real things in their physical presence. These thoughts may be thoughts *about* physical things or aspects of reality, but they are nevertheless the soul's own property.

2. Judaeo-Christian Monotheism

Now I come to the second moment, Judaeo-Christian *monotheism*. As psychologist I do not look at monotheism theologically or in terms of religion and piety, but instead psychologically.

The monotheistic God is the *world-external* creator of the world and all-knowing, all-seeing. The idea of the monotheistic God is psychologically the explicit notion of the I. As the maker of all he is the concretely imagined *concept* of *absolute* autonomy, unconditioned self-determination, and unrestricted freedom, and as the all-seeing eye he represents nothing else but the "*absolute* VIEWPOINT *as such*". (We had seen the connection of "VIEWPOINT" and "I" when we realized that in the shift from "Paul is hungry" to "I am hungry" the VIEWPOINT of experience is internalized.) The soul's move to monotheism therefore also means that the soul has all of a sudden and for the first time become *explicitly conscious* of the standpoint of reflection, fundamentally impersonal reflection *as such*, in other words of that standpoint that in early Greek philosophy had only been innocently and unconsciously acted out in philosophical thought. For example, even Aristotle's *noêsis noêseôs* had been only a semantic content of thought and as such had the form of *object*. In monotheism this thought has obtained the form of subject, active subjectivity.

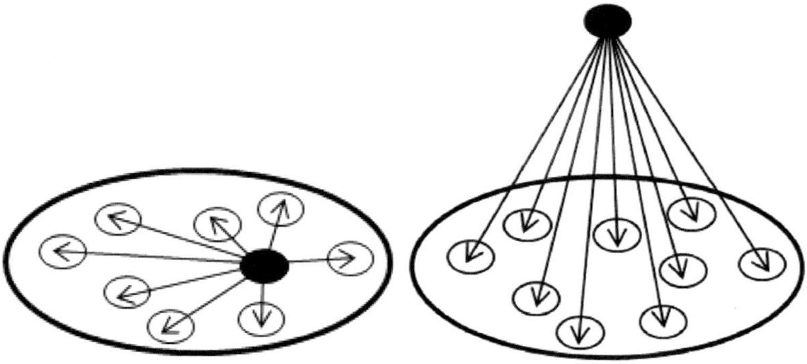

From the I as world-internal VIEWPOINT *to the world-external* VIEWPOINT *of the monotheistic God*

As world-external creator of the world God is the absolute counter-image to consciousness's primordial in-ness in nature. God has the world as a whole, the cosmos, in front of and vis-à-vis himself, and although he is said to permeate everything in it with his omniscience, this "meta-level" knowing is the exact opposite of the self-presentation of natural things in their eachness that prevailed during the times of the consciousness's in-ness in the world and of the mythological and ritualistic mode of being-in-the-world.

Jung gave his book on UFO's in German the subtitle: "Of things seen in the skies".[63] We could say similarly that qua God the I is one of the things imaginally seen in the skies, up there in Heaven. As much as in the monotheistic God the standpoint of reflection has obtained the form of active subject, God as a personal God is nevertheless still a projection. In conventional Jungian psychology projection is usually understood as throwing some internal, but unconscious content out upon something external as a projection screen. As a consequence of this view one thinks that projections

63 The English translation merged Jung's title ("*Ein moderner Mythos*") and his subtitle ("*Von Dingen, die am Himmel gesehen werden*") into one single phrase: "A modern myth of things seen in the skies". But Jung does not speak about a myth *of* things seen in the skies. For him it is the other way around. Because things are seen in the skies, the UFO's seen there have the character of the appearance of a myth.

should be withdrawn; what is "seen" out there should return into the inner of the psyche of those persons whose projections they are and should be recognized by them as aspects of their own personality. The problem is that this view is due to the prevailing personalistic perspective, and that it is itself a projection (upon people)!

A real psychology sees at least cultural or collective projections as the soul's, not people's projections. Projection in this sense is the first appearance, the first dawning, of the idea of something as yet still unthinkable. As such it is necessarily only the first immediacy of this totally new idea, that is, this idea not in its proper soul form of concept, of logical or mercurial spirit, but in the externalized form of object-thinking, substantiation, personification, in other words, as *imagined* content. The imagination is a usual, but fundamentally deficient mode of the soul's self-manifestation. In this sense projection is certainly the first-time awareness of an entirely new possibility, but the awareness of it only in its first immediacy, that is to say, in its inauthentic form. The authentic form would, in our context, be veritable subjectivity. About God we can say that as highest being and personal God he is, to be sure, the *idea of* the absolute VIEWPOINT, of the "I" as subject, but he is this idea, this "I" or "subject", precisely only in still imagined form and thus conceived as an "object", a being or person ("God"), and thus he is, in obvious self-contradiction, the "I" decidedly *as* not-"I", *as* "He" or "Thou", the *impersonal* standpoint imagined *as* tied to a supranatural *person*.

Rather than being the throwing out of a content from a person's inner upon something external projection should be comprehended as the form change called hypostasis, substantiation, reification, or personification. Why is projection in this sense necessary, what function does it have in the soul's life? For the soul to become explicitly conscious of the new standpoint of reflection it needs to envision this standpoint very clearly and distinctly in isolated form, experience it as a separate, independent reality vis-à-vis itself that it could focus on. This is why it needed to project and hypostatize the new idea of absolute viewpoint, and it is what happened through the soul's invention of the idea of the monotheistic God.

We need to understand projection as a preliminarily envisioned but still transcendent future goal. Accordingly, it is not people's, not our task, to integrate what had been projected into *ourselves*. Projections need to come home to *themselves*. They need to be interiorized into their truth, *alchemically* decomposed and sublimated into logical form. Therefore, the monotheistic God, too, is to be comprehended as a *project* or task that the soul assigns to itself for the future. But why did it have the have the form of highest *God*?

In order to give itself a distant goal, in order to set for itself an enormous task to achieve, the soul has to project it up to heaven as an absolute ideal, as something to be wholeheartedly worshiped and aspired to. The move to reflection in Greek antiquity initially affected only one special area of life, that of philosophical thought, and in social regards only a few intellectuals, leaving at first most other areas of life (such as concrete social customs, religious practice, private and public life) as well as the majority of society intact, only slowly seeping down and reshaping them to some extent. By contrast, monotheism a priori claimed all areas of life and all people for itself. It necessarily, by definition, had to be all-comprehending, for how else could the monotheistic God be the world-external creator, sustainer and upholder of everything in existence? And conversely, it had to be the one and only God in order to be the ideal and absolute value that could muster all the striving and passion of the soul and harness them for the realization of its project.

What the soul has set up for itself with its invention of the monotheistic God is the historical *project* or *task* of inwardizing the all-seeing eye or world-external absolute VIEWPOINT for everything in the world from its reified and imagined form as an existing being in spatial reality into soul, into the spacelessness of logical form and true subjectivity, thereby for the first time making it really conscious. In other words, the task is to alchemically decompose, distill or vaporize its preliminary self-alienated form of supernatural object and of "He" and to convert it into its true form of "I", into a *general principle of seeing*. We could also say that it is the project of alchemically distilling or vaporizing what at first appeared as *semantic* content into *syntax*, logical form, spirit.

3. Filippo Brunelleschi's experiment

The realization of this project took centuries and it finally surfaced during the period that we call the Renaissance. Here I first need to clarify difficulties arising around the word "modern" and "modernity". In German, additional terms allow for a distinction within what in English is "modernity". We distinguish "*neuzeitlich, Neuzeit*" as the historical period from roughly 1300 or 1400 to 1800, for which in English we must use something like "early modern", from "*modern, die Moderne*" for the time from around 1800 onwards. Within modernity we must in turn distinguish two phases, "industrial modernity" and, starting around 1970, "medial modernity". (The expression "post-modern" does not make sense, since medial modernity is simply modernity on the way to its coming home to itself, to its full, pure development.)

I will *illustrate* the explicit emergence of the I by means of a small example, a marvelous "symptom" (in the sense given). It is an experiment executed by the Italian artist, architect, and engineer Brunelleschi who was instrumental for the discovery of the mathematical, geometric laws of central perspective. Brunelleschi made this particular experiment between 1415 and 1420.

On a small square wooden panel he painted the Florentine Baptistery San Giovanni from a central front view. The artist then drilled a little hole through the middle of the *back* of the painting and asked his test subjects to hold with one hand the panel close to one eye with the painted surface facing outward away from the viewer and with his other hand hold a mirror so that it faces the painting at a prescribed distance. While peering through the little hole, the observer was supposed to look at the mirror reflection of the painting. Then the Baptistery, Brunelleschi said, would appear to him "as if he saw it in its complete veracity".

It is a surprisingly complicated arrangement. One wonders why the mirror was necessary. Why was the viewer not shown the painting directly, straight on? Why did he need to put the blank wooden back of the painting to his eye and force his gaze through a tiny hole as a narrow channel?

If we do not take this experiment as Brunellischi's mere playing around, but as a "symptom", that is, as an unintentional self-manifestation of an otherwise invisible soul truth, a new world-relation or mode of being-in-the-world, than we must take note of the fact that it represents an utterly unusual and artificial form of seeing, one that has absolutely broken with the immediacy of seeing and the "natural" direct experience of reality itself.

a. The empty backside of the painting as reflection of the emptiness of the world-external space. Let me first concentrate on the one crucial feature of this new form of seeing, the subject's peering through a hole from the back of the painting at the mirror reflection of the front side of the painting, in order to determine what new soul stance or soul truth expresses itself in it. Making someone take a painting and put *its naked back* to his eye in order to gaze through a small whole at a reflection of the painting is absolutely unexpected, *contra naturam*, at first glance even absurd. What necessitated this weird arrangement?

The empty, barren back wall of the painting represents a forbidding, excluding barrier. The actual event of "seeing" takes place within the relation of painting and mirror. The mirror is the primary viewer; *it* "sees" the painting the way in which under the normal conditions of natural seeing a human viewer would see it. The interplay between mirror and painting represents ordinary seeing, the natural form of human experience in the world. But here this natural way of seeing is precisely bracketed, so to speak, firmly enclosed within itself, and thus *sublated*. Inasmuch as the mirror is an inanimate object and not a conscious subject at all, its seeing is in itself dead, blind, obsolete. It needs a living human viewer *outside* in order to come to life and be turned into a meaningful, consciously aware seeing. The *second* viewer, the human person who sees from a *superordinate* point of view, is now the actual viewer.[64]

---

64 This is analogous to the relation of the alchemical adept to the *vas*. About the latter Jung pointed out that " it had to be made of glass, and had also to be as round as possible, since it was meant to represent the universe [*Weltall*, the All]..." (*CW* 13 § 245, modif.). The adept looks at the universe from an extramundane standpoint and has the world as a sublated object in front of himself. And since what is inside the vas "has everything it needs within itself" and he must under no circumstances "let anything from outside, that does not belong, get into it" (*CW* 14 § 749), the adept has symbolically his position in the nothingness of empty space.

The back wall of the painting objectively bars and excludes this human viewer from the real process going on "inside" between mirror and painting. The fact that only by, so to speak, secretly peeping through a peephole he can get access to what the mirror sees makes his seeing a secondary, meta-level seeing. The natural world-internal mode of seeing and experiencing has been left behind. In fact, what the viewer sees through the peephole in the mirror is twice removed from the real Baptistery. First, there is the painting of the Baptistery and then the mirror image of the painting of the Baptistery.[65] The human viewer's seeing is one from an expressly external point of view, and as decidedly *second* viewer he sees from a *meta-level* point of view.

Psychologically seen, this superior point of view is the objective representation and symbolization of the *world-external* absolute viewpoint of the monotheistic creator God. Brunelleschi's turning his painting around so that his viewer now faces the naked back of the painting expresses the soul's turning its back to the visible world and natural experience. We must read his experience like a dream or other soul image, which means that we must stick to the image, enclose it, so to speak, in an alchemical retort and not "let anything from outside, that does not belong, get into it..." (*CW* 14 § 749). It has everything that belongs within itself. Therefore we must not allow ourselves to be misled by the obvious fact that all around the viewer there are things and people. This experiment took place in the middle of busy Florence and near that very *real* Baptistery of which he saw the painting in the mirror. *Within* the experiment, there is nothing, indeed, nothingness around him; the empty, barren back wall of the painting symbolizes the worldlessness in which this viewer logically finds himself in this experiment and from which he now looks at the world. It reveals the soul's now having its place as viewer in the absolute empti-

65 For centuries, it was thought and deeply felt that the sciences, above all physics, had the purpose of presenting the true picture of the world as it really is. This is what gave to science its almost divine dignity. However, during the 20th century it dawned on the advanced scientists themselves that they were not at all talking about the world as it really is, but only about their own *models* of the world and that even Newton's classical mechanics had only been dealing with an idealized system, not the real world. The most modern science seems at long last to have caught up with the idea, already inherent in Brunelleschi's experiment, that science studies its own "already *painted* picture" of nature, not the world itself.

ness, loneliness, and isolation of the sphere outside the world as such. This stance is in little what the position of the extra-mundane all-seeing God is on the large metaphysical plane.

It signifies that the *world-external position* of the monotheistic God as all-seeing eye of the world has been deliteralized as imagined personal God and supreme being and alchemically distilled into a *general methodological principle of seeing*, indeed, a *principle of the very constitution of consciousness as a whole*. As a methodological principle it was from now on available to man. The "absolute VIEWPOINT as such" does not need any longer to be projected onto heaven, totally outside and beyond the universe. The projection has been caught up with, the projected idea has come home to itself. The notion of "absolute viewpoint as such" that before had been imaginally reified as a supernatural being, the literally transcendent God up there, had become inwardized into itself and thus vaporized into a spirit, into consciousness's logical form as "I". It has turned into early-modern man's stance or mode of being-in-the-world.

Jung already once pointed out that "every spiritual truth is gradually objectified and turns into a ... tool in the hands of man" (*CW* 13 § 302, transl. modif.). But what we have here is qualitatively more than a tool or method that can be used at will. It is early-modern man's new invisible truth, the objective stance that from now on *defines* him in his innermost depth. It is his inevitable mode of being-in-the-world.

b. Excursus on inflation. It is crucial not to misconstrue this withdrawal of the projection as man's identification with God, his usurpation of an exclusively divine position. Man did not, as it were, absorb the transcendent position of God into his own breast. We must not diagnose an inflation. Understanding it this way might suggest itself to us if we follow Jung's view concerning Nietzsche's "God is dead". Jung said, "The tragedy of *Zarathustra* is that, because Nietzsche's God died, he himself became a god [...] He to whom 'God dies,' will become the victim of 'inflation.'" *CW* 11 § 142 (transl. modif.). In a letter to Victor White, 10 April 1954, he likewise claimed that, "Through the negation of God one becomes deified, [...]", (*Letters 2*, p. 168). During the Renaissance and the whole early-modern period it was of course not at all a question of the denial or death of God. What really happened was that God suffered a radical form change, a transformation, but *remained* (as I will show later). But even the decidedly *modern* "death of God", as expressed by Nietzsche, is not a denial the way Jung presents it. It is recognizing and paying heed to the discovery that "God" had simply disappeared from the soul's inventory.[66]

Nietzsche and modernity at large are not our topic here. We are concerned with the early-modern rise of the I as subject through the distillation of the projected "absolute viewpoint as such" in the form of a literally transcendent highest being into logical form or the syntax of consciousness. To interpret this change as man's being inflated by the God-archetype would first of all be a personalistic, anthropological fallacy. Nothing of this historical change was man's doing, and man did not confuse himself with God. It was a revolutionary change in the soul, and it shaped him, not he it. This change *happened* to him, he found himself in it.

Secondly, it would be a grave misunderstanding of, or even a defense against, the real insight that what had happened here was precisely not a simple relocation of the transcendent God into the human breast, but an "alchemical" transformation of the projected and hypostatized *form* of "God" from substance or being into spirit or logical form, in other words, a distillation. The *numinous*, substantiated content (God) was transformed into a general *principle*. A principle is characterized by two facts. The first is that it has lost the numinosity of the divine figure who used to demand human upward-looking and worship, and instead turned into a rational truth that can be fully insighted and comprehended, and in this sense become the human mind's own property. The absolute distance between man and the projected God is abolished. The second fact is that a principle is a law or rule that man can adopt as his own rule to be obediently and consistently followed. This having to abide by a principle is the distillation-form of the former *worship* of the numinous God or gods.

Inflation is something totally different. It means that the numinosity and fundamental structural otherness between human, on the one hand, and divine or "archetypal", on the other, is

66 Nietzsche himself was also guilty of an egoic interpretation of his observation by accusing man of having killed God.

retained. The structure of "projection" is not dissolved. Instead, human consciousness is, as it were, directly short-circuited with the *projected* wholly other numinous content, becoming infected by, infused with it. Worship is replaced by the inflated consciousness's being in the grip of and driven "from behind" by the numinous content,

Jung's thesis that "He to whom 'God dies,' will become the victim of 'inflation'" ignores the possibility of such a death possibly having the form of a distillation, vaporization, through which the numinosity and thus the inflation-producing agent is simply decomposed and the structural gap between the human mind and the formerly projected content is removed. It ignores the possibility of the transformation of God into an abstract committing, obliging principle. One's adopting the idea of man's identification with God would really amount to a counterfactual (neurotic?) attempt to keep intact and rescue the old logic of the *projected* God, to *post factum* "prevent" his fermenting corruption and vaporization as substantial being and semantic content of consciousness into spirit or syntax: the interpretation in terms of inflation as a neurotic defense against the already real alchemical decomposition of God, one's own consciousness as the last asylum for the *substantiated* God. For this attitude, where "He" was, there "I" is obviously not allowed to be.

c. The conquest of the world-external "absolute viewpoint as such" and the camera obscura. What has been achieved by the inwardization of the projected and as such substantiated idea of God *into itself* is the real ability of consciousness to take a fundamentally transcendent, world-external standpoint in its *world-internal* and thoroughly *finite* seeing and experiencing the world. It is consciousness's conquest for itself of the *logical form* of a seeing that in fact sees from an "absolute viewpoint as such". It is that viewpoint that with the invention of the monotheistic God had been projected literally outside of the world, altogether beyond the universe, as a semantic content of consciousness and object of pious devotion.

The temptation to interpret the acquisition of the absolute viewpoint as such as man's identification with God is one problem. Another major difficulty is that one needs to have risen to the psychological standpoint and thus to the insight into the psychological difference if one wants to understand what we are concerned with here. Habitual consciousness tends to think only in terms of human behavior (human thinking, feeling, imagining, and acting), with what is immediately empirically accessible, easily imaginable, and familiar to ego-consciousness and thus with semantic contents and human behavior. But psychology is only concerned with the "hinterland of the soul", with the *transcendental* invisible *logic* informing, from "behind" or within, the major course of events. The fact that the world-relation of early-modern man is from a logically decidedly *world-external, transcendent* standpoint may induce persons who stay on the level of empirical behavior to think that it must be something absolutely fantastic, mysterious, if not simply impossible. This is despite the fact that in reality it is no more than the all-pervasive truth in which we all still inevitably live, the truth of our scientific, technological civilization. The difficulty is similar to that expressed by Heraclitus with respect to the *lógos*: "They divorce themselves from that with which most of all they are in continuous contact, the *lógos*, and what they come across every day, that appears foreign to them" (Fr. 72 DK)

In a way, the arrangement of Brunelleschi's experiment has some similarity with the device called a *camera obscura*. It consists of a closed and thus internally dark box into which rays of light coming from things outside fall through a centrally placed tiny hole in one wall so that an image of the things outside is thrown upon the back wall. This image can be made visible to an external viewer through additional technical means and then copied on paper. The camera obscura became popular with artists from the Renaissance onwards as an aid for correctly drawing and painting objects such as buildings with the exact foreshortening of the lines in linear perspective. Shigeru Tsuji has even argued that Brunelleschi already painted his picture of the Baptistery by means of a camera obscura.[67] Here we have again a tiny hole in the wall, the reflection of a picture inside the camera, and the external viewer. It is again testimony to the new type of seeing. What happens by means of the camera obscura is not world-inter-

67 Shigeru Tsuji, "Brunelleschi and the camera obscura: the discovery of pictorial perspective", in: *Art History* 13 (1990), pp. 276-292).

nal seeing, direct seeing, but seeing from a methodically established "world-external" viewpoint and seeing a literally "boxed-in" picture of a piece of "the world". I think that the popularity of the camera obscura in early-modern times gives even more weight to my claim that what Brunelleschi's experiment signifies is not only an isolated event and personal whim, but a "kind of document of the soul", that is, a self-manifestation of the new logical status of consciousness. This new logic of seeing is not only relevant for painting. Brunelleschi's experiment is evidence of something invisible and larger, namely the hidden logic of early-modern man's mode of being-in-the-world, his world-relation as such.

An even broader base is given to my claim by the general success in painting of linear central perspective. We will learn more about perspective in the following when we now begin to look at the kind of seeing that happens from the new world-internal world-external standpoint, more specifically: at the inner logic informing that seeing.

d. The peephole or: Representation (*Vorstellung*) as *not-natural* experience of the world. What is seen by Brunellischi's viewer from his logically (not empirically) "world-external" viewpoint beyond the back wall of the painting is fundamentally removed from archaic experience. The latter had been an experience in which man is, as it were, "hit" by the inner divine essence shining forth as face or voice from within the phenomena he is confronted with. What we have in Brunelleschi's experience is instead a seeing that proceeds exclusively from the human subject for which *what* is seen is on principle utterly passive and mute. Only the seeing, studying subject is active. All spontaneity is on its side. This seeing is, furthermore, a completely self-contained artificially constructed mode of seeing that has its *real* referent totally outside of itself beyond the back side of the painting. The viewer looks at the purposely, methodically produced reflection in a mirror of a likewise *man-made picture* (of something real). It is not one's seeing the natural reflection of *real* buildings as in a lake or river or a shiny surface.

Very important for the new form of seeing is the little peephole in the back of the painting. The single precisely placed hole turns the viewer's viewing into a *methodically disciplined* and *fixated* peering, not an ordinary, natural looking. As the drawings and paintings of children and medieval or ancient peoples show, ordinary seeing sees things from different viewpoints at once. It does not see like the lens of a camera sees and therefore it remains ignorant of the geometric laws of perspective. The tiny hole in the back of the painting shows that it is felt to be crucial that the viewer's gaze is channeled. The peephole produces the fixated eyepoint in which all rays of light coming from what is to be seen are drawn together into one single point. This concentration or assembly point is the I. The fixed hole guarantees that the viewer's eyepoint represents what I called "absolute viewpoint as such".

That the rigid fixation of the viewpoint through the tiny peephole is necessary can be interpreted as the inevitable compromise that alone turns the contradiction of a world-internal world-external viewpoint into a real possibility.

By peeping through the peephole you have to use one single eye and sacrifice the other eye as organ of seeing. The Germanic God Odin had to sacrifice one eye in order to obtain his shamanic knowledge. Early-modern man sacrificed one eye to achieve something very different, but likewise fundamentally "higher" and precious, namely the finite human, world-internal realization of the world-external absolute VIEWPOINT as such. From then on, his (*essential*) seeing is, figuratively speaking, a one-eye seeing, camera-lens-like. His second eye is lost. But the word "sacrifice" puts this loss in the right perspective.

In Brunelleschi's experiment there is a *literal* peephole. But the soul as early-modern I does not need a literal board with a peephole to look through. It *is* the methodologically disciplined and fixated seeing. This is its inner logic. Brunelleschi's experiment merely makes this hidden logic visible for us.

The world-external viewpoint has consequences for what is seen, for the logic of "object", which is the "subject's" own other.

Stefan Winter[68] connected Brunelleschi's experiment with Heidegger's insight that it was in Western history only since the

68 Stefan Winter, "Ruin der Repräsentation", in: *Reality strikes back II: Tod der Repräsentation?* Ed. by Kathrin Tiedemann / Frank Raddatz, Berlin (Theater der Zeit) 2010, pp. 24-31.

Neuzeit, the early modern period, that a subject arose that "represents" (*vorstellt*) its objects and the world, where to "represent" means, as Heidegger put it, "*das vor sich hin und zu sich her Stellen*" (the subject's placing [its objects] before itself and referring them back to itself, or, more precisely perhaps: making them face the subject).[69] Winter suggested, and I think we can agree, that far beyond what this experiment's immediate purpose for Brunelleschi was, namely a demonstration of linear perspective, it is also a precise illustration of "*Vorstellen*" (representation) in Heidegger's pointed sense. Thus this mode of seeing and experiencing is also the illustration of what the modern I, what "subject" and "object" mean in the modern sense. Brunelleschi's painting of the Baptistery is the object placed before the subject and, by being reflected in the mirror, referred back to the subject. And "object" as ob-ject, the *Gegenstand* as *Gegen-stand*, is from now on only what is seen in this way: as representation, as the *reflection* of the from the outset already *"painted"*, i.e., always already *apperceived* and at bottom mathematically structured, phenomenon, not the original phenomenon itself, in our case the Baptistery. The "object" seen is, as it were, boxed in between painting and mirror. This at the same time implies the systematic exclusion of anything external (including the original object) from what is boxed in. In Brunelleschi's experience this is the real Baptistery. And what along with the original real sight is on principle excluded is the active penetrating gazes and demanding voices that things would have had for archaic experience. Kant, more than three centuries later, would call the "what" of this new seeing the "appearance" (*Erscheinung*) in contradistinction to the "thing in itself", which by definition is out of reach. And modern science, above all physics, knows that it only deals with *models* of reality, that physics is the representation of the world in mathematical terms and not the description of reality itself.

69 Martin Heidegger, "Die Zeit des Weltbildes", in: *idem*, *Holzwege*, Frankfurt a.M. (Klostermann) ^{5}1972, p. 85. There are two English translations of this essay: "The Age of the World Picture," in: Heidegger, *Off the Beaten Track*, trans. and ed. by Julian Young and Kenneth Haynes, Cambridge 2002, pp. 57–86, and Heidegger, "The Age of the World Picture," in: *idem*, *The Question Concerning Technology and Other Essays*, trans. by William Lovitt, New York 1977, pp. 115–54.

Having gained the insight into the nature of the object as "ob-ject" and representation and from the outset already "painted" allows us to return to the topic of the sacrifice of one eye and raise (and answer) the question: What does one-eye seeing mean in a not figurative sense and what is lost through the loss of the second eye? Natural seeing with "two eyes" is, to say it with one word, "phenomenological". It is one's apperceiving whatever is to be seen as the sight of phenomena in their individuality and eachness, namely each with their own inherent truth and dignity. Early-modern man's one-eye seeing is, by contrast, "cosmological". By this I mean that whatever is seen is a priori apperceived as an integral part or segment of the world or universe as a whole and in terms of the concept of this whole. The *concept* of the systematic, coherent whole comes first; all details are subsumed under this whole. We can illustrate the difference between the two stances with the difference between the Biblical view that God created "*every* living creature ... *after their kind*, and *every* winged fowl *after his kind*" (Genesis 1:21, my emphasis) and the modern theory of evolution.

If we want to review the whole soul movement described here once more we can say that the first stage was the emergence of the real, but *unconscious*, *presence* of the logical status of reflection. The second stage was the explicit *awareness of the principle* as such that makes reflection possible, but this awareness was itself still unconscious since it was objectified and hypostatized as the monotheistic God. The third stage is that consciousness has explicitly become aware of this awareness.

III. The distillation of Infinity and the Spirit-nature of the I

1. Infinity

Brunelleschi's painting is a particularly good example of this sense of "object" because it showed the Baptistery in geometrically correct linear perspective, which, as I said, is not how natural seeing sees things. The painting was *mathematically constructed.* And the very point of his endeavor was to demonstrate the laws of linear perspective in general and in particular the fact that "the convergence of [...] parallel lines in nature seems to occur always in line precisely with the viewer's eye level. In other words, if the viewer looks straight ahead, he will see that any set of parallel lines retreating from eyepoint and also parallel to his own axis visualis always seems to converge on the horizon." (Edgerton p. 176). The point of this seeming convergence on the horizon is the so-called vanishing point.

This seems to have been Brunelleschi's revolutionary discovery, and it has fundamental metaphysical and psychological implications. In empirical reality parallel lines, for example, train tracks, never converge. If they did, trains would be derailed. And according to the thinking of classical and medieval philosophy the thought of the convergence of parallels in finite earthly reality was not thought, indeed, was not allowed to be thought, because the convergence of finite things could only happen in the beyond, in infinity, and the laws of Earth and Heaven were, and *had to* remain, separated by a hiatus, personally and practically speaking by one's death.

But Brunelleschi showed that for the (fixated) human eye, i.e., optically, parallel lines in fact *do* converge at a vanishing point. For us this means that, as attested to by his discovery of central perspective, for early-modern consciousness the absolute gulf that used to separate the empirical world from the ideal realm, from the Infinity of God, had been overcome. The vertical separation (sublunar world vs. celestial sphere) was replaced by one continuous horizontal plane of both eyepoint and vanishing point that showed that, ideally perceived and comprehended, there was in finite reality itself an inherent tendency to be oriented toward and to vanish in infinity. Infinity was no longer absolutely transcendent, it had become accessible. To be sure, not directly, practically, in a hands-on way. The parallel lines still do not physically converge. The convergence was visible only for the mathematically constructing mind and on the basis of the strict fixation of the one single eyepoint. It belonged to a decidedly *ideal* plane, an abstraction from the empirically, physically real. The point of convergence was not for nothing called the *vanishing* point. Nevertheless, by mentally continuously following the vanishing lines to

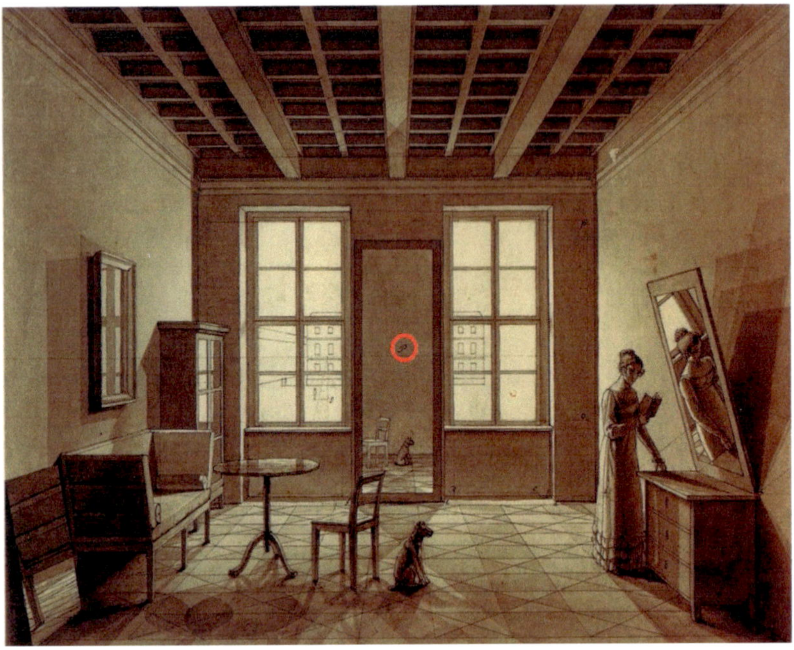

Interior, by Johann Erdmann Hummel (around 1820).
The red circle added by me marks the place of the vanishing point.

their very end, linear perspective allowed man to *see into Infinity* (or at least to the point where it begins).

For the mind committed to this mathematically informed ideal type of seeing, Infinity had become really accessible. And in the long run this had even downright practical consequences, for the notion of infinity could be put to practical uses, not only by painters, but also in science, engineering, and later in economics through the likewise revolutionary invention of infinitesimal calculus in the 17th century by Gottfried Wilhelm Leibniz and Isaac Newton. Now it had become possible to *quantitatively* determine *infinitely* small intervals. The precise quantitative calculation by the finite human mind of something infinitely small is an intellectual *coniunctio oppositorum*. A way had been found to overcome the absolute contradiction between the infinite and the finite.

Semantically, the new paintings show static objects or scenes. But syntactically the *form* of depth perspective presents a dynamic, a pull, the seemingly static objects' zooming into the depth of the distant background, into Infinity. The painting by Hummel (p. 168) demonstrates this suction quite literally. But it does not need such obvious representations of central perspective; even landscape paintings without any explicit vanishing lines, indeed, the whole world experience as such of the early-modern soul bear witness to depth perspective. The third stage is that of a fundamental *dynamization* in the very notion of reality as a whole and of substance as such.

After so much emphasis on Brunelleschi and linear perspective it may perhaps be necessary to remind the reader again that the thesis presented in this paper is not that Brunelleschi's experiment, the discovery and use of linear perspective and of the *camera obscura* in painting, and the invention of infinitesimal calculus, *caused* a psychological change in man's basic attitude to the world. It is the other way around. The phenomena mentioned are merely tiny "symptoms" of a fundamental and otherwise invisible change in man's being-in-the-world that had happened in the depths.

2. The Spirit-nature of "the I" as subject

Central linear perspective shows that the human eyepoint and the vanishing point both lie on one and the same horizontal level. The one corresponds to the other, both are, so to speak, the two endpoints of one and the same line. Thinking back to the mirror used to see the painted picture, we could also say that the human eyepoint and the vanishing point are the reflection of each other. This corresponds to the early-modern idea that ultimately the human mind (*mens humana*) is of the same nature as, and a part of, the *mens divina*, the divine Spirit. It is the limited, finite version of the infinite Spirit. And the lines that vanish in the vanishing point depict, in anticipation, the dynamic and direction of the movement of the human spirit (*mens*), the movement of its infinitesimal approximation to the divine Spirit; Nicholas of Cusa explicitly expressed the early-modern principle of infinite perfectability. Psychologically, this pull towards Infinity is behind the enormous motive power and the accelerating internal dynamics that propelled modern science forward and gave it its extraordinary elatedness and nearly divine esteem.

For the early-modern period, God was by no means dead the way he is for modernity. Infinity had not at all disappeared altogether. But the relation to God and to Infinity was completely new, different from what it had been in the Middle Ages, for whom, as I indicated, the vanishing point was unthinkable and for whom the fact would have been even more unthinkable that both the human eyepoint and the point of the convergence in infinity would be on the same *horizontal* level, connected by an unbroken continuity from the finite to Infinity. For the Middle Ages and Antiquity the finite and Infinity had been vertically and thus on principle separated. For the medieval mind God had mainly been substantiated as a highest being and imaginal figure, God Father or the redeeming Son. Meanwhile, however, "God" himself had become distilled, vaporized into Spirit, and Infinity, once a transcendent location or realm high above the sublunar sphere, had become *dynamized* into a forceful movement towards the *infinite depth* of the visible world itself. The word "vanishing" in "vanishing lines" does not imply absolute disappearance, vanishing into nothing. It is a determinate negation and means the dynamic "vanishing" of substance into infinite depth and spirit.

Equiprimordially with God's sublimation and deliteralization, there was the exactly corresponding transformation on the human side, inasmuch as there was a fundamental shift of emphasis away from the definition of man as physical, substantial existence, as *ens creatum*, to his being predominantly defined by his innermost nature as *mens*, soul, and thought (Descartes' "*res cogitans*"). The dynamic of the *vanishing* lines rushing into the *vanishing* point is itself an objective pictorial representation of the general distillation/vaporization process that for the experience of the early-modern I transforms the logic of "physical being or entity" into the logic of "spirit", i.e., mainly into mathematical formulas of the laws of nature.

"The I" is not a psychic part of the personality and not only the logical structure of people's consciousness. It is not only on the human and not only on the subject's side. It is a general form, a mode of being-in-the-world that gives subject *and* object, empirical reality *and* God its ultimate, innermost form: the form of spirit. In fact, "subject" in the new sense is not only the one side of the pair of opposites, but much rather the opposition of subject and object as a whole.

3. The Spirit-nature of the I's "object"

The world as object appeared in between these two poles; if we stay with Brunelleschi's experiment we can say it stayed between painting and mirror, or in terms of central linear perspective between eyepoint and vanishing point. Although I had said earlier about the early-modern object that it is dead and mute, I must now specify that it is true only by comparison with the experience of nature in the mythological and ritualistic worlds. Seen in its own terms, the "object" in the early-modern sense, the world, is also an expression of the divine spirit. As such it was in itself dynamic. Nicholas of Cusa had already interpreted the world as *explicatio dei*. In this sense it was by no means dead and mute. But of course, what appeared from within the world in the new form of "object" was its inner spirit, its intelligibility, its rational, mainly *mathematical* form; it was not, as in mythological times, imaginally individualized divine presences as concrete face, figure, or voice. The nature spirits of old in the plural had been distilled into the *generalized* awareness of the *intelligent* inner construction of the universe.

The inner divine spiritual quality of the early-modern "object" expressed itself in painting in the demand that a painting should be the oneness of trueness to life AND aesthetic *pulchritudo* (beauty). Trueness to life because the intelligent mathematical design of the world had to be seen *in reality*. The aesthetic *pulchritudo*, on the one hand, was the divine spirit's shining forth from the inner truth of the things of the world. It could be seen as the successor to the former *claim* that the presences shining forth from things of nature in archaic experience used to make on the person seeing them. At the same time it presupposes (or attests to) the early-modern "subject" looking, out of its own innermost essence as *mens humana*, at what for it has become "object".

The dynamic of the "vanishing" movement is not only expressed in the works of painting and their *pulchritudo*, the depth of feeling into which the extraordinarily, *almost religiously* appreciated works of art seduced. The pull into Infinity found later also its supreme and purest expression in music, such as the music of Mozart and Beethoven.

IV. The modern Western I that *as* the psychic or linguistic I has assumed the *general form* of the psychological I

I cited Jung's speaking of every spiritual truth's gradually becoming objectified and turning into a tool in the hands of man. But this objective representation, this objectification, is only one effect that a major soul truth has. The other effect is just as significant. The longer man lives with an idea or soul truth as the determinate logical form of the world and his interchange with the world, he himself also becomes slowly more and more assimilated to this form in his own logical constitution. In this sense it is not surprising that the form of "I", as *subject* in the eminent sense that the early-modern period had conquered for itself, in the course of time also retroactively re-shaped the very definition of man. In the long run we always become redefined in the image and likeness of the tools, methods, views, and categories that we use and the products that we produce. In the beginning of the early-modern period, the newly conquered notion of the world-external viewpoint as a possible general principle of human seeing the world had only been the first inkling of the exciting discovery of a theoretical idea, and had been explicit only as an object and content of no more than a few learned people's consciousness. In the course of time what at first was a principle in the realm of ideas high above existing people turned more and more into the general mode of how the world was seen and related to. And at the end of the period what had been a mode of man's seeing and relating to the world had entered also the inner logical structure of man himself. He no longer needed to "apply" this principle. He has *become* it. He now *was* subject.

1. The dynamic, inherent in the revolutionized mode of seeing,

towards the *realization* of "subject" in the *existing* concept

One aspect of what made this transformation possible was that there is a dialectic inherent in the polar relation between God's spirit and the human spirit (*mens*). At first and explicitly for consciousness, the Spirit of God (*mens divina*) is the all-important ultimate and infinite reality, and human *mens* is fundamentally secondary. Although it is of the same kind, it is essentially derivative of the *mens divina*, a definitely finite version of it.

But in practice all depended on *man's* active use of his spiritual power. The human exercise of his mental powers was the important factor. To describe the ensuing historical development with our example of eyepoint and vanishing point, the whole psychological weight slowly shifted to the eyepoint, and this meant that in the course of time God turned more and more into *the human spirit's* vanishing point, so that later, in modernity, God had indeed literally vanished from the soul's household. This shows the ultimate distillation that happened to him. From the beginning of the early-modern period, God was on the way to being dissolved into the absolute "principle of principles" of *human* reason.

There is another and even more important aspect that facilitated the shift from general principle of seeing the world to the redefinition of the constitution of man himself, and it too involves a dialectic. It concerns a more immediate feature of Brunelleschi's experiment, namely an aspect of the tiny hole in the back of the Brunelleschi's painting. First we need to realize that the viewer or rather his eye (the viewer could use only one of his eyes, not both!) looking through this hole was not himself/itself the eyepoint. The eyepoint was not his personal property. The eyepoint was much rather this tiny hole in the painting. As such it was something objective, not personal, not subjective. The apparatus created the one single eyepoint. Only one single person at a time could look through the hole, but the human persons looking through the hole were exchangeable. For each person looking through it, the eyepoint remained one and the same. This reveals the decidedly not personal, not subjective, but transcendental eyepoint to be the successor of the one single all-seeing eye of God.

Each human individual could potentially look through the hole, that is, adopt this objective eyepoint for himself. Whoever does so, does it in isolation, as a single individual, which corresponds directly to the absolute loneliness of God's all-seeing eye in the no-space beyond and outside the world. Brunelleschi's experiment reveals to us the enormous emphasis on the individuality of this seeing. Precisely the seeing of the objective sciences is fundamentally the seeing of individuals,[70] each separately in his or her singularity. There is no room here any more for any *sensus communis*, for *quod semper, quod ubique, quod ab omnibus creditur*. This communality of experience is replaced by *intersubjectivity*, by all the separate single individual's seeing the same thing through this hole in its eachness. Intersubjectivity means *each subject*, each I, completely alone for itself, but at the same time *all alike*. External sameness, because the viewpoint for all is the single the world-external absolute position. It is not the sameness of the "We" of communal seeing.

Now I come to the dialectic mentioned. Looking through a tiny hole prevents natural seeing, which is the seeing with two eyes and changing eyepoints and informed by the *sensus communis*, by collective knowledge. The absolute fixation of the eyepoint in turn means that the rays of the viewer's gaze go out in a cone-like shape to what is to be seen (in Brunelleschi's experiment: out to what the mirror shows of the painted Baptistery). After all, early-modern seeing was not passive beholding, but the human spirit's productive, mathematically-constructing seeing. But this cone-like shape of the arrow-like rays of the viewer's gaze going out to the mirror is at the same time also the opposite, namely, the cone of light coming arrow-like from the objects seen in the mirror to this one single eyepoint. As I pointed out, all rays of light coming from seen reality are gathered together and converge at this eyepoint (just as parallel lines in paintings converge at their respective vanishing points). What is to be *seen* acts in this sense like a huge spotlight aiming at and "hitting" the eyepoint. All reality to be seen or experienced seems to "focus" on the viewing subject. In this scheme everything in the world becomes concentrated in one single point. This point has now become the real (and the one and only) center of the world. Seen reality is *logically* no longer infinitely spread out before the viewer, with each thing having

70 And the one-eyed-ness of this kind of seeing.

its center, dignity, and self in itself and taking up the room that its own inner needs demand. The eyepoint—and this means the human mind that is behind it—becomes instead, so to speak, the vanishing point of reality; it "swallows" into itself, as if into a black hole, what is to be seen.

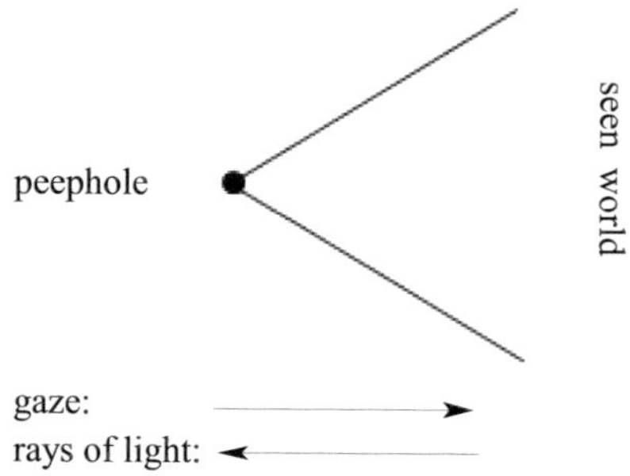

At this point in our discussion I am only interested in the dynamic and psychological impact that this concentration has upon the human subject. This assembly of the rays of light all directly *heading for* this single point give the individual subject logically a singular importance. All the energy of reality becomes *psychologically* concentrated with full force in the seeing and thinking of the individual viewer as person.

If we take fully into account the dynamic force of the transference of the weight of reality from things in their eachness to the one eyepoint gazing at the world, we can assume that inherent in the logic of the early-modern general principle of seeing there is a powerful tendency for this principle (i.e., for the logic of 'subject') to go beyond the *objective* eyepoint or the general early-modern mode of being-in-the-world and take hold of the real viewer as human person himself and reform the definition or logical constitution of "person" in terms of "subject" and center-point. The new mode of being-in-the-world had ultimately also to come home to man himself. The more the transcendent God as the "vanishing point" became de-emphasized and the *divine* spirit vanished, and, along with the growing emphasis on the human productive, the more the constructive side the eyepoint gained in importance over against the vanishing point, the more the *concept* of individual man could itself adopt the form of "subject", of the "psychological

I". In early-modern art "the eyepoint" rightly belonged to the painting, *not* the painter. But now it inevitably had to become individualized and go over from the *logical generality* of art (painting) and the science of the world to the self-experience and self-understanding of really existing man.

Even more striking than the two features suggesting the development from general principle of seeing to the redefinition of man himself as individual in terms of this principle is a third observation or argument based simply on the concept of "I" itself. The new early-modern I or subject *as general principle* concerned only consciousness-as-such. So far in our description it hovered *above* real people, having its place in an ideal sphere and on the purely intellectual, conceptual level, the level of reflection and *generality*. It was one single "position" for everyone, just like in Brunelleschi's experiment theoretically *all* individuals could, one at a time, have looked through the one single peephole in his painting. But such a singleness of one I that all individuals have in common contradicts the very concept of I, which is the demonstrative pointing to each speaker in his eachness, in his individuality. As long as I is something abstractly universal, a "common" much like the village green of old, I or subject still has the form of "it" and is not the first person demonstrative. For this reason, the early-modern subject had to come home to itself, that is, to the "linguistic I" as existing concept in the plural, as embodied in individuals in their multiplicity and eachness. The I had to come down from the heights and purity of the abstract generality of "logical principle" and *enter the realm of existence*, of actually lived life and *personal* life, the realm of the *psychic* I, where it would inevitably also get entangled with all the concrete diverse human feelings, desires, and behaviors. It was not enough for man to "apply" this principle. He had to *become* it, *be* it. The individual had to make it its own.

Whereas the linguistic I used to prevail innocently and unconsciously, it now had to become actively conscious and explicit—I "to the power of two", applied to *itself*, and thus the individual's own identity.

2. The actual historical appearance of man's *redefinition in terms of* the psychological "I"

There are a number of "symptoms" of this change that illustrate what the general principle of the early-modern subject's having come home to itself amounts to. I will describe a few of them briefly. The first example refers to art and poetry. In them the idea emerged at the end of the early-modern period that the artist was a "genius" (and *had to* be a "genius" in order to be a true artist). Formerly one might have said about certain artists that they *have* genius, just as we say that someone *has* wit, esprit, intelligence. But now a great artist *is* a genius. This change came to the fore especially during the late 18th century in the Storm and Stress period and continued in the Romantic period.

What does this change show? The former diction ("he has genius") betrays that speaking about the artist is, although on a higher level, really much like the little child's referring to himself by his name rather than saying "I". In "He has genius" man is apperceived in terms of third-person language. Man is viewed as an entity, a substance that in addition to its existence also has the quality of genius as its attribute. This description is no different from that of a dead thing, for example, a stone: "this stone has great hardness". By saying, "he *is* a genius", however, he is no longer first of all a substance, an existing entity, a human *being* that in addition to its existence has also as one of its properties the quality of "genius". The *person* is no longer comparable to a clothes rack ("substance") on which numerous items of wearing apparel ("attributes") are hanging. There is no longer the duality which is inherent in the idea of a "thing" *plus* its many properties as its attributes. Instead the artist *exists* as "genius". He has all of a sudden been comprehended from within himself, so to speak appreciated as an "I". What he used to "have" and what used to be the attribute of an entity, him as a (human) *being*, has come home to the very definition as his own inner reality. He *is* spirit, *mens*. The spirit, genius, is what exists, is the true existent reality, *not* an entity or being that happens to have spirit. The artist is now truly *subject*, a full-fledged I (not merely the first immediacy of I).

This is only one small "symptom" of a fundamental change, although an exemplary one. There are many other "symptoms." Very interesting in this regard is the reversal in the political meaning of the word "subject" itself. Formerly it used to mean the king's or ruler's subject, *Untertan*. The king used to be the sovereign. Ever since Enlightenment thought and above all the French Revolution, the human individual himself had also in a political sense become "subject", that is to say, a priori *free*, autonomous, self-determined, self-responsible, while the predicate "sovereign" had been removed from the king and was now assigned to the people as a whole. Also during the 18th century, the Enlightenment developed the ideas of the Dignity of Man and Human Rights, which apply a priori and unconditionally to every individual.

Psychologically more important and revealing as a "symptom" exemplifying the character of the new I is another phenomenon in the history of the soul. It comes best out in the philosophy of Immanuel Kant. Kant developed in ethics and in theoretical philosophy the idea of the absolute autonomy and self-determination of man. He demanded of the individual in his behavior as well as his thinking not to be heteronomously guided by inherited and thus always already *given* religious dogmas and traditional social customs or convictions, nor by the dictates of people and institutions as authorities (parents, rulers, the government), but rather exclusively by general principles and rational reasons *directly* accessible to him through his own intellect as faculty of judgment, that is, by the insight into what is right and reasonable. Kant thus spoke of man's necessity to emerge "from his self-incurred immaturity (*Unmündigkeit*)" and to make use of his own power of thought on his own responsibility. Autonomy also implied the individual's self-mastery, being in control of *his own* desires, impulses, and drives, inasmuch as being determined by these internal forces would be just as heteronomous as being determined by outside influences. Authority was not at all altogether abolished, but moved from outside to inside, to the person's self-relation, that is, to the I. The I had, Janus-like, to have a critical distance to both the inner and the outer sphere.

What Kant referred to as self-incurred immaturity was precisely the psychological situation of what I had called the linguistic I, the situation of people who all were correctly able to say "I", but were psychologically not explicitly what "I" actually claims, promises, and demands. They lived *psychologically*[71] as particles or integral parts in society, in family, tribe, as well as group spirit. The whole came first, *it* possessed priority. This also means that the whole was ultimately the determining factor. For the psychological understanding of the linguistic I it is essential to realize that what is meant here by the dominance and priority of the whole is not oppression of actually free citizens like in modern or ancient dictatorships, but a logical constitution of the I according to which this I *itself* feels as a subordinate particle of the whole and decidedly secondary over against the whole—and ipso facto does not really feel as I, but as an "it". The real I has to be self, self-determinded, guided only by the principles of its *own* reason, and thus (logically, of course not necessarily empirically) free and primary, having its center and logical origin *as* self *in* itself and *not* in the communal whole. The I is *a priori* self-relation; to be this is, as it were, its *raison d'état*, whereas the relation to others as well as to the community or group is secondary like foreign affairs in the politics of a nation. *Emancipation* from social group, from natural instinct or powerful inner feeling, and from body is a precondition of being autonomous I.

The full-fledged I is emancipated, free, its own origin, and a center. But this is to be taken only in a logical sense and is not necessarily also true in an empirical or positive-factual sense. This fact of the possible divergence between logical constitution and empirical situation indicates that I is not a natural entity, a fact, something given, but something psychological, the result of the soul's having emancipated itself from the *unio naturalis* with the community as well as with its own natural impulses or powerful inner emotions and fantasies, its natural base[72]. It is the result of its *establishing* itself as self. It comes about through a logical

71 "Psychologically" needs to be emphasized and contrasted with "empirically", "socially". Socially we always need to be well-adapted and this also means integrated into the group or society we belong to. But the question for us today is whether one is *psychologically* fully adapted to one's social environment *as* a self-determined I, or merely *as* a linguistic I that *in its very definition* IS first of all a member of the whole (the group, society) and only secondarily also an individual.

72 What I mean by this natural base is what Jung might have called the individual's rootedness in "the collective unconscious".

act on the part of the soul. Because of the dissolution of the *unio naturalis* and the emancipation from man's unconscious natural base, Jung could identify the I with modern man as such, with civilian man, or with the ego-personality: "the ego—that is, the empirical man" (e.g., *MDR* p. 346), "the I, i.e., the empirical, ordinary, present [*bisherige*] man" (*CW* § 233, transl. corrected) or, the other way around, "man—that is, his ego" (*ibid.* p. 337), where "ego" should in each case be replaced by "I" as in Jung's German diction.

In literature, also starting in the late 18th century, the type of novel called *Bildungsroman* concentrated on the character development and inner formation of a young individual, his growth into true maturity, into a well-rounded personality, a self-contained organic whole, indeed into a world unto himself. The individual had become a self that has logically everything it needs within itself. Mind you, we are here not speaking about *having* a self, but *being* self. The result of the development described in the novel is a firm personality, well-grounded in itself, resting within itself, and responsible for itself. What needs to be added is that "self-contained organic whole" and "self" may furthermore even involve a certain aesthetic quality of personality, that is, the ideal of character formation as forming one's personality as if into a work of art, so that everything in oneself is permeated and animated by spirit and one and the same spirit. The ideal is the inner *freedom* of the soul or mind [*Gemüt*] in the living play of all its faculties.[73] The thus developed personality is in life at large what the artist as genius is in a specialized sphere.

The individual's having become a world unto himself makes it clear that now the "world-external" absolute viewpoint is applied to man himself. Only from a logically external, superior standpoint can "I" perceive itself as a world unto itself, as a self-contained organic whole. This comprehending itself as a world contrasts sharply with the logic of the linguistic I, which is defined, and understands and feels itself, first of all as a *child* of parents,

73 This idea was forcefully expressed by Friedrich Schiller. We can remember in this context also his statements quoted by Jung: "For, to declare it once and for all, man plays only when he is in the full sense of the word a man, and he is only wholly man when he is playing" and "Man shall only *play* with Beauty, and only with *Beauty* shall he play" (*CW* 6 § 171).

Creature of God, *member* of the community, tribe, or social group, in other words, as fundamentally derivative. For it the whole (as well as the individual's true self) was precisely the larger units (family, the created cosmos, the social group). Just as the ultimate authority was transferred from external authority (heteronomy) to inner authority (autonomy), so also the qualities of true wholeness and self were taken away from the larger encompassing units and inwardized into the individual.

The difference becomes obvious when we compare the *Bildungsroman* with the earlier Picaresque novel (mainly later 16th and 17th centuries). As allegedly autobiographical narrator, its hero, the *pícaro*, is usually an I-saying person, but precisely not a well-rounded, uniform personality, but merely a type, an abstract figure, who is more driven about than himself moving through the series of many different adventures in the world that he becomes exposed to. He does not undergo any character formation whatsoever through the events and situations he becomes *subjected* to (which is why we could hardly speak of these events and experiences as his *experiences*). Although practically shrewd and tricky and in this sense resourceful, the *pícaro* is *psychologically* more object of circumstances than true subject. There is no sense of self. The actual subjects in this type of novel seem to be the conditions of (usually corrupt) society and fate. If we leave many other characteristics of the *pícaro* aside and concentrate only on the aspect of personality and character, we can see in him an exaggerated caricature of the logic of the linguistic, merely implicit I.

By contrast, the hero of the *Bildungsroman* experiences the world in the fullest sense of the word. He is inwardly touched by his experiences, learns from them something about himself and has to give his personal answer to them, mainly in his inner judgement but in addition perhaps also in his behavior, rather than merely muddling through and trying to survive as in the case of the *pícaro*.

With all the features described in this section we see how "the psychological I" (the general principle of "subject" that belonged to consciousness-as-such and had its logical place in the ideal sphere) had come down from the heights of abstract generality to the reality of the concrete individual as the linguistic I and transformed the latter into the full-fledged psychic I. The psychological I has become embodied in man as empirical individual, as psychic I. Already the linguistic I is, as I insisted, the existing concept. But the psychic I as linguistic I had still been dormant, merely been an empty claim or promise of I, merely a shell. Now it has awakened, come home to itself. With what we have seen in the present section, the existing concept of I has become fulfilled. Fulfilled in two senses: (1) it now has a real content (self-determination, self-discipline, rootedness in itself, etc.) and (2) the claim or promise inherent in the meaning of the word "I" has become realized. From early childhood on, people found and find themselves as linguistic I without knowing what brought it about. It (*it*, third person!) had of its own accord (*sua sponte*) happened to them. But the fulfilled psychic I, i.e., the linguistic I informed by the psychological I, is *active*, *explicit*, and *conscious* self-relation, self-reflection, self-determination, self-responsibility, self-reliance, autonomous deliberate decision-making, and self-development. It is the general logical constitution of modern Western "empirical man", of "civilian man" as so-called "ego-personality" (*Ichpersönlichkeit*).

E. The subject's own self-objectification and the emergence of "the ego"

With what I described in the foregoing discussion, the soul's historical project of the development of the "I" has been completed. What remains to be seen now is the further fate of this I.

The fulfilled psychic I as *Ichpersönlichkeit* was essentially subject and self, or to be more exact, the unity or oneness of subject and self. Inasmuch as "subject" had self-character, its relation to itself and to the world was uroboric self-relation, that is to say, the relation was not that of a subject to an object as absolute other, but a relation of decidedly *speculative* character; the I or subject was permeated and informed by spirit (*mens*, *Geist*) and as such in itself also the extension of the finite into infinity in the same way as we could see it directly portrayed in Renaissance paintings with linear perspective. The real world with its finite character opened seamlessly up into infinity. The medieval hierarchical relation and strict separation of the finite and infinity had thereby been overcome through the early-modern period's general move from substance to spirit as the dominant mode or nature of human world-relation. It is spirit that made possible the uroboric, speculative unity of the finite and infinity, as also of subject and object, I and world, and this unity is also the inner character of that "personality" that arose at the end of the early-modern period.

But a rupture, a revolutionary change, took place with the end of this period, with the end of the age of classical Western metaphysics, and with the entrance into modernity heralded by the Industrial Revolution. Heaven and Earth collapsed into one. It is like clapping a book shut, which thereafter can no longer be read, can no longer be the presence of the infinity of mind, meaning, spirit, but only a three-dimensional thing, a physical object in space. The fundamental metaphysical difference between the finite and Infinity, the sublunar world and Heaven as the sphere of the divine, was abolished altogether so that the universe, the All, became leveled into one uniform sphere of positivity. "The Earth"—empirical reality in the sense of positive facticity—now extended over and encompassed also what once upon a time had been the wholly other starry heaven, the realm of the eternal Gods. As Jung said, "the blank barrenness of the world reaches to the very stars", and "Heaven has become for us the cosmic space of the physicists, and the divine empyrean a fair memory of things that once were" (*CW* 9i §§ 29, 50). Transcendence became a meaningless word. Not only the dimension of verticality, the whole vertical metaphysical difference that prevailed during Antiquity and the Middle Ages, but also the early-modern inwardized dynamic continuity of the finite into the depth of Infinity had to make way for that absolutely congealed and condensed character of everything that exists that we call "fact".

Along with the closure of the difference and the vanishing of God, Infinity, and the beyond, Spirit (*Geist*) as such also disappeared as the medium and inner form of man's world-relation. The speculative or uroboric unity became impossible (and the word "speculation" even lost its proper hallowed meaning, degenerating into now meaning "wild fantasizing about things beyond possible human experience" or "engaging in risky financial transactions"). Above I mentioned that early-modern (*essential*) seeing was fundamentally one-eye seeing, the second eye having been sacrificed. With the entrance into the stance of modernity the early-modern one-eye seeing had become literalized, applied to itself. The moment that Infinity, transcendence, the metaphysical difference between Heaven and Earth have become eliminated, the loss of the second eye makes speculative, uroboric, or Mercurial seeing altogether impossible. One-eye seeing *under the conditions of modernity* is inevitably direct, immediate, linear seeing[74] and monomaniacally leads to the one-sided translation of everything, everything qualitative, into exclusively quantitative terms.

Becoming immersed into this new logic of being-in-the-world meant consequently for the "personality" that its previous uroboric unity necessarily fell apart. It ceased being a self; it as subject and I all of a sudden stood radically vis-à-vis itself and had to apperceive itself as object, as entity, as positive fact without depth. What used to be its "depth" degenerated into the so-called "the unconscious".[75] (Having just now spoken of degeneration and

---

74 This was fundamentally different during the early-modern period. Here the one-eye seeing precisely *made possible* the awareness of the dialectical unity of the finite and Infinity, in contrast to the absolute hiatus prevailing between the sublunar world and the realm of the eternal gods or God during the earlier periods. It is the abolishment of the metaphysical difference that pulls the rug out from under speculative thinking.

75 Jung, as we all know, made the desperate but futile attempt to counter-factually give precisely to the positivistic concept of the modern individual's "unconscious" the meaning of the lost true depth and Infinity, *inflating* "the unconscious". Despite his clear awareness that nowadays "the blank barrenness of the world reaches to the very stars" and that the former Heaven has become the by definition meaningless universe of the physicist, in other words, that "Earth" conquered and *assimilated* "Heaven" to *itself*, he nevertheless tried to make us believe, in denial of the real phenomenology of the soul seen by himself, that what happened was only that the stars, Heaven, that spirit "has descended from its fiery heights" and has therefore become "heavy" and turned "to water" (*CW* 9i § 32), the "living water" of the unconscious (*ibid.* § 50). Spirit *as spirit* did by no means disappear. The opposites did by no means collapse into one, eliminating the difference between them altogether. No, for Jung it was just a "phase change" of one and the same spirit and a change of location of the stars. The living water of the unconscious is itself still authentic *spirit*, only that it is now "*spirit* become nature" (*ibid.*, transl. modif., my italics), become heavy, become water. And because it is still true spirit, Jung can insinuate "that the treasure lies in the depths of the water" (the unconscious).

before of disappearance and loss, I need to dispel the possible misunderstanding of interpreting this negative development as regression. Rather, as reductive and impoverishing as it semantically indeed is, syntactically it is nevertheless a historical *forward* move on (or pushing off from) the basis of the high, previously achieved level of the personality as subject and self.)

The loss of the uroboric, speculative spirit has two complementary implications. On the one hand, it means the absolute loss of the metaphysical difference in favor of a logic of universal uniformity of the world and the absolute inner closedness of everything as positive fact. On the other hand, it brings at the same time the logic of the unbridgeable difference, of absolute otherness between subject and object and between mind or soul and reality. This means that the difference did not disappear altogether. Rather, it was, as we could almost say, itself "positivized" or literalized, having been transferred from the verticality of metaphysics to empirical, civilian man's (or the human animal's) horizontal world-relation. The result of this loss with its double consequence led to that logical form or cultural constitution of consciousness that I call "the ego", in contradistinction to the former full-fledged psychic I.

As an aside I mention that the "ego" as a cultural form of consciousness at large needs not only to be distinguished from the "psychic I", but also from the "ego" as a *complex*[76] or *dominant* of consciousness in the *personal* psychology of individuals. People can be, and often are, in the grip of this "ego". It is characterized by one-sided self-centeredness and it is a sign of childishness, immaturity, and lack of adaptation. Its first manifestation in a person's life is therefore in childhood, e.g., in the temper tantrums of little children when their will is crossed. But it is also common in adults, basically in all emotional outbursts, such as the ones that frequently occur between spouses. Such outbursts show that their training in childhood or their self-education has been deficient so that they lose their self-control and thus succumb to such boorish behavior. As Jung rightly stated, "And you always have emotions where you are not adapted. If you are adapted you need no emotion; an emotion is only an instinctual

76 Here the notion of "the ego complex" has its legitimate place, whereas I had to reject it ("*der Ichkomplex*") at the very beginning of this paper when it was supposed to refer either to the psychological or the psychic I.

explosion which denotes that you have not been up to your task. When you don't know how to deal with a situation or with people, you get emotional. Since you were not adapted, you had a wrong idea of the situation ... ... to be emotional is already on the way to a pathological condition."[77] As "instinctual explosion" the ego in the sense of a *complex* has its roots in the human animal and not in the soul and *its* history. It is, so to speak, pure "biology" and therefore *not really a topic for psychology*.

Nevertheless it is to be surmised that the lack of adaptation and the possibility of the sudden loss of self-control have a psychological and cultural-historical aspect, too. For this ego seems to make itself felt especially in modernity in the Western world, in fact mainly during the last few decades (let's say since the 1960s). In former times and in other cultures, in archaic or primitive societies, in antiquity, in the Middle Ages, during the early-modern period, in the Islamic world and the Far East, people were generally much more adapted, civilized, and possessed much more self-control. From childhood onwards they grew into an intact system of traditional social mores and clear-cut social roles that held and constrained them; personal dignity and "one's not losing face" were far too precious for the individual to let himself or herself lose self-control; people were basically sober, down to earth and realistic about life to become subject to personal fancies, illusionary demands, and wishful thinking; the dominant motivating powers were to a higher degree than in modernity collective (traditional cultural values and religious ideas) rather than subjective. Adaptation was normal. In modernity, above all medial modernity, the individual has become emancipated from a major part of collective restraint. Individualistic modern man has lost much of any former civilized (and civilizing) polish. The sense of personal dignity has pretty much disappeared. Authority is scorned. Children grow up in a permissive society. Almost "anything goes". This means that subjectivity is let loose to absolutize one's personal feelings, desires, and ideals, which is at the bottom of the occurrence of "instinctual explosions". As a compensation for the loss in the *culture* (or should we say: for the cultural pathology?), meditation courses are lately being offered to the (biologically) already grown-up *primitive egoic individual* in his private subjectivity to learn what is called "mindfulness" or "*Achtsamkeit*".

---

77 C.G. Jung, *Nietzsche's Zarathustra*. Notes of the seminar given in 1934–1939, edited by James L. Jarrett, vol. 2 (Princeton University Press: 1988), p. 1497 f.

The ego, having become in itself distanceless, inevitably takes itself absolutely literally. Taking itself as subject absolutely literally means that it becomes literally subjectivistic, as individual strictly individualistic, logically isolated, i.e., cut off from its previous internal dialectical connection with the generality. It is essentially abstract. It has become identical with the "absolute viewpoint as such" and exists (for itself) as *the* center of its world. It can no longer recognize itself in the other. The ego is the now "divorced" "I as subject", cut off and isolated from its uroboric, spirit-permeated wholeness as self and from the infinity of its self-relation. Subjectivity is now the empty insistence on itself, the empty and endless saying: "I, I, I". As such the ego becomes concretely manifest in an attitude of self-interest, egocentricity, and self-importance.

The fact that the uroboric circle of speculative selfhood is broken has also consequences for the ego's self-relation. The subject having become literalized and reduced to the insistence on the empty, naked "I" has itself as qualitatively determined individual necessarily outside of itself and strictly vis-à-vis itself. It must paradoxically precisely *objectify* itself (and "man" in general). What "myself" now, in this objectified sense, refers to is fundamentally estranged from the ego. The very definition of "subject" is reverted into the opposite. "Subject" in the early modern sense was the result of the distillation of substance or entity into spirit (*mens*). Now it has become object, entity, fact again and is thought of as something or some processes located or happening in the brain. As *ego* in the emphatic sense I am for myself strictly positivized, I logically look at myself as a "dead" object, a thing, namely, as body, organism, brain, hormones, genes. "*Life*" having lost its sense of being the first immediacy of spirit has become reduced to biologically understood so-called life as purely objective biochemical processes and literal behavior. As nothing but a thing, I also appear to myself as nothing but the product of, and fundamentally conditioned by, biology, my social environment, events and circumstances. With "the ego", the old dream of de La Mettrie, namely *L'homme machine*, has come true in a new, more refined, and scientifically certainly more informed and complex way.

These are the two halves of the broken circle: here the literalized abstract subject with its cult of the only-subjective and egocentric, and there self-objectification, self-positivization. The circle has broken apart, but the two broken halves nonetheless remain counterparts and reflections of each other.

The ego's objectifying itself also leads to its one-sidedly positivistic orientation to the world at large. The commonsensical, human-all-too-human, what we call the day-world, becomes for it the exclusive horizon. The ego is committed to strictly pragmatic and utilitarian concerns, to the will for "survival" in the widest possible sense (self-assertion, self-protection, self-enhancing). It is dominated by the wish to have everything under control and to solve problems in a strictly external, purely technical way. Only the literal and positive-factual has validity. Soul, depth, the night-world, are for it by definition excluded.

The breaking apart of the uroboric circle of self meant the loss of the spirit and speculative life as that which used to tie the opposites together to "self". As a compensation for this loss and for man's qua ego having *logically* become a dead thing, as well as for the ensuing estrangement from himself, *subjectivized* emotional *feeling* becomes all-important. As ego, I have to have feelings in order to feel alive. And as ego, I have to have the utterly subjective feeling of love to have a marriage relationship. Feelings, emotions have in this context the purpose of making me feel *myself*. On account of the immediacy and intensity of their physiological effects, they provide me with the momentarily convincing fiction of being alive. But feelings subside, they are valid only for the moment, therefore more and more feelings and feeling-producing things or events are needed: glamour, thrillers, computer games, sensations, excitements, reports of disasters, sport events, new love relationships, music festivals, drugs. Under the rule of the ego, works of arts and the inherited treasures of our cultural past in museums necessarily become subject to cultural consumerism; they exist only for "consumption" by people: they have to be presented as means for one's getting subjectively involved, even excited; the viewers are invited to say or write what they feel and think about them. Forms of presentation that allow for interaction are preferred. There is a shift of emphasis away from the object or work of art to "what *I* feel (when faced with it)" and to my showing *my* presence (just like sprayers want to put their visible mark on buildings or public vehicles). The ego cannot any more just look and appreciate a work of art for what it *is*, because having ceased to be self, it cannot find any more *itself* in it (in what *it* presents) and so it must intrude with its own activity and emotion.

What also gives to the abstract subject, as which "the ego" exists, the *feeling* of being alive (as a substitute for or simulation of the lost spirit) is one's subjective wishes, desires (and their immediate gratification), ideas, fantasies. The more I am ego, the more my desires, my imaginings, what I think, what pops into my mind, become all-important. This is especially so, because the abstract subject that takes its subjectivity literally is fundamentally uprooted. Being radically emancipated, an atomic individual in mass society (the mass of abstract egos), it has lost, in essential regards, its a priori embeddedness in religion, metaphysics, in a living faith in God, in Mother Church, in a social class, political party, or guild. It is cut off from its psychological groundedness in traditional lore, customs, and other collective ideas, in what Jung meant by "the collective unconscious", and so has psychologically nothing to stand on. This makes the ego susceptible to all sorts of movements, fads and crazes, fashionable (political or ideological) ideas, the belief-systems of so-called gurus or obscure sects, etc.

Another reaction to, and ipso facto admission or confirmation of, the loss of *being* self is the above all Jungian idea that one has to experience *the* self, has to *become* self.

This observation takes me to the key example for the fact that the ego means man's having become an object to himself, namely to the rise of psychology in 19th century and the popularity of psychotherapy in the 20th century. All schools of psychotherapy make the person into an object (most obviously, of course, cognitive behavior therapy) and/or force the individual to take himself as an object to be analyzed. Man becomes a problem for himself and as such a topic of prime interest and importance. He has to work on himself, to develop, to individuate. His hidden secrets have to be unearthed and he has to be explained, and learn to understand himself, in terms of his complexes, the traumas he experienced, etc. Of course the substantiated concepts of "the unconscious", of "the psychic apparatus", as well as of "the ego" itself as a complex or agency or as the center of consciousness (I mentioned it at the very beginning) are part of the ego's positivistic "self-relation". Karl Kraus said about psychoanalysis that it is that very illness that it wants to cure. In a deeper sense than one might expect, this is true of all psychotherapy. Psychotherapy is part of the problem, not just the solution.[78] It is the preferred ritual of the cultivation of ego.

F. Concluding comment. The objective *obsolescence* of the I and its *subjective* indispensability

The ego was in the history of the soul's logical life the dominant logical form of consciousness during the 19th century and most of the 20th century, the age of Industrial Modernity. But this domination in the soul's general logic of that time does not mean that the ego had totally replaced the foregoing psychological I continuously and that it was also the form of the psychic I of all real individuals in the West living then. As a soul truth of a particular era, it ruled in the depth over Western culture in general, but not exclusively and throughout. The cultural as well as personal ideal that individuals should have a firm character and be autonomous personalities was still present and consciously often in effect, although logically already superseded by the ego. Both forms, the ego and the fulfilled psychic I, coexisted, each in individuals or in society at large coming to the fore partly at different times or in different situations and partly to differing degrees in different persons.

Meanwhile, at least beginning with the last three decades of the 20th century, the soul has left Industrial Modernity behind and openly entered Modernity's second phase, Medial Modernity, that is, the phase of modernity's at long last coming home to itself, and with this phase the logical form of I has become altogether obsolete.

This present age is the time of the Web, the essentially decen-

78 Which, however, does not mean that it is unnecessary.

tralized Internet. People are networked in multiple ways, via mobile phones, different social media. Teamwork is hailed. In the sciences interdisciplinary studies and cooperation between different scientific institutes or between universities and companies are preferred. We orient ourselves in the world via GPS. Car-sharing becomes possible, which is logically a small attack on the previously sacred notion of "my own car" as symbol of individuality and personal independence, indeed ultimately, on the privacy of property. In philosophy the ideas of "author" and "center" have become discredited. Marriage as a commitment for life has become challenged as people go through different partnerships during different phases of their life and reinvent themselves and experiment with their identities. One's traditional clear-cut self-definition as *either* male *or* female as well as the unambiguous definition of these terms themselves has been decomposed. Memory is outsourced to databanks; cloud computing more and more takes the place of traditional stand-alone PCs. Vinyl records, CDs, and DVDs, i.e., existing things as permanent sound or video carriers, are more and more replaced by live streaming—a move from entity or substance to sheer movement as such. Intelligence is becoming outsourced to the self-teaching algorithms of Artificial Intelligence, people's personal data and the information contained in their use of the Internet and their cell phones are digitally and automatically "tracked" and accumulated by companies on a planetary scale, behind people's back (even if they once consciously had to agree to this practice). The loss of shame, so essential to the traditional sense of the autonomous personality as self, and the large-scale renunciation of "privacy", the self-display and self-marketing in the social media, in Reality TV, and in advertizing, reveal that the notion and value of "self" and individual(ity) have disappeared culturally (in the logic of the age, of course not in each individual), even if the words still exist and may even still be popular (just think of "selfies": a clear *objective* mockery of "self").

A permanent I has no place in the logic of this modern world. The soul is already somewhere else. The notion "I" as "self-contained organic whole" is simply incompatible with "Cloud", "Web", "networking" and outsourced psychic functions. I, self, and individual are slowly being dissolved and dispersed and can be no more than *sublated moments* in the network world. (Again, this is a statement about the present status in the soul's logical life, not about empirical reality and the reality of all individuals.)

Particularly revealing and pertinent for the fate of the I is the following phenomenon. It may be considered as a powerful "symptom" in the sense given above. In former times, portraits were painted or drawn, and the expectation was that not merely the looks of the person would be shown, but that also his character, his personality, his self—his true identity and inner essence—would be captured in the portrait. This is also why those who sat for their portrait carefully chose which clothes to wear, in which pose and position they would be painted and which objects or attributes should be included so as to reflect their dignity, rank, achievements, pious attitude or the like. During the Baroque age, for example, many persons had themselves painted with their hand on a skull, or a skull lying in front of them, to indicate their awareness of the ultimate vanity of existence in this world and their hope for the coming true life in the beyond. Now, in the age of snapshots and smartphone selfies, there is no thought of trying to capture the true character of a person. On the contrary, the emphasis is precisely on the absolutely contingent chance appearance in this one moment. The external positive-factual looks in trivial or casual situations are to be captured, not anything deeper, expressive of a more permanent truth. Indeed, often snapshots are taken that show people precisely with a momentary untypical, funny or awkward facial expression or position. Even more important and more telling than this move in picture shooting away from deeper essence to the accidental is, however, what happens with facial recognition systems. Being based on self-learning algorithms and big data, they decompose the very sense of personal "identity" as inner essence by reducing it to *biometric* "sameness". Another fundamental new phenomenon pointing in the same direction and complementing facial recognition is the construction of artificial "identities" of people through commercial companies and secret services by letting big data algorithms use the pictures in social media, emails, contacts, movement profiles, etc. of individuals for the calculation of correlations between them and thus patterns that allow to predict these individuals' future intentions and actions. Here "identity" is not the inner truth of a personality, but fundamentally composite, put together: calculated on the basis of a mass of intrinsically unrelated external data.

In view of this analysis of the obsolescence of the I, I introduce my thesis, advanced elsewhere,[79] of the necessity for one's personal emancipation from the soul. The general logic of the respective status reached in the soul's history must not go to our heads. No doubt, as a matter of course we must pay tribute to it. And we will do so inevitably, since nobody can escape the logic of his time. *Vocatus atque non vocatus* not only *deus aderit*, but also the present form of the soul truth will prevail. But this inevitability does not mean that we would personally have to identify with it, become completely absorbed by it. On the contrary, it is always necessary for man to distinguish himself from the unconscious images, from the gods, the archetypes, and from the ruling cultural truths and to free himself from their suggestive power.[80] And indeed, in the course of history man has on a collective, cultural level conquered and reserved for himself more and more of a small free-space of private life amidst and underneath the larger sphere of the logic of the soul's life that allows us to become aware that we are "*only* that!" (*MDR* p. 325)—individual creaturely human beings with to a large extent the same needs that people also had in former ages, not only the obvious needs for food, drink, sleep, shelter, safety, etc., but also the psychic need to stand on our own feet, to become and be self-determined, self-reliant, self-responsible persons with a firmness of character, power of judgment, decision-making ability, and a certain well-rounded wholeness.

In this sense I conclude this paper with the assertion, especially important also for the field of practical psychotherapy, that *for the private individual* the time of the fully developed psychic I, of subject and self is not over, even if it can, of course, not be anything more than a sublated moment within the soul's new logic of a fun-

79 *What Is Soul?* New Orleans, LA (Spring Journal Books) 2012, now London and New York (Routledge) 2020, pp. 317 ff.

80 Cf. "The aim of individuation is nothing else than to liberate the self from the false wrappings of the persona on the one hand, and from the suggestive power of unconscious images on the other" (*CW* 7 § 269, transl. modif.).

damentally supra-individual reality, no more than a kind of "sanctuary" of privacy that passes, if I may say so, under the radar of the inexorable soul. ❦

Chapter Three

The Discovery and Production of the Ego. A Chapter from the History of the Western Psyche

The title of this paper may surprise you. Is the ego something that was discovered like America was discovered by Columbus? Is it produced, that is to say, manufactured or *fabricated*, like tissues of lies are manufactured? Let us leave these questions and the puzzling nature of the wording of this title aside for the moment. I hope that in the course of this paper, when after some theoretical preliminary discussion we will turn to Renaissance drawings and paintings to demonstrate the production of the ego, it will become clear what is meant.

At any rate, in this paper we will be concerned with the ego, with a central notion both of psychology and practical psychotherapy. To realize how central it is we just have to remember how often we speak of the ego complex, of ego consciousness, ego development, of ego strength and weakness. Daily we make use of these very concrete concepts, and this may lead to the idea that we also know what we are talking about. But as always when one wants to do psychology, psychology *with* soul, so here, too, it will not do to present a few clear-cut definitions and descriptions about the ego, as if the psyche could be studied much the same way as we learn what a car is and how it functions. We cannot dogmatically set up a theory of the ego and apply it to whatever psychic material, but start out from this material and delve into the matter in order to slowly derive our theoretical notions from it. As all discussion of the soul, so also our discussion of the ego will have to be an exercise in stretching the mind.

In the ego we approach a dark and most difficult topic, one that makes high demands on our capacity to comprehend. With the ego we touch on some of the deepest mysteries of the soul itself. The ego is not a ready-made object in the psyche. It goes far beyond being a mere component in the psyche. In one way or another, what we call soul involves self-awareness, self-relation, reflection and self-reflection, and this means *subjectivity*, and therefore without some form of ego, or let me rather say, some form of "I", there would not be soul at all, neither the subjective nor the objective psyche. Mythic images, although certainly not ego concoctions, nevertheless presuppose a reflecting, interpreting soul, a soul that is not physical in the sense of biological and causal stimulus-response automatisms, but has gained a distance to the physical, established itself vis-à-vis the world as a subjectivity and that only for this reason is capable of perceiving the world and life in images, images of its own making. But these fundamental questions will not be our topic today either. I mention them only because it is good to be aware of them as a backdrop to our discussion even when it is dealing with a much more limited, specific question of the psychology of the ego, with one particular phase in the ego's history.

Part I.
On the difference between "the ego" and "the I"

I have been speaking of "the ego," but I also already once used the term "the I," which is not at all a standard English term in psychology. But in their own German texts both Freud and Jung generally did not speak of "das Ego," but of "das Ich." It would have easily been possible in English too to use the ordinary-language term "I" instead of the Latin, and thus more scientific sounding, "ego." But in the English translations of Jung's text the term "the ego" has been chosen and has become the standard term. In the *General Index* to the *CW* there is only one single reference to the word "I," and that refers to sentences that are merely quoted by Jung from Ramakrishna, but the moment that Jung in that passage makes his comments on what Ramakrishna says, his own term "Ich" is by the English translator again rendered by "the ego."

Two discourses

This near-exclusiveness of the term "the ego" is problematic, but it also holds one advantage for us, because the English language thus offers two distinct terms for our use. By availing ourselves of both terms, we can now easily make a terminological difference between different psychic realities, (a) the modern ego as a particular style of orientation, of an egoic attitude, on the one hand, as well as the ego as a specific clearly defined *construct* or fantasy in modern psychology on the other hand, the ego, e.g., in the sense of the "ego complex," as a part of the psyche in contrast to other components of the psyche, such as the unconscious or the shadow or the anima. Just think of Jung's early book "The Relations Between the Ego and the Unconscious." By contrast, we can (b) reserve *the term "I"* for those cases where we speak of the real sense of I that each of us has, of a person as a whole insofar as this person can make use of the general human capacity to linguistically refer to itself as "I" and to experience itself as such, as a person and subject. The ordinary-language word "I" can signal linguistically that with it we do not want to operate with a technical scientific term, with a construct already appropriated by a particular theory about or conception of the psyche.

In German, where we normally only use "das Ich," this term is ambivalent, equivocal, which is why Jung, when he did not mean it in the narrow technical sense of the ego complex had to qualify the expression by some addition, e.g., he said, "das Ich, d.h. der empirische Mensch" *Erinn.* p. 349 (characteristically *MDR* p. 346 has: "the ego—that is, empirical man—"). What Jung means here by "I" (or according to the English version by "the ego") is the whole person as it understands and experiences itself ordinarily, in the context of everyday life and practical reality. He does not refer to one of the complexes or organs or agencies in the person. "The ego—that is, empirical man—" means the human being as a whole inasmuch as it is not aware of its own other, the soul, in other words, the whole person—however that particular form of whole person that is perceived and perceives itself as a positivity under total disregard of the soul, under complete abstraction from soul. "The ego" thus means a particular *mode of being-in-the-world* (and not at all a component of the psyche). This is the mode of being-in-the-world of modern man, modern man who does not so much *have* an ego, but *is* ego, exists as ego, i.e., *is* this soul-less mode of being-in-the-world (where "soul-less" does not mean the value judgment "soulless," but is a descriptive term pointing to the disappearance of soul from man's priorities). By contrast, premodern man existed to a large extent *as* soul. We can see this, namely that in former ages the care of the soul had top priority, e.g., from Jung's comment about the Australian Aborigines, namely that they "sacrifice to it [the symbolic life] two-thirds of their available time—of their lifetime in which they are conscious" (CW 18 § 649), or we can see it from the fact that in most parts of the world in former times enormous riches were used to be expended for pyramids, graves, temples, cathedrals, and so on, and a large portion of both public and even private life was—*contra naturam*—devoted to cultic or religious services, in other words, to activities that from a strictly practical point of view were useless, but that gave satisfaction to, and were indispensable for, the soul.

We have to be very clear about the fact that the talk about the ego complex and about ego strength, ego development, on the one hand, and the idea of "The ego—that is, empirical man—," on the other hand, belong to two fundamentally different discourses. The second idea occurs only in the later Jung and has not really been followed up by the Jungians, whereas the former notions have their place predominantly (but not exclusively) in the earlier Jung and have become part of the general jargon and thinking of analytical psychology. The difference is crucial. It comes out very clearly if in each discourse we think what soul means. Within the first discourse, the discourse in which the ego is a complex in the sense of a component, the discourse of personalistic psychology, paying attention to your dreams and going into analysis would mean to devote yourself to the soul.

But from the point of view of the second discourse, going into analysis to discover your shadow, observing your dreams and trying to work with them would generally still belong to the *ego* and by no means transgress the sphere of the ego in the direction of soul, because it is done by "empirical man" and exploring oneself, one's inner life and one's hidden motivations, is a very normal thing to be done in modern life. As a compensation for the complications and pressures of modern life, it is fundamentally integrated into the pragmatics of modern life and one of those things "empirical man," i.e., the ego, does. To some extent, to go into analysis and to be interested in Jungian psychology and New Age things may even be fashionable. In the sense of the second discourse, working with dreams and being interested in myths and symbols is unmistakably ego work. The soul that late Jung, Jung when he is psychological and is not trying to be scientific, has in mind when he speaks, e.g., of the ego as empirical man is something very different, very alien, a true other; the soul's demands and concerns lie outside this entire sphere of professional psychotherapy, although Jung did not explicitly say so himself.[81] So we see that the term ego is highly ambivalent or equivocal, all the more so if we keep in mind that I here restricted myself to pointing out merely two different specific discourses to be found in Jung. There are yet other discourses that would complicate matters still further.

The popular notion of the ego

I will begin my particular discussion with the first-mentioned discourse, that is, with the most popular notion of the ego as it occurs in personalistic psychology, the ego in the very narrow and rigid sense, according to which it is a *complex* OF a person's psyche or a kind of *organ* IN the psyche, rather than the psychological constitution of the empirical person as a whole. We get the most concise and precise articulation of this conception of the ego from Jung himself, when he tried to explain to his students the make-up of the whole psyche. He did this in his Winter-Semester 1934-35

81 But compare the following statements by Jung: "It is the smallest part of the psyche, and in particular of the unconscious, that presents itself in the medical consulting room" (*Letters 2*, p. 307, 17 June 1956, to Nelson); "... analytical psychology has burst the fetters which hitherto have tied it to the consulting-room of the doctor. It transcends itself ..." (*CW* 16 § 174, transl. modif.).

Seminar on *Modern Psychology* at the Eidgenössische Technische Hochschule in Zürich, Lecture XVI of March 1st, 1935. In his own context, he is not at all interested in our topic, the *ego*. However, since the ego happens to be mentioned by him in passing, his explanation is important for us here. Jung's own focus is on something else. In previous lectures he had discussed a dream in his own amplifying way. And because a "large number" of his students "are still wondering why it was necessary for me to bring forward so many mythological associations in order to understand this dream," he wants to explain this to his bewildered students. Jung continues, "I have already explained this, but I will try to do so more clearly. We will do this by means of a diagram." His earlier explanation obviously did not get through. So Jung now resorts to a diagram in order to make his explanation *foolproof*. The use of diagrams is comparable to how elementary school teachers use apples, fingers, and pies to teach children basic arithmetical operations. And since these are university lectures, it is understandable that Jung here tries to be *scientific*—and thereby is in danger of compromising psychology, making something logical (and thus irrepresentable) representable to the optically envisioning mind of the ego, i.e., to ordinary empirical man.

According to this diagram (see Fig. 1), the whole psyche is depicted as a number of concentric circles. In other words, it is

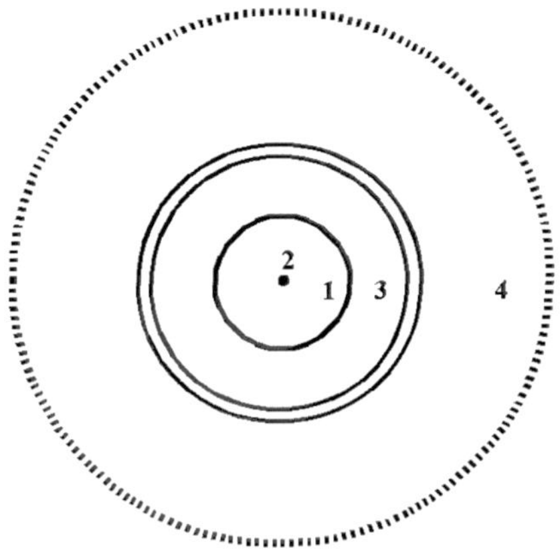

Fig. 1. Diagram of the whole psyche (top view) *according to C.G. Jung*

envisioned as so many regions. As Jung explains in his *Seminar*, "(1) is the smallest circle" and represents "the conscious" (= consciousness). "(3) is the personal unconscious—a dark zone on which consciousness rests like an island in the sea. The contents of the personal unconscious are mainly attainable, we can with great effort remember the things which it contains, but there is a trench set round this, beyond which is: (4) the collective unconscious. I will only represent this by dots, because it is impossible to set boundaries to it. It belongs to humanity in general and also to the animal world." Then Jung continues, "I will also draw the diagram in section in order to show that each circle lies deeper than the last" (see Fig. 2 [and 3]). We see that for Jung the two diagrams show one and the same, represented from different viewpoints. The top view shows a kind of map of the psyche with

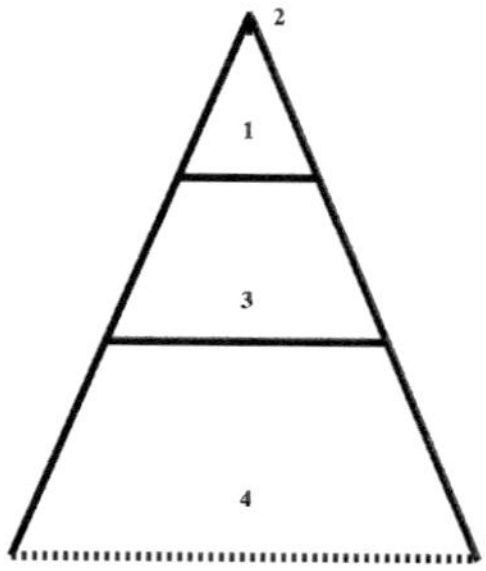

Fig. 2. Diagram of the whole psyche (front view) *according to C.G. Jung*

its different areas or regions, while the front view or cross section shows it as layers, in the case of Jolande Jacobi's depiction (from her *Die Psychologie von C.G. Jung. Eine Einführung in das Gesamtwerk*, Olten (Walter-Verlag) 1971, p. 48) layers of a cone. In connection with the first figure I spoke of a map, which shows us that underlying it is, as it were, a *geographical* fantasy, which also comes out in the metaphorical imagination of consciousness as an island floating in the sea. The cross section, by contrast, gives us the corresponding *geological* stratification. Geology was also present in Freud's thinking, namely when he fantasized that the psyche rests on the "bedrock" of the biological.

Clearly, these are terrible fantasies about the psyche, absolutely misleading. We should immediately forget these diagrams. The only excuse for them might be, in the case of Jung's situation, that Jung wanted to make things foolproof and thus simplistic. But *this* is precisely the mistake. Jung thereby did psychology a disservice. He should not have lowered his standards in order to fraternize with the foolish level of ordinary consciousness, its simple-mindedness. It is the early, pre-alchemy Jung who does not live up to the standard of true psychology. A real psychologist does not address the ego, does not want the ego to understand, and thus fraternize with the ego.

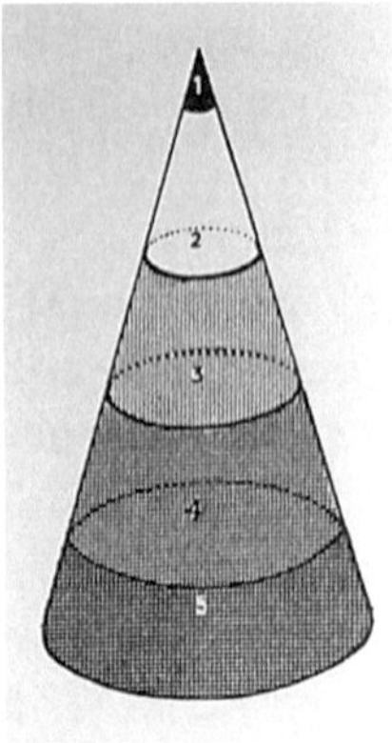

Fig. 3. The same as seen by Jolande Jacobi. Note, in Fig. 3, the different numbering and the addition of a fifth very dark layer for "the part of the collective unconscious that can never be made conscious".

What in particular is wrong with these conceptions? They are naturalistic. They support the naturalism and concretism, indeed positivism, of the everyday mentality. The naturalism consists in or involves several features, all of which are different but related aspects of the same. (1) The psyche is imagined as if it were an object in space. It is extended, a *res extensa*, with a top and a bottom, with width and breadth. (2) This entails that it is conceived in analogy to physical things, treated as if it had somehow thing-like substantiality, as if it were a body. (3) Like physical things, *this* psyche is compartmentalized, it has parts, namely clear-cut, neatly demarcated regions or layers, similar to geographical areas and geological strata or to how the human or animal body has clearly distinguishable layers of different tissue. (4) The regular-geometric nature of the model used in the diagrams—concentric circles, triangle, cone—suggests a thinking in terms of a rigid and very simple structure. The psyche as a whole is well-circumscribed, has clear, definite *linear* borders; it has an outside, is surrounded by something external. (5)

This imagined simple structure of three separate layers or regions is implicitly viewed as timeless, just as biologically the anatomy and physiology of the human body has been and will be the same from prehistoric times to the present and into the future. (6) The psyche is ontologized, that is to say, the impression is created as if it were an existing entity, something ontic, like a piece of nature.

One could here of course object that all these naturalistic, positivistic conceptions are meant only metaphorically, merely as an "as if." They are precisely not to be taken literally. This is true. Jung did of course not suggest that the psyche is indeed a triangle or cone with layers. But *psychologically*, what counts is precisely the *metaphors* that in fact inform and dominate our thinking and imagining in the back of our minds. The metaphors, the style of our thinking, betray how we actually think. Psychologically the difference that we may make between the metaphoric and the literal, the difference between our merely metaphorically picturing something in a naturalistic way and our by no means actually believing that it indeed *is* this way is only an intellectual, rationalistic trifle. The assurance that we do not mean literally that the psyche is a cone with so many layers is psychologically as good as when we have said something to somebody that hurt his feelings and immediately afterwards apologize by stating, "But I did not mean it this way!" Even if this excuse may be subjectively true, objectively what counts is what the actual meaning of the unkind words that we said is, not what the ego means or how they are *supposed to be* understood. Our declared subjective intentions are psychologically relatively unimportant. Merely ego-stuff. The psychologically real dominants are precisely the metaphors and "as if's" that we use.

So we can in good conscience forget the objection that the positivistic fantasies are merely metaphors and take those fantasies seriously, regardless of whether they are intended as metaphors or literally.

Beware of the physical in the material

The ego in Jung's diagrams partakes of this naturalism. It is conceived as the point in the center (1), as the in-itself extensionless center-point within the extended "smallest circle," consciousness. It is like the axis of a wheel. Even if it is imagined as extensionless, it is nevertheless a *real* part of the existing psyche, the psyche imagined as an entity. But we have to ask: does the ego exist? Does the soul exist? Do we *have* an ego, a soul? Is there, as Erich Neumann thinks, an Ego-Self axis? It is true, we do have a heart, a stomach, a liver, a brain. You can show these organs through X-Rays and they can be cut out and demonstrated to exist. But an ego, a soul?

Already Hillman insisted that the soul is not an entity. He thought that it is much rather a perspective. And alchemy warned us: beware of the physical in the material, which we might translate today by "beware of the positivism which is normally the starting-point of how we imagine whatever matter at hand" or "do not imagine psyche and psychic phenomena as positive facts." Alchemy also warned us: Do not begin any operation before everything has become water, i.e., become liquefied, fluid. This warning is directed against any substantiating in our thinking and against a simplistic, primitive thinking. If we heed the advice of alchemy, our thinking has to become fluid, more sophisticated, more subtle and sublimated than the crude mechanistic thinking in terms of entities, parts, layers, regions, agencies. There *is* no such thing as an ego or a soul. Jung's diagrams amount to a fundamental reduction of the *nature* of the psychic, a great simplification. It is obviously wrong, a category mistake, to think of ego as well as of psyche or soul in ontological terms. With Aristotle we could speak of a *metábasis eis állo génos*, but it would be more correct to speak of a *katábasis eis állo génos*, a taking recourse to a more primitive set of categories and mental instruments. Our thinking needs to become more complex in order to do justice to soul and ego. Rather than entities, natural objects, soul and ego are ideas in the mind, thoughts, concepts, theoretical fantasies, fictions, at best *interpretations* of certain demonstratable facts, but in no way pieces of nature, as if man could be seen as a package consisting of two parts, body plus soul, and as if body and soul were two entities on the same level, although of course each of a different nature, the one visible, the other not. With the object-thinking underlying

Jung's two diagrams, he commits a metaphysical hypostasis. As concepts, fantasies, interpretations, both soul and ego are logical *negativities*, not positive facts of nature. This understanding fits well to the alchemy-inspired idea that our whole thinking in psychology has to be *contra-naturam* thinking.

By speaking of negativities, I do of course not suggest that ego and soul are nothing at all, and that we should therefore dismiss these ideas. The importance, and in this sense also the reality, of both of them is not disputed. What is disputed is the style of conceiving them and of speaking about them. What needs to be categorically rejected is the naturalistic, ontological, positivistic approach that perceives of the ego as an object. I already claimed that ego and soul are ideas, concepts, fantasies. This might lead us to think in terms of the opposite standpoint, according to which they are subjective. But obviously, this is, although it is a move in the right direction, also not sufficient.

It is true, the ego is *contra naturam*, it is not a natural entity, it is a thought, a concept. But it is that particular kind of a concept that produces its own reality. It makes itself objective. We see this already clearly in small children. The moment they can say "I," they have become and are an I. They did not all of a sudden receive from somewhere an "I" the way they are given a doll or a tricycle. They now do not *have*, possess, an I. No, the point is that they *are* I. Their having become able to *think the thought I* instantaneously turned them into real I's. "I" is the *existing* concept. It is a concept, not an entity, and as such a negativity, and yet it is existing. Here we already see one instance of how I is both discovered and fabricated. The child discovers the possibility to speak in the first person singular, and *ipso facto* it fabricates the I, constitutes itself in fact as an I. It is a particular logical, mental *act* of self-constitution. The I is performative. It is not 'something'.

The question arises of course, who is the actor or agent who performs this act. Is it the child? I would say, not really. All the child as a natural, existing entity does is to *discover* this possibility; but the self-constitution of the I's reality is the concept's own work. It is the concept "I" which is the true actor, *it* produces its own reality and existence. It *is* the power of the concept I discovered by the child that allows the child to in fact be an I. If this production of the reality of the I were the child's own achievement, then one would have to assume analogously that merely by saying "cow" or "tree" or "dragon" a child, or any human being for that matter, would also be able to produce a real cow, tree, or dragon.

Younger children refer to themselves in the third person singular, by their name. They cannot use the first person singular, despite the fact that they already hear everybody else say "I" and despite their understanding what is meant when the adults say "I." Why are small children not able to say "I"? Because they are not yet capable of really *thinking* "I." The concept I has not dawned on them yet. But the moment they manage to comprehend the concept "I" they instantaneously have become "I."

The counter-natural thought-status of "I" can be seen from the fact that I has no external referent. The small child who refers to himself or herself by saying "John (or Mary) is hungry" only implicitly refers to *himself* or *herself*, but explicitly refers to an external referent, to John or Mary as an Other, to an empirical object, a natural being. But the real self-reference by means of the thought I does not refer to me as the bodily existing being, to the entity me, but to me as the thought "*myself*," the thought "the *person* me, the person that I am." Person and self[82] are not visible objects. They exist only as thoughts and in thought: as the execution of the logical act as which the thought "I" exists.

The *psychic* I and its varying *psychological* garb

Now I have to come back to my distinction between the ordinary-language word "I" and the technical term "the ego," a distinction which expresses the "psychological difference," and state that *it is part of our HUMAN NATURE that we have the logical, CONTRA NATURAM potential to say "I."* We do not have an I, like we have positive-factual body organs, but the I is also not nothing. It is an idea in the subjective mind. Rather, *by nature* we are capable of referring to ourselves in the first person singular, of actually thinking and comprehending the concept I, of thereby *counter-naturally* performing, sort of *"out of the blue,"* the special

82 "Self" as the reflexive pronoun, not in the sense of the Jungian "Self."

mental, conceptual act of constituting ourselves as I. And for this reason it is also *by nature* that we *are* I, we *are* soul, *are* consciousness, all three of which, however, are in themselves *by no means* natural. Human *nature* is *not* natural. It is *contra naturam*. Or to put it a bit differently: It is human *nature* to be not natural. Inescapably we are I, as long as we stay in fact human. We cannot help it.

In this sense, the I is something psychic, anthropological. However, this I is also something psychological, not only because of its thought and concept rather than entity nature, but also inasmuch as in its particular form it is not fixed, but can be constituted or defined in different ways. In this sense, the I is essentially historical. In the history of the soul there were many different forms of the I. The I can be dressed in different garbs, it can give itself different self-interpretations, self-manifestations, and it always must give itself some interpretation. For example, the form that the I had in the people at the archaic time of myth and ritual was fundamentally different from that of the time of classical Greece, which in turn was different from that of the Christian Middle Ages and again different from that of the 19th century, and so on, just as there can be different styles of I in an individual's lifetime, the young child's I, the adult's I, the old person's I (to mention only these crude distinctions). Jung's early main work was entitled, "Transformations and symbols of the libido." We could use this phrase in our context and speak of *transformations and symbols of the I* or of metamorphoses of the I's self-manifestations, historical changes of the I's self-interpretations.

Now "the ego," the way this term is used in analytical psychology, is one particular *form* that the I may take at a certain stage of its history, one fantasy according to which the I, or consciousness, may have defined itself. And it is that constitution or form that the I or the soul mostly in the Western world gave itself in modernity, in the 19th and a major part of the 20th centuries, during the time of positivism. As a general form of consciousness it is a mode or style of perceiving, thinking, and experiencing the whole world and anything in the world. That is to say, it is not merely and not so much something *in* us, but much rather the whole world itself if it has been seen and construed by this style.

It is the logical constitution or the syntax of this world.

"The ego" is precisely not individual, but universal, Jung might have said "archetypal." An individual may be dominated by "the ego," but "the ego" is not his.

So we have to distinguish between the I and "the ego." But in addition we have to introduce another distinction concerning the second element, the ego, so that we get a tripartite distinction: (1) the I, (2a) the ego in its first sense, and (2b) the ego in its second sense. For, the ego is (a) the I's true self-interpretation *at a certain stage* of the soul's cultural-historical development, but also (b) the *fixation, codification* of this particular form of the I into a technical term of the theory of depth-psychology, a rigid construct, and the hypostatization of this construct by this theory as a constituent part (complex, agency) of the psychic apparatus.

In the second version of "the ego," a cultural phenomenon is taken at face value and turned into a theory. The mind of the psychologist has become identical with the ego in its first sense and, instead of seeing through it, takes it literally and blindly acts it out, makes a dogma of it, projects it out into empirical individuals so that it becomes reified, hypostatized as the center-point or axis of a person's consciousness. In conventional analytical psychology, "the ego" is taken literally, is believed in as if it were the true and one-and-only nature of the I. It is substantiated. And because the ego is taken by its word, it is as a matter of course reductively stuffed into the positively existing individual, imagined as something that is each person's own property. It seems logical that since the ego refers to *me*, it must be exclusively *my* ego, my most private and personal possession, something in me. But it is false. Thereby something *psychological* and as such universal is reduced to something *psychic*: psychologistic psychology undoes the psychological difference. The difference between the I and the ego disappears. They are merged into one and in this merged form have lost their status of being something universal. Jung's diagrams are examples for this. They are the self-portrayal of the literalization of the modern "the ego"; they show its codification, positivization, and privatization at work, they show what psychological theory you get if "the ego" is believed in.

But the diagrams can also make us aware of the dialectic of the ego. For in them, the ego is its two senses at once, and yet in a contradictory way. What the diagrams explicitly *teach* is that the ego is only the tiny center-point of the smallest circle in each individual and that there is much, much more to the psyche beyond the ego, namely the wide range of the unconscious, especially the collective unconscious. In this sense the *semantics* (the message) of the diagrams show the unconsciously acted-out, projected, and reified ego.

But at the same time, the *syntactical form* of the diagrams themselves and as a whole breathe the spirit of "the ego." The form of the diagrams is the self-display of the ego in its true soulful sense as one of the self-definitions of the I, namely its modern, rigid, positivistic self-interpretation. This whole theoretical way to imagine the psyche as consisting of all these clear-cut components (consciousness, the personal unconscious, the collective unconscious) is an ego fantasy. The fantasy of "the unconscious," of there being such a thing as "the unconscious" and of consciousness being only a small island surrounded above all by the collective unconscious is paradoxically a *product* of "the ego." It is an ego fantasy. It is precisely the fact that this theory unconsciously acts out the ego as the now prevailing self-definition of the I resulting in its setting the ego reductively up as the tiny center-point of each private individual's consciousness. It is this fact which made the invention of "the unconscious" as the universal ocean around the alleged island of consciousness necessary. The invention of the theoretical construct "the unconscious" as a literal region of the psyche is the reflection *within* this theory *of* this theory's own unconsciousness about itself as a self-portrayal of "the ego." Its own unconsciousness consists mainly in its falling for and taking literally its own semantics, its acting the latter out, being incapable of seeing through to the ego as one syntactical form of the I, a form of the whole psyche, namely as the very logic prevailing in its, modern personalistic psychology's, own theorizing.

The soul does not have parts. We cannot split up the soul into consciousness, the personal unconscious, and the collective unconscious. As I showed somewhere else,[83] at times Jung himself re-

83 W.G., "First Shadow, Then Anima," in: *idem*, *Soul-Violence*, Collected English Papers vol. III, New Orleans, LA (Spring Journal Books: 2008), here pp. 84f.

jected this thinking in terms of parts with the unmistakable statement, "This is all nonsense!" In that case he was aware that what we conventionally consider parts of the psyche (the shadow, the anima, the ego, etc.) are *each* the *whole* psyche in a different garb or self-interpretation or syntax.

Let me briefly summarize the main results of our investigation so far.

1. Like everything psychological, the I and the ego are nothing ontological, not positive facts of *nature*, but thoughts, mental acts, performative, *contra naturam*, the counter-natural contradiction of an existing concept.
2. The I semantically sets up the sense of individuality, but logically *is* nothing individual, personal (not "mine"). It is universal. Everybody is I.
3. We need to distinguish between
   (a) **the I** as a *psychic* fact—as the biologically (naturally) given need of human beings to exist as (counter-natural) concept or thought,
   (b) **the ego**,
   and again within the ego between it either as
      (α) the **phenomenal** ego or
      (β) "the ego" as a **technical construct** of psychological theorizing, namely that construct that—as the blindly acted-out and thus semanticized phenomenal ego—substantiates, positivizes, and reifies the ego.
4. The phenomenonal ego exists again in two completely different forms.
   (a) as a *psychological* reality, namely as one particular syntactical and historically real form or garb of the soul or the I, a *style* or *constitution* of consciousness,
   (b) as a primitive *psychic complex* rooted in human nature, in the biology of the human animal (the self-preservation instinct), and thus quite visibly manifesting above all in outbursts of emotion, e.g., when an individual's will is crossed, but also in "the will to power" and selfish acts. As a merely psychic fact it does not fall within the precincts of psychology.

5. The former, "the ego" as a *psychological* reality, is not an anthropological constant, not a product of nature. As one particular self-definition or syntactical form of the I it is a product of history, the history of the soul, and a very late product at that.

The title of this paper speaks of the discovery and production of the ego. But it only speaks of "the ego" because I could not burden the title with the terminological difference between the ego and the I. This distinction first had to be introduced. But our actual topic in the following will be the discovery and production of the I, that is to say, that point in the history of the soul where the I, which is the naturally given and as such the only implicit necessity of human beings to exist as the existing concept, also became explicit, conscious, came home to consciousness and accordingly was expressly taken over by the mind as its own responsibility. From then on it was no longer that the soul merely *was* I. From then on the soul also *knew* itself as I, had explicitly comprehended itself as I and thus made the I or subjectivity the I's self-interpretation, self-definition. Consciousness had become self-consciousness.

So we see that we have to introduce an additional distinction in our scheme. I distinguished the ego as one of the self-interpretations of the I from the I. Now we have to realize that the "I" in its turn can mean two different things. In one sense it is that *which* is dressed in one of various garbs. In another sense "I" can also mean one of these *garbs* or interpretations of the I. But if we want to investigate the discovery and production of the I in the sense of one of the soul's self-interpretations, this conversely means that the I that existed all the time from the beginning of truly human existence did not always understand itself *as I or subjectivity*. And in fact, merely looking at the times of the ritualistic and mythological mode of being-in-the-world, we see immediately that then the I had no inkling of itself as being I. The further back in history we go, the more the I was completely enwrapped in soul; it was only implicit, had not yet become born out of its containment in soul. It had *as* I its sense of I or subjectivity much rather in an other out there, namely in the gods. The gods are an early form how the I appeared to itself, how it *implicitly* appeared to itself, just as "the ego" is a late and now not merely explicit, but on top of it also literalized, positivistic form. "The ego" became only possible once the sense of I had become explicit and, after centuries, had fully, exhaustively come home to I.

It is therefore a serious fault to try to understand "the ego" in terms of the solar hero of mythology. Mythological categories cannot explain modern phenomena. The modern ego is not heroic at all, but positivistic; it does not have a solar consciousness, but a rationalistic one. A fundamental difference. It is not threatened by underworldly monsters, because it is not threatened at all. At least logically, although not empirically (in practical reality), it has everything under control. But by now, since we have entered the age of television and the world-wide web, of the media in general, even the time of "the ego" has already become a thing of the past.

		the gods
		the one God
The (psychic) I	*garbed as* (e.g.):	
		(the psychological) I
		"the ego"

What I want to discuss and illustrate in the following is the discovery and production of the I in the sense of its becoming explicitly aware of its being I or of its giving itself the definition of "I," which happened beginning with that time in history that we call the Renaissance. And I want to illustrate this by means of the invention of linear or central perspective in art, because thereby it becomes most easily accessible. We can visibly see the emergence of the I as the self-definition of the psychic I. In what I will present I follow Jung's insight that if we truly want to find out something about the soul, we have to leave the consulting room behind, the always already prejudiced experience gained from work with individual modern patients, and that instead we have turn to history, to the great cultural phenomena of the past. "It is the smallest part of the psyche, and particularly of the unconscious, that presents itself in the medical consulting room" (*Letters 2*, p. 307, to Nelson, 17 June 1956), on the one hand, and "... it became clear to me that without history there can be no psychology" (*MDR* p. 205), on the other hand. We even have to go a step further than this cautious wording of in the former of the two quotes and say: by psychologistically looking at *people* and what is going on in them, we do not study the soul at all, do not do psychology at all, but merely explore the modern structure of "the ego" (that is, empirical man) in its/his inner complexity. (And of "the ego" as a sunken, sedimented cultural heritage at that. The ego is psychologically no longer "state of the art." Historically, the soul has already moved beyond "the ego.")

Excursus on "the self"

Above I stated that "The gods are an early form how the I appeared to itself." In the Jungian tradition it would of course be customary to see in the gods "the self," rather than the I. But I and self are really the same person. In many contexts both words can be used synonymously. In grammar, "self" is called a reflexive pronoun, because it indicates that I returns to itself ("I myself," "he himself"). For this reason I, too, would not really mind calling the gods "self," i.e. selves, *if* in the Jungian tradition the self would not imply an other, to some extent even a wholly other. In other words, if I and self were not usually dissociated. The self is supposed to be *experienced* by the I. They are divided by the subject-object split. In Erich Neumann's "ego-self axis" this dissociation of the actually uroboric unity has become solidified.

It is a question why Jung had to set up the self as an other. Why could he not say that the Gods or God are an early form of the manifestation of the I? Probably because at a historical time—in modernity—when the I had already come fully home to consciousness, when consciousness had long realized itself as I, nay, more recently even as being more than that, namely as "the ego," and when *ipso facto* "God was dead," the soul having already comprehended its *essential* relation to be uroboric self-relation rather than relation to an other, Jung felt he still needed, against the truth of the age, to rescue our having a God or gods and thus the logic of otherness. So he not only split up the soul into consciousness and "the unconscious" as its veritable other, but also "I myself" into two ("the ego" and "the self") and reserved "*das Ich*" or "the ego" for the human subject and "the self" for God (or the God-image in the unconscious). It is the *word* "self" alone that now still retained a faint trace of a reminiscence of the actually uroboric relation of "I myself," but this reminiscence was of course contradicted by the explicit meaning attached to the word.

By extracting the self-character from the soul's movement of reflection, in which "self" is an integral moment, and by substantiating it as *the* self vis-à-vis the I and as the latter's object[84] of experience, Jung left the precincts of psychology and trespassed into theology, the traditional discipline of *essential* otherness.[85] Psychology, by contrast, is the discipline of (logical) interiority and *essential* "sameness" (uroboric self-relation).

At the same time, Jung obscured the psychological difference, substituting for the difference and relation between the *psychic* I, which is given with human nature, and the *psychological* "I" (or "ego"), which is a psychological garb or self-interpretation of the psychic I, the difference and relation between the ego and the self. Both "the ego" and "the self" are conflations of something psychological with the psychic: particular historical forms of the soul's self-*interpretation* are taken as positively existing and timeless components of the human personality in analogy to body organs. If on the basis of this ahistorical scheme one views the ancient gods as expressions of the self rather than as an early self-interpretation of the psychic I and as such only as an *implicit* precursor of the psychological I, then one probably also retrojects the modern ego into the past, thereby blinding oneself to the crucial insight that psychologically there was no I as yet at all (let alone "the ego") in the archaic situation. For calling the gods the self in Jung's sense makes only sense if one believes that there was already the counterpart of the self from which it had to be distin-

84 I do not wish to obliterate the fact that there is in Jung's thinking a dialectic concerning this object. This object of the I's experience is precisely thought, and experienced, to be the true and downright overwhelming "subject" whose "object" we as ego-personalities are. But no matter how the roles of subject and object are distributed, in either case the dissociation remains.

85 The natural sciences are disciplines of ordinary otherness.

guished.

But archaic man was without I or ego. The only I (in the psychological sense) that there was for archaic man he had precisely "outside" of himself in his gods or, in an even earlier situation, in his ancestors (and their earthly representative, the shaman or king), in other words, in an other and as an other and as such precisely *as not* I (as He, She, or They). But if so, it is even more impossible to assign to the gods the predicate "the self," which would express an already existing objective awareness of the fact that the gods are the I's self-reflection.

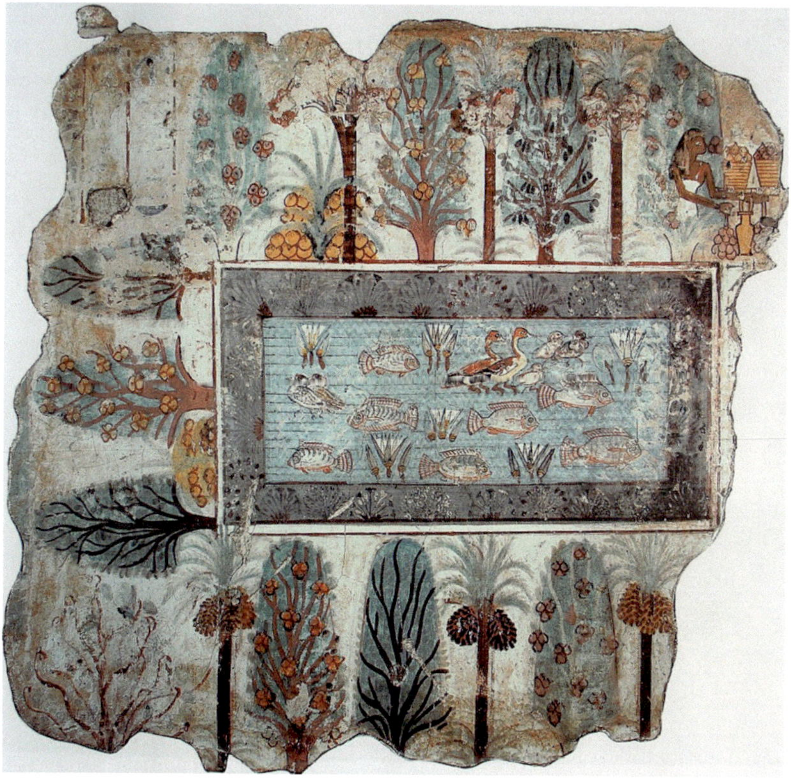

Fig. 4. Egyptian pond surrounded by trees (1). Le jardin de Nébaoun

Part II. Linear perspective as one self-display of the I

In order to be able to appreciate what the special achievement brought about by perspective is, it is helpful to contrast it with depictions that are not in perspective. Some Egyptian pictures, on the one hand, and small children drawings, on the other hand, may serve us as the most extreme contrast. (Fig. 4–6).

Painting what we know versus painting what is optically seen

In the first Egyptian picture (Fig. 4) of a pond surrounded by trees the pond is shown from on top, from bird's-eye view; the people who are standing in the pond or at its edge are represented in

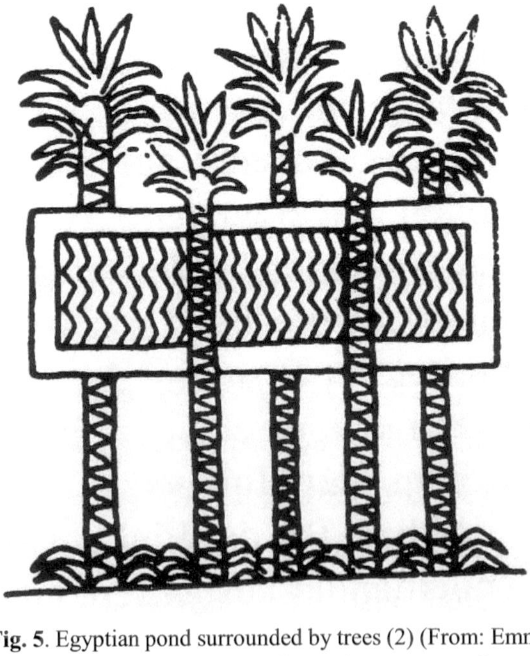

Fig. 5. Egyptian pond surrounded by trees (2) (From: Emma Brunner-Traut, *Frühformen des Erkennens am Beispiel Altägyptens*, Darmstadt (Wiss. Buchges.) 1992, p. 20.)

front-view, whereas the trees surrounding the pond are seen on each side from another standpoint, the trees in the back from the front, the ones in front from the back, those on the left and the right of the pond each from the opposite side. Analogously, the second Egyptian pond picture and the drawing by an eight-years old girl show the same principle at work. In each picture, one and the same picture, we get numerous viewpoints.

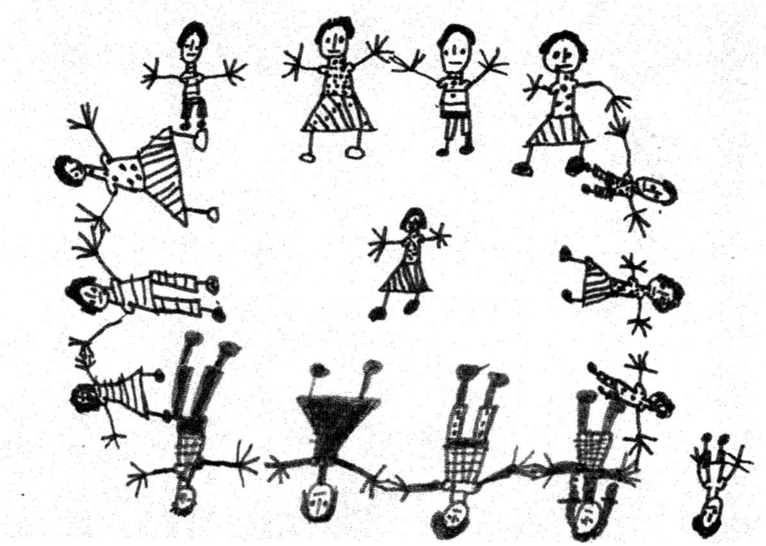

Fig. 6 Drawing by eight-years old girl. (From: Emma Brunner-Traut, *Frühformen des Erkennens am Beispiel Altägyptens*, Darmstadt (Wiss. Buchges.) 1992, p. 45.)

Drawings or paintings in perspective, by contrast, are characterized by the fact that everything in them is seen from one single viewpoint. In this regard, they show a scene much in the same way as a camera would show it. The field of vision has one center, one eye-point, which functions as a superordinate ordering principle and organizes the *whole* space for everything that appears in the picture. The whole reality depicted is subsumed under and made obedient to one system, the manifold of reality is drawn together into one totality. (Fig. 7, Tintoretto, Last Supper; Fig. 8, Mantegna, St. James on the way to his execution).

The invention of perspective in art is the move from a multitude of standpoints to the singleness of one standpoint.

The question arises what the reason is for the fact that, for example, the Egyptians and small children showed things in one and the same picture from different standpoints and what this entails. Each object or group of objects has its own standpoint. In this sense we could speak of an "objective" (object-centered) depiction in contrast to the subjective pictures in perspective. Each object here sort of owns its own viewpoint, *it* determines from which standpoint it has to be seen. In other words, in this type of representation the things shown have a much greater dignity and independence over against perspective pictures, in which everything is integrated into and subservient to one single scheme. In the one case, the soul is in each object; each object has or is its own soul within itself. In the other case, the soul is in the total picture, in the systematic whole. The soul has moved out of the individual objects, in which it had been their inalienable property, into the viewing, into the artist's and the viewer's seeing and conceiving. We could also say it is a move from an ontological standpoint to a more subjective one.

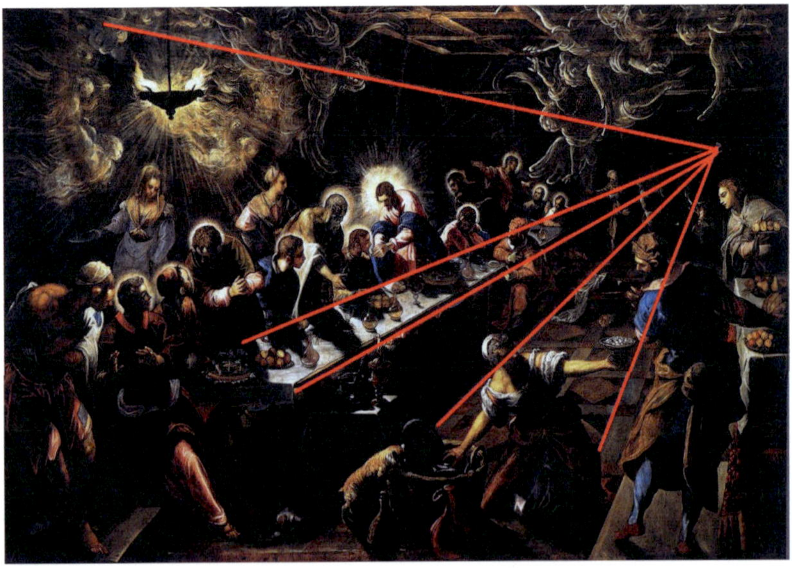

Fig. 7. Tintoretto, Last Supper (1494, Venice)

What is meant here by "ontological" becomes perhaps clearer if we look at one particular object, the pond in the Egyptian picture (Fig. 4, pond). If it had been shown in perspective, it would have been foreshortened. Depending on how low the eye point had been, its depiction would have approached a mere line rather than a rectangle. You could still have seen how long it is, but not how wide or deep it is. And what in truth is a rectangle with two sets of parallel lines would have been shown as a trapezoid, the left and the right sides being no longer parallel and the top side being shorter than the bottom side. So we can say that from the Egyp-

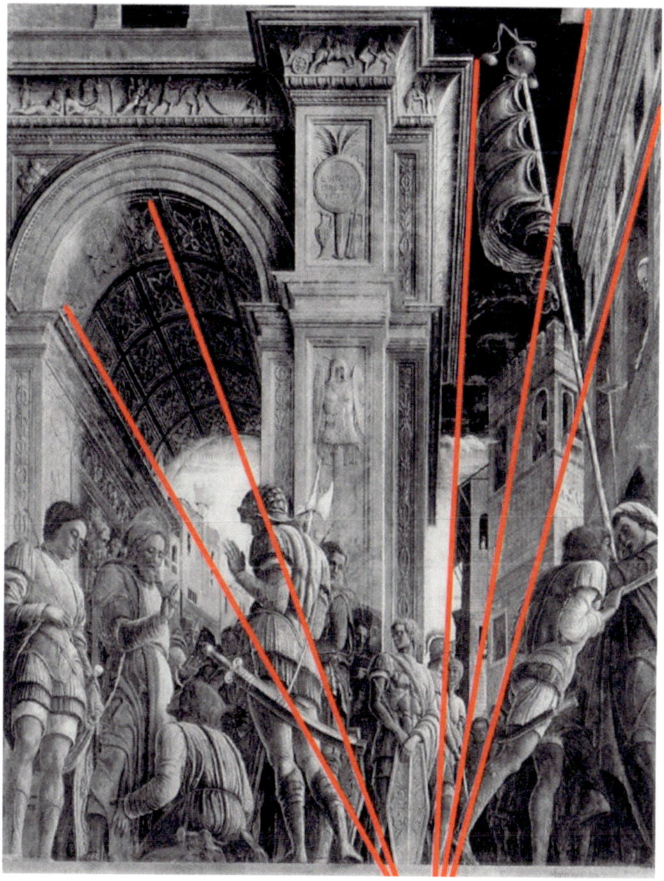

Fig. 8. Mantegna, St. James on the way to his execution (1455, from a mural in Padua).
The eye-point lies outside the depicted scene.

tian or from the child's point of view, perspective would have meant doing violence to the object and its truth. The pond IS rectangular and not a trapezoid. So you also have to *show* it as a rectangle. You must not foreshorten, curtail the object's truth. The object needs to be protected from the violence that such a distorting foreshortening would amount to. It is here, we might say, felt to be an insult to the true nature of the things. The Being of the object (how and what it in truth *is*) is here more important than how we actually see it. The *object* is what counts; *it* is what is dominant here, and the seeing subject is oblivious of itself and a priori abstracts from its seeing. In this psychological situation, it is the real, the things, that have a self or are a self. Each thing is treated as an individual with its own rights. The viewer who sees all the things is comparatively forgettable, merely of secondary importance. The seeing subject is fully given over to the objective world. We can diagnose here a kind of infatuation with objective reality, provided we do not understand "infatuation" as an emotion but as a logical relation.

In the case of the girl's drawing of a number of children standing in a circle around a single girl, perspective would have meant that only the backs of those children who are standing in front would have been seen. Their faces would be hidden. But the face and especially the eyes are the most essential features of a person. Showing only the children's backs would have deprived them of their personhood and reduced them to things, which highlights once more the insult done to the real by perspective.

In addition, from behind people look pretty much alike. It is not so easy to recognize an individual without seeing his or her face. This takes us to another aspect of this kind of drawing. Emma Brunner-Traut, an Egyptologist, spoke in her insightful cited work (*Frühformen des Erkennens am Beispiel Altägyptens*) for this style of depiction of "*aspective*" in contrast to "perspective." Her term is not meant as a simple negation of "perspective," but is much rather derived from "aspect." Instead of "aspect" we could also say "face." "Aspective" pictures want to show the face of each item depicted, its principle side, its physiognomy. But the terms "face" and "physiognomy" are ambiguous. We think when we hear the word face of the actual likeness, the visible appearance. But we see that the girl's picture is not interested at all in the real likeness. For her, "face" in its literal sense means nothing more than "two eyes, a nose, and a mouth, surrounded by a circle or oval." She precisely abstracts completely from the visible concreteness and graphicness or plasticity of each individual child's face.

What she draws is thus only the abstract-universal *concept* of a face, the concept represented by its *differentia specifica* eyes, nose, mouth. All individual features of the different noses, eyes, mouths, etc., i.e., the concrete facial expression, are erased, which is why all faces look basically alike. It is by no means that this is due to the fact that the little girl is technically not yet capable of presenting the actual likeness of the individual children. No, she is perfectly satisfied with her depiction. For her, nothing is missing or deficient. She did not *want* to draw anything else but the abstract concepts of the real. She draws *types* of things, not individual things. Or she draws the things *as types*, *as* their *concepts*, not as their actual visible appearance in their singularity.

Another way of putting pretty much the same thing is to say that she draws what she *knows* and not what she actually sees. She is guided by her conceptual knowledge, not by sensory perception. The whole richness of the facial expression that we actually see is fundamentally *reduced* to a few *abstract signs* that stand for characteristic features of the *generic* type of thing. She uses a kind of shorthand, abbreviations. It is mental, noetic drawing, not sensory drawing, not even imaginal drawing. And this is why I think that Brunner-Traut's term "aspect" is not hitting to mark. "Aspect" contains the same root "SPEC" that we also find in perspective and that means to look. So it still refers to seeing and to sensory perception, whereas in truth this type of picturing is basically intellectual, a secondary *notation in signs* of contents and properties of the mind. While drawing the girl is enwrapped in her mind. She depicts her *memory* of the real scene, and not her memory *images*, but the concepts of what she remembers. She is not informed by what she sees, but by a fundamentally *sublated* seeing that distilled the few characteristic distinguishing marks of a type of thing from out of what can be seen. She does not look outwards at the real scene in order to capture in her picture what is actually to be seen out there. She does not want to *portray* the children. We have to make a difference between portraying and notation.

Our girl is still dwelling in the world of the mind, the ideal world. She is, as it were, a Platonist, painting Platonic Forms or Ideas. And this is why *psychologically* she herself is ultimately still living in paradise, in heaven—paradise and heaven not in the sense of a place of milk and honey and of literal perfection and absolute happiness, but in a strictly logical/psychological sense. ("Psychologically she is living..." means her soul is living...) Everything experienced by her still has its place in the ideal, not the

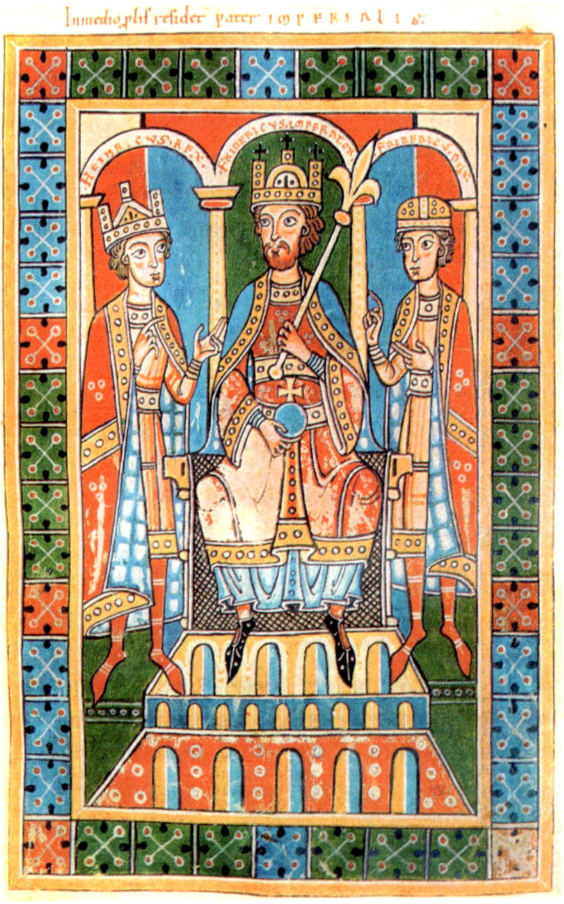

Fig. 9. Emperor Friedrich Barbarossa and sons.
From the *Welfenchronik*

real, world. Her soul is still innocent. Even while factually having been born and living on this earth and *psychically* being aware of empirical reality, *psychologically* she is still up in the clouds, has not yet been born, not yet come down to earth, into empirical reality. This is what she documents in the style of her drawings.

The medieval soul's being as a being-in-heaven

The result of our reflections can be applied directly to the earlier Middle Ages, from which Renaissance painting pushed off to its own style of representing the world in perspective. Even when real concrete persons like an emperor or a knight or bishop were depicted, the medieval artist had no interest in the specific visible looks and particular facial expression through which the depicted person would be recognizable in his singular individuality, in the photographic sense. They had no interest in portraits. (Fig. 9 "Emperor Barbarossa"). A picture showed the generic type, the concept, not the individual. The picture of Emperor Barbarossa could just as well serve as representation of any other emperor, except maybe for one specific feature, his red hair. And the fact that most pictures produced during the earlier Middle Ages showed the figures to be represented against a gold background (Fig. 10, Crucifixion; Fig. 11, Enthroned Madonna on Throne; Fig. 12, Lochner, Madonna of the Rose Bower) is a reflection and evident self-display of the fact that the soul is still residing in heaven. This is also underlined by an additional feature.

The topics almost exclusively deemed worthy of being depicted were religious ones, ones that showed the eternal sacred truths; there was hardly any interest in the visible, the sensory, in natural reality and in the temporal world. The soul related to the eternal and divine, to its (the soul's) heavenly truth, and it related to it directly, without needing this truth to be mediated via the sensory world. (Jung might have said it related directly to the archetypal world.) The truth was revealed truth. It had been revealed to man, and so he was in possession of truth. While medieval man *empirical-factually* lived in the harsh reality of this earth, in a world of wars, feuds, corveé, and rather miserable living conditions, *psychologically* he still lived, that is, the soul lived, in paradise, in the Garden Eden, where it is possible to be, like Adam and Eve, in direct contact with God. The soul had not yet come down to earth, and for it, for the soul, God had not yet become utterly transcendent, divided from the empirical world by a fundamental rift. The soul was completely given over to its celestial mysteries, and in the paintings and sculptures of that time it could immediately *see* and *participate in* those mysteries, just as it could directly experience and live them in the Church's rituals.

The psychological expulsion from paradise, the soul's departure from existence-in-heaven began historically with (and is reflected

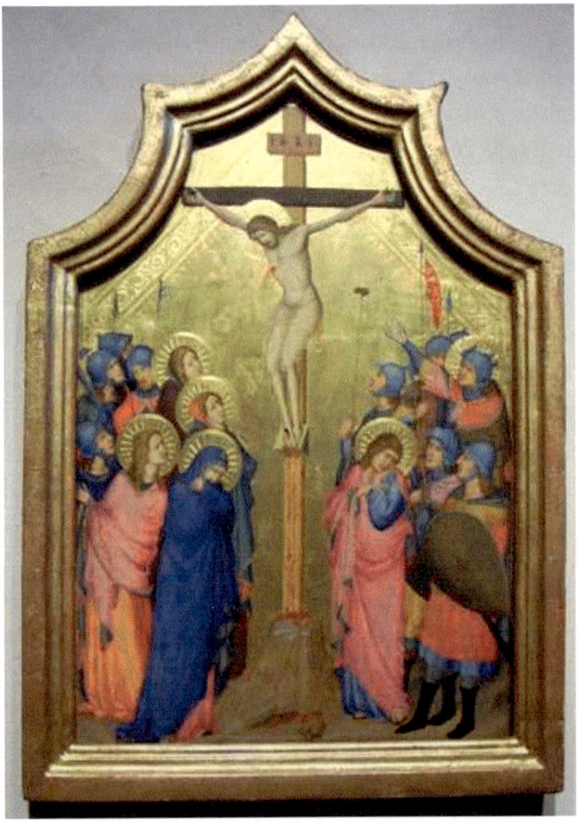

Fig. 10. Master of the Codex of Saint George: The Crucifixion, *c*. 1340-45.

in) the invention of the idea of purgatory, which introduced a third, *intermediate* space *between* heaven and earth, and with the rise and growth of the various Orders of Preachers (Dominicans), of mendicant friars, of the preachers of repentance. According to Jacques Le Goff, the "birth of purgatory" dates from 1170–1200. Psychologically, the invention of purgatory expresses the fact that now the soul had lost its innocence. A distance had come about. The soul was no longer directly in contact with God, no lon-

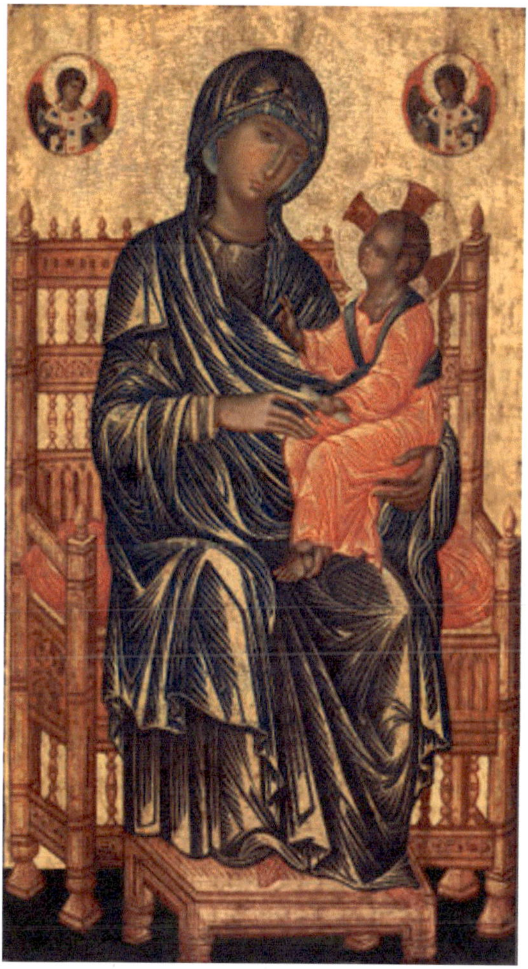

Fig. 11. Enthroned Madonna and Child.
Byzantine, *c*. 1250/1275

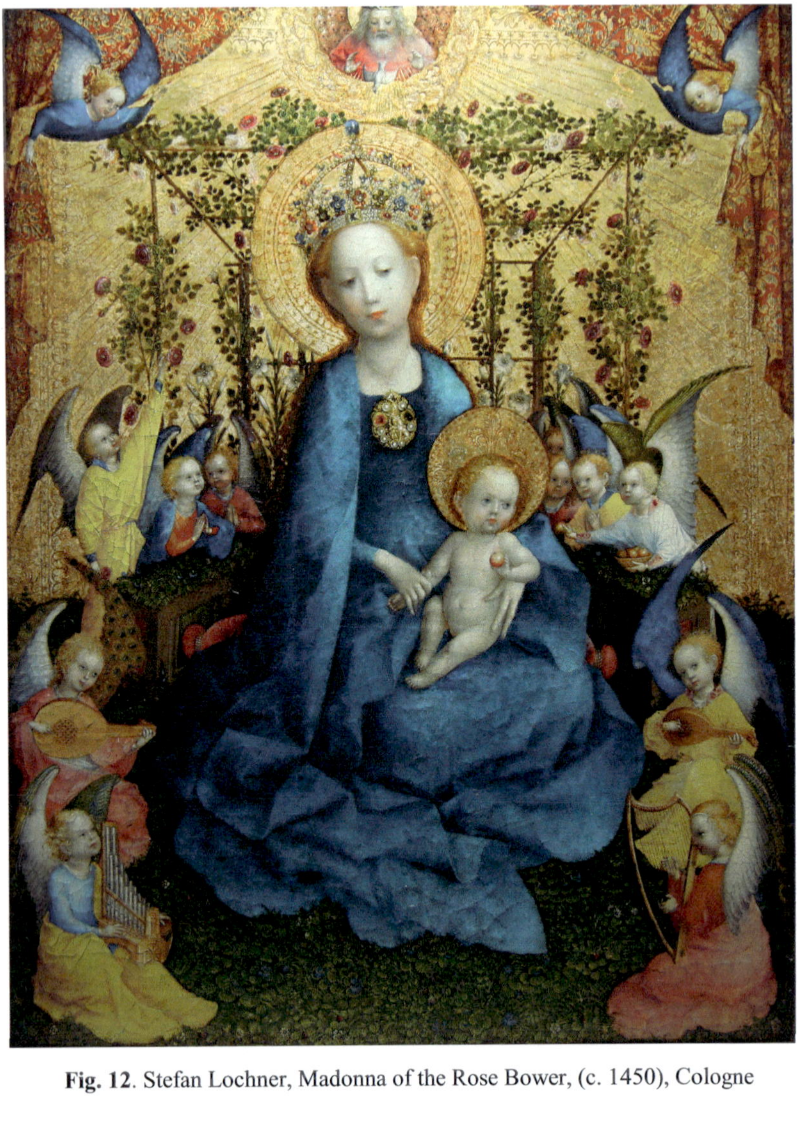

Fig. 12. Stefan Lochner, Madonna of the Rose Bower, (c. 1450), Cologne

ger already dwelling in heaven. This is why repentance became culturally so overwhelmingly important and popular during the next two or three centuries. Repentance is *man's* work to compensate for the *soul's* fall from heaven. The soul now knew that it was outside paradise.

But only with the Renaissance and the Reformation had the

soul psychologically come really down to earth. For the time being it was neither in heaven nor on this earth but in an in-between state, namely in purgatory. Purgatory is psychologically a compromise-formation. It documents the soul's full awareness of its factually having lost its existence-in-heaven and of therefore being in need of terrible works of repentance, but at the same time it also documents that this fact has not fully come home to the soul, has not been integrated and taken to heart by radically having changed its categories and orientation. Rather, the soul's thinking keeps clinging to its former mode, that very mode that has precisely been overcome. It holds on to "existence-in-heaven" as the one and only standard and measure, as what ought to be, so that it forces man into repentance, in the hope of thereby undoing its actually already experienced fall.

But this is part of the normal process of psychological change. Psychological change realizes itself in a double-step (Latin *passus*[86]). First, consciousness becomes aware of the obsolescence of its old truth and of the fact that something else (here, the soul's expulsion from paradise) has become the new truth for it. This is a change that its historical development has sprung on the soul. It had not been not asked for or desired. However, at this point consciousness is aware of this prevailing new truth only *semantically*, as a *content* of consciousness. It perceives and assesses this new truth with the old *syntax* or logical *form* of consciousness, with its old categories and expectations, which is why it is unable to ap-

86 A Roman *passus* ("pace") was not, as for us, the distance in walking between the one foot and the other foot, but the distance from the place where the one foot had originally been to the new place where it, the *same* foot, was set down again, e.g., the whole stretch from left foot to right foot plus from right foot to left foot. What we mean by step, the placing of one foot in front of the other that stays in its old position, in other words, the compromise between holding on to the old and venturing forth to a new position by means of a distribution of the one task to the one and the other task to the other leg, is therefore only the first half of a *passus*. The second half consists in letting the other foot, which had been left behind at the starting point of this move, give up its initial position and find its new *standpoint, its new "home,"* as it were, *in front of* the one that has already moved. A *passus* is one and the same foot's full swing around the other already advanced foot, a movement required to take the person as a whole fully to (or even a little beyond) the new position reached by this already advanced foot, whereas before the person had merely extended this one foot forward to the new place.

preciate its new truth *as* its *truth*, but is forced to view it as no more than the new external conditions of life and to evaluate them as a mistake, a faulty development, a fall, a sin to be corrected or undone. Only in a second step and over a longer period of time, the newly acquired content of consciousness gradually comes also fully home to consciousness, which means that the new content fundamentally transforms the logical form of consciousness, its categories, expectations and outlook, its value system, so that ultimately what had factually all along already been its new truth is now also logically (psychologically) turned into its acknowledged truth. Its truth has become true '*for* it' or, as we could also put it, what had been viewed as mere experienced fact has now been released into its *being true*.

Both types of examples, the Egyptian depictions and those of the Middle Ages that I showed, although they certainly do not express the same psychological status, nevertheless betrayed that the style of painting or drawing was essentially *intellectual*, the secondary notation (representation in pictorial signs) of what the mind *knows*, rather than being authentically informed and guided by sensory perception, by what the eyes see.

We could think that this implies that there was an unbroken continuity from the ancient Egyptian style to the medieval style. But I have to remind you, without here being able to go into it, that, for example, classical Greek art which precedes medieval art was not intellectual in style. The works of such artists as Polyclitus or Praxiteles are clearly based on the careful focus on the actual sensory looks of the real. They certainly produced *idealized* statues, but this idealization was a secondary work performed on the eyes' sight as its primary material. They did not pictorially represent an intellectual knowledge that the mind had; not abstract types or concepts, not so to speak Platonic Forms. On a much more naive, more innocent, more harmless[87] (namely "nat-

87 I am of course only speaking of the ancient Greeks' *psychological* innocence and harmlessness, which is something totally different from literal behavioral harmlessness or naivety in the sense of a life in Arcadian bliss and peacefulness. Anyone who has read the *Iliad* and Thucydides and takes into account the fact that ancient Greek culture was based on bloody sacrifices and on slavery will be aware of the brutality and treachery in war as well as the ruthless egotism of individuals and states that prevailed in antiquity.

ural"[88]) level of consciousness than the Christian medieval one (Christianity is the explicit overcoming of "nature" and the "natural world"), it was already possible for ancient Greek art of the classical period to be down to earth. And conversely, the medieval soul began with a form of art that showed that *on a much more advanced and complex level of consciousness*[89] it was nevertheless much more innocently and radically up in the clouds.

But then one might question whether it is legitimate to speak of the Greeks' being down to earth, since in the context of the *unio naturalis* and within the first status of Pseudo-Democritus' dictum[90] ("nature delights in nature") there is not really yet any "earth" in the pronounced psychological sense. The earth in the psychological sense comes only into being when it has been left (Pseudo-Democritus' "nature subdues nature"), when a radical rift between nature and spirit, a conflict between aesthetics and morals has brutally opened up. Which is why a real coming down to earth could only happen on the basis of the Christian overcoming of nature.

At any rate, the Renaissance that imagined that it gave rebirth to antiquity did no such thing. Rather, on the much more complex level of consciousness than within the Greek world and on the shoulders of its *Christian medieval* predecessors it conquered a completely new soul situation, a situation of having fully arrived in the empirical world. Renaissance painting displays a situation that because of some external likeness merely gives the impression of being a revival of what had already been achieved by the Greeks. As new research has shown,[91] the invention of perspective during the Renaissance was inspired by Alzahen's new Arabic

88 The level of the *unio naturalis*. Just think of the naturalness of the Greek gods, the idea of the *kalokagathia* (the unity of the beautiful and the good, which according to Jung is what "the anima believes in," "a primitive conception that antedates the discovery of the conflict between aesthetics and morals," *CW* 9i § 60), the power of sensuality and aesthetic seduction as well as the close religious relation to the natural world (*CW* 5 § 113).

89 The progressive achievement of Christianity over the world of antiquity was discussed by Jung, e.g., *CW* 6 §§ 107 ff., CW 5 §§ 104 ff.

90 (Pseudo-)Democritus' complete axiom on nature reads: "nature rejoices in nature, nature subdues nature, nature rules over nature" (e.g., CW 9i § 234).

91 Hans Belting: *Florenz und Bagdad. Eine westöstliche Geschichte des Blicks.* Verlag C. H. Beck, München 2008.

mathematical theory of seeing, his measuring the gaze and the rays of light. His work on this subject had already around 1200 been translated into Latin in Spain and was known at European universities as early as the 13th century. In the West, this theory of seeing was later transformed into a new theory of depiction, of the mathematically correct projection onto a plane. Even the term "perspective" is due to this philosopher from Bagdad. It was one of the titles of the Latin translation of Alzahen's book.

Another feature worth giving some weight to is the fact that the early medieval artist generally did not feel the need to sign their works of art and that society did not feel the need of recording their names for posterity. The artist stayed anonymous. This indicates the fact I mentioned earlier that the subject in this type of art (and soul situation) is not all that important. What *is* important is the object, the real, that is, the soul's truth. The painting subject, the artist, is merely the servant of this truth.

Artificial construction

All this changes with the Renaissance invention of perspective. In order to visibly demonstrate the essential features of perspective, I could start out from paintings which use perspective. But it is even more helpful for our purposes to turn to a woodcut by Albrecht Dürer (Fig. 13, Dürer, Draftsman of reclining woman) which not only makes use of perspective but also has the construc-

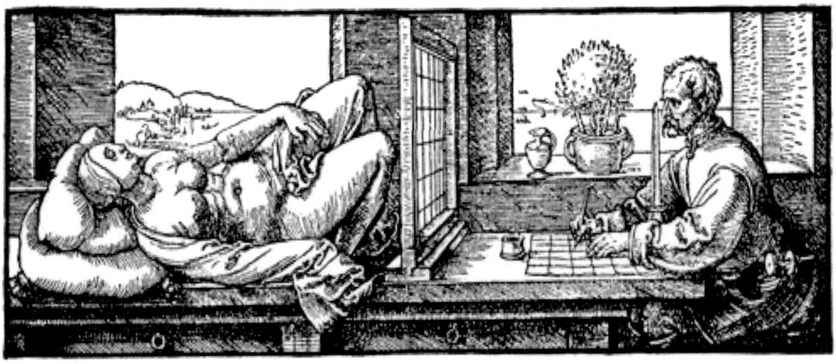

Fig. 13. Albrecht Dürer, Draftsman making a perspective drawing of a reclining woman. Woodcut from *Unterweysung der Messung*, Nürnberg 1525.

tion of a depiction in perspective as its explicit topic. In psychoanalysis we distinguish between acting-out and remembering or interiorizing. Dürer's woodcut does not merely act perspective out by applying its laws, but it also consciously reflects it. In this way perspective sort of lets us in on its secrets. It reveals its own internal logic, which is otherwise hidden. This logic becomes visible.

The grid in Dürer's picture allows us to realize that the perspective view must be artificially constructed, despite the fact that our eyes have unwittingly seen reality according to the laws of perspective all along. It is not inherent in the nature of the *perceived* world, in our natural perception. It takes lots of effort to master linear perspective. The grid is the artist's contribution to the situation of seeing. He brings it with him from outside and applies it to reality. That is to say, the artist no longer looks naively, innocently into the world. He has stepped outside the situation of ordinary or natural seeing and is now vis-à-vis it. His viewing is now in itself essentially reflected viewing. The world has become his object in an emphatic sense. Psychologically, the artist is no longer inalienably contained, embedded in nature, in an immediate and natural exchange with it. This means that now the condition of the a priori possibility of mythic experience, namely the soul's *in-ness* in nature, has been left altogether. In order to apperceive the inner image of real situations, the mythic truths animating them from within, their gods, you have to be logically inside them, contained in them. The artist in Dürer's woodcut sees fundamentally from outside.

The grid through which the world is captured in a *systematic* view of it only appears as a literal grid here, in this woodcut that is *about* perspective and reflects it. It is not visible in paintings that *apply* perspective. The type of technical construction represented in our woodcut is only an aid for the preliminary studies in preparation for a painting. This aid is not in the depicted final result. Much like in the construction of a house the scaffolding is removed once the house is finished, so also the final Renaissance painting would delete all traces of its artificial construction and the effort it required. On the contrary, the final product of the artist depicted in Dürer's woodcut would create in us the beautiful illusion of an absolutely natural looking, sensuous woman. The grid exists in the mind. Perspective is in this sense a schematic mental design, a style of thinking and perceiving. Nothing real, but strictly ideal. The same applies to the eye-point. The painter does not paint it along with everything else in his picture. Although it structures everything in the picture, it has no real existence. It is an ideal point outside the picture. What exactly the place of the eye-point is needs to be reconstructed from the lines in the painting. (Fig. 8, Mantegna, St. James on the way to his execution)

Disciplining both our seeing and the seen reality

The grid in Dürer's depiction in a certain sense also functions like the bars of a prison or cage in which reality is locked. The seen phenomena are disciplined. Only for the purpose of this disciplining is there a need of the grid in the first place. If the soul would by nature see the world in perspective, we would not with great effort have to learn to draw in perspective. Even when a view in perspective of something real does no longer have to be painstakingly constructed in an empirical way, dot by dot, according to the method portrayed in Dürer's woodcut, because an artist has mastered the geometric rules and can construe the perspective view freely, nevertheless the same disciplining or domestication is inherent even in his free, commanding construction. His free mastering of perspective merely shows that he has totally integrated this disciplining. We can see that in the production of perspective there is an execution of a not physical, but logical violence or force at work.

This logical violence and this disciplining show that what is happening here is part of the soul's *opus contra naturam*. The soul pushes off from an earlier stage of its historical development.

Dürer's woodcut also allows us to see that it is only possible to subject everything appearing in the picture to the one single eye-point if the eye of the artist is fixated with absolute stability by means of a fixed sharp-pointed instrument. Seeing in perspective thus also presupposes the self-disciplining of the subject. The subject must be domesticated, too. (Or what we call the early-modern subject *is* this self-domestication.) It must force itself to see not like a human being naturally sees, not like the soul sees, but like a camera sees. The artist must train himself to systematically relinquish his natural human seeing. Natural human seeing is one in which several varying standpoints are at work at the same time and in which our *knowledge* about what the things seen are, what color they have, what they look like, etc. is essential. We do not so much see what the eye physically sees, but what we know. The disciplining necessary for perspective has therefore two tasks: (a) it has to force our natural seeing to become constricted to the limited apparatus-like seeing of a camera-lense, and (b) it has to drive out or suppress our always-already existing knowledge about the looks of the real. This underlines once more that the seeing in perspective is artificial, a construct, because it needs artificial crutches, namely the grid as the not physical but logical cage for the world and the pointed instrument for the firm fixation of the subject's gaze at one single eye point that is supposed to be immovable and *rules* over everything seen. It also underlines the fact that the move to perspective is the move away from *noetic* seeing to *sensory* perception. Our seeing is cleansed and stripped of the mind's and soul's knowing, be it mythical or conceptual knowing.

Every painter who in the time to come would paint in perspective had this pointed instrument as well as the grid as mental realities in his seeing. He did not need to make use of the instrument and the grid for each new painting as *literal* aids. But he nevertheless still made use of them, having inwardized them, integrated them into the form of his seeing. And today, after a century-long training, every person, we all, carry those instruments interiorized in ourselves as our mental property and the *mode* of our looking into the world. We do not even need to be great painters any longer in order to see that way. In fact, the real painters already left this mode of seeing at least one-hundred years ago. We ordinary people, the proverbial man on the street, always needs a couple of centuries longer to acquire what the artists, philosophers, poets, scientists first developed. Modern art has already left behind the I conquered and developed during the early-modern era, the time from let's say about 1400 to 1800 A.D.;

however, it has not only left the I, but also "the ego" behind, "the ego" first developed during the 19th century.

Neutralization of reality: mere appearance and model

A very striking feature of Dürer's woodcut is the optical partition of the picture. On the right the artist, sitting upright, working in total concentration and dedication to his rational concern, and on the left the provocatively voluptuous woman in her naked beauty. Let us read this picture as if it were a dream image. What this image shows, all the more so because this is by no means intended by Dürer, is the form prevailing here of man's relation to the soul. The woman could be seen as a representation of the anima. Now what is the specific relation prevailing here? The "relation between the I and the unconscious," to use Jung's wording, consists here in their fundamental separation. A grid, i.e., a fence has been interposed between them and keeps them neatly apart. In other words, the relationship has the character of a dissociation. There is no seduction, no erotic fascination, no love-making, despite the fact that a potentially seductive sight clearly offers itself to the I. The sensuous and voluptuous reality remains on the one, the strict rationality, ascetic soberness, and business-like seriousness on the other side. The I has become a professional; his is a professional look at what is to be seen. The *medieval* subject had not been a professional. It had an immediate pious relation to the soul's truth. The character of this image excludes the possibility that a spark might jump across the fence from the sight of her to him and ignite a fire of desire in him. The artist, so much is certain, will remain unaffected, immune, in complete control. This separation and the I's nonsusceptibility is again an expression of the *opus contra naturam*.

In this scheme, there cannot be a relation between the two because he precisely does not see *her* at all, but is conversely and only interested in the *sight* of her, her optical *appearance*, merely the *image*, which he wants to capture in *his* grid or scheme and on canvas. He has completely abstracted from her as person and woman and natural reality. In Kantian terms we can say that the division between the woman as mere "appearance" and her as "thing-in-itself" has here irrevocably been performed and she as "thing-in-itself" or rather as "person" has been eliminated. Extrapolating from the interpersonal relation to the general relation to the world that is reflected in the relationship between the artist and the anima in our woodcut, we can say that in this sphere, the sphere of the I, there cannot be an in-ness (*Inständigkeit*) in the world, not any being reached by and won over to the real. The possibility of being hit by the real's ultimately numinous flash and claim, by its archetypal image, does not exist. All this is systematically filtered out. The direction of the gaze is reversed: instead of our being struck by the gazes that come from the real and penetrate us in the depth of the soul, we have now a *construction* of the world in its optical visibility. The condition of the possibility of a mythic experience of the world is once and for all over.

The anima has been reduced to being an object of the subject's seeing. She has become a priori neutralized as a mere "model" to be studied, we could also say with our psychological jargon, a mere "image." As a model or image, she is no more than the "sublated" anima, the reflected, mediated anima. She is no longer taken seriously as she herself. With all her erotic charms she now has her place in what we might call the (scientific, not alchemical) "laboratory" of the subject as artist. He is the distanced experimenter or scientist. Although in the woodcut they still appear on the same level, logically he is standing above her, on a higher level of reflection.

The firm fixation of the eye by means of the pointed instrument has a significant function in this regard, too. In addition to fixing his gaze, it also gives him stability, it helps to make the painter immune against the tempting character of what there is to see and at the same time against his own receptivity for this seductive sight.[92] Only if he stays immune can he succeed in his project of

92 We may remember in this context how Jung once contrasted the consciousness of primitives and our modern consciousness. About the consciousness of the primitive he said that it "lacks the firm coherence of our own. We have control of our will power, but the primitive has not. Complicated exercises are needed if he is to pull himself together for any activity that is conscious and intentional and not just emotional and instinctive. Our consciousness is safer and more dependable in this respect ..." (*CW* § 9i § 213). Medieval man's consciousness can certainly not be identified with that of primitive man. Nevertheless, it too did not have yet that kind of "safety", i.e. immunity, that

the foreshortening (both in the technical and in a wider sense) of the real. This foreshortening of reality consists in the translation of its *known or revealed truth* into its mere *sensory appearance* as well as in the translation of its inherent mythic or archetypal depth or metaphysical-religious claim into a subjective experience.

The painter seems to focus on the lady in high concentration and dedication. She is what his eager efforts are about. However, it is precisely not the lady herself that he is concerned about. All his striving is for success in managing to capture in the geometric system of his grid something as ungeometrical, human, alive, and sensuously seductive as this woman or as the anima and thereby to subject her to an essential foreshortening. This foreshortening is required for him to portray her on the plane of his canvas. What is depicted in a perspective painting is more than its explicit subject-matter. It is also, through and by means of it, the reality of the grid, that is, the centralist ordering system as which "the I" exists, a general and superordinate ordering system which itself, however, remains invisible.

The artist's drawing or painting a picture in perspective is implicitly a ritual act in which always anew the proof of the complete subjection of whatever reality to the one freely chooseable eye-point is furnished, or rather, the proof for the on principle existing possibility of subjecting whatever reality to this viewpoint. Thus it is also the triumph of having foreshortened reality by one whole dimension: the dimension of its truth and its concept character and of being on principle *capable* of achieving this foreshortening. To be sure, this proof is always a partial one. It is each time furnished only for the one in-fact-depicted specific *part* of total reality, of the whole of geometric space. But it is the proof of the fact that one possesses the *principle* which, if need be, can be applied to any and each reality.

Looking at our woodcut with its clear-cut division between the anima and the artist-subject, Jung's early, pre-alchemy work on *The Relations between the Ego [the I] and the Unconscious* immediately comes to mind. Early Jung's title establishes the same vis-

---

Jung discerns in modern consciousness and that is probably the inherited product of the cultural process of the subject's self-disciplining depicted in Dürer's woodcut.

à-vis situation, the same dissociation. The irrevocably separating grid that is expressly visible in Dürer's picture exists in Jung's scheme in a more hidden form, too: in the word "unconscious." "The unconsciousness" by definition assigned to the soul a priori divides the soul by a fence from consciousness. We also find the same immunity of the subject. Jung insists that the unconscious must be "carefully observed" by us. As observers we are logically distanced, irrevocably outside, vis-à-vis. We take on a professional stance toward the psyche. Jung even restricts the meaning of the Latin term *religio* to "careful observation" (from *religere*) and systematically rejects its other possible etymology from a word that implies "binding obligation" (*religare*). Obviously, there must not be, or rather can no longer be, a direct and committing encounter with the psychically real. Just as the anima in the case of the Renaissance artist is metaphorically speaking placed into his "laboratory," so she is in early Jungian psychology also primarily placed into and confined in the artificial laboratory of the consulting room. We "*work*" on our so-called unconscious. And in much the same way that the artist relates to the mere appearance of the woman and not to her as real person, the psychologist's relation is to "images," dream images, fantasy images, archetypal images, symbols. With our term "image" we show that we do not relate to the soul as a free reality, but only to it as a priori neutralized (logically neutralized).

A brief look at another woodcut by Dürer helps me to make another point (Fig. 14, Draftsman of the lute). The I, as it emerges during the Renaissance, is an objective universal concept, not an individual and stricly subjective possession.[93] We see this in this woodcut because here the eye-point is not the artist's or his assistant's real eye, as it was in the other woodcut, but it is the objective point on the wall, the place where the string is attached. But of course, we could say much the same about the earlier woodcut. In its scene, the artist could be exchanged by any other seeing person. The I is precisely exchangeable. Anybody is I. To be I is nothing special, nothing individual. It is a universal logical standpoint. The real representation of the I in this first woodcut would

93 I am of course speaking of the *psychological* I as one historical garment or self-interpretation of the *psychic* I, not about the latter.

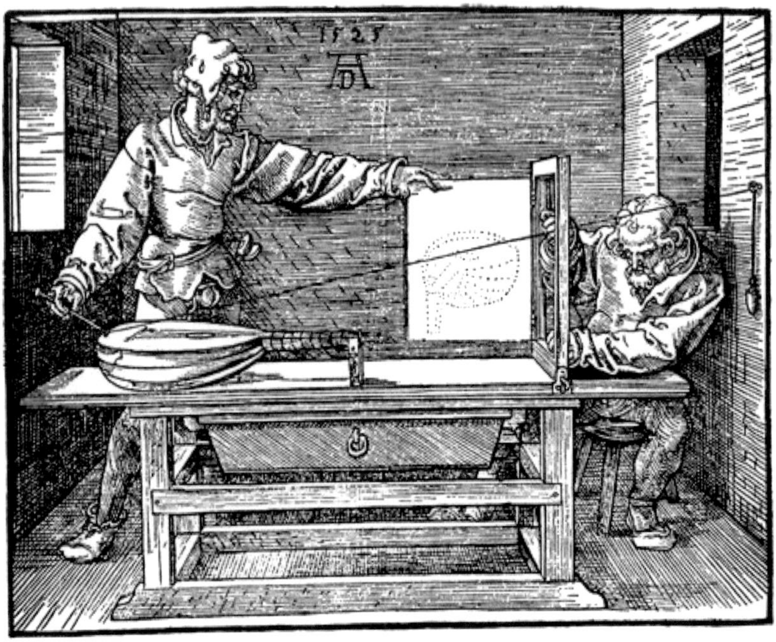

Fig. 14. Albrecht Dürer, Draftsman of the Lute. Woodcut from *Unterweysung der Messung*, Nürnberg 1525

therefore have to be comprehended as being the sharp point of the fixed instrument that enables any viewer to hold his gaze in a fixed position.

A revolution concerning the ownership of the gaze

The subjugation of reality under the ordering system given with the single eye-point also amounted to a revolution of the conditions of ownership. Prior to perspective in painting each thing or person carried within itself its own measure and truth and laws. *It determined* how it had to be presented. The Egyptian pond had to be shown from on top because it was characteristic of it to be square or rectangular. Not how the pond would incidentally *appear* to the subject from an arbitrarily chosen standpoint was what was painted, but what is inherent in its own essence. Each person or object possessed independence, a dignity of its own, sort of a will of its own. The things made a claim on the painter. It is not so much that the artist looked at them, but much rather that they gazed at him, showed themselves to him, confronted him, addressed him, similarly perhaps to how in the beginning of some stage plays, the *dramatis personae* step forward and introduce themselves before the actual drama begins. If we keep in mind that in early medieval paintings what was painted was almost exclusively divine scenes and saints, it is immediately clear that the figures depicted did not exist for the purpose that there would be something beautiful to look at, but rather conversely as something that demanded submission, namely piety and devotion, from the viewer.

When, however, all phenomena have been subjected to the one single eye-point and have to submit to the total scheme established by it, then they turn to pieces or sections of the one homogenous geometric space and as such literally to the *res extensae* of Descartes. Space as such, as an abstract universal and as pure extension in its mathematical sense, comes logically first, and all things or persons are now placed into it, have to fit in it. They have to divide up among each other the available total space, so that in some cases they necessarily overlap. There may not be enough space to show each figure in full. The figures in medieval paintings were not placed in geometric space. They *were* their own space.

Now the seeing I, the subject, is logically (of course not empirically) the lord over everything depicted, whereas in the earlier medieval situation the viewer of a picture would conversely feel penetrated by the gaze of the sacred figures. *They* looked into his life and demanded something from him, which means that they were the true subject and the viewer was "the object" that was looked at. But now that with perspective the viewer and the artist have appropriated ownership of the gaze and the power of looking and that paintings *ipso facto* have become what is only looked *at*, the viewer has become the true subject and the painting an object. At the same time art has become *aesthetic*, a matter of aesthetic appreciation, that is, of an inner feeling.

This revolutionary change is also reflected in language in a reversal of the meaning of certain words. Thus the very words "subject" and "object" reversed their meaning. The old medieval meaning of "subject" (*subiectum*) was "substance," the real, whereas *obiectum* meant precisely only the content of consciousness or perception, that which is known in our knowing, our ideas or representations, in other words, what from our point of view is subjective. For us it is the other way around. The subject is the sovereign I, the lord of the gaze, and the object is what is (passively) seen or dealt with. The English language preserved the ambiguity of "subject" that arose with the reversal. This word can mean either the subject-matter, i.e., what we usually mean by object, and politically (as in "British subjects") the subject of the king or queen, or it can mean the autonomous seeing subject, such as when we speak of the subject-object split or that something is merely subjective (the I's private opinion or fancy).

There are a number of similar reversals in meaning. *Hypóthêsis* originally meant that which has been put underneath and thus is the foundation of something, like the a priori principles of mathematics. When we, by contrast, speak of "hypothesis" we mean a subjective assumption on a trial basis that still needs to be tested. Medieval *informatio* meant the process of giving form to matter, especially God's creative act of giving each thing or being in the world its own specific, determinate form or essence. It thus referred to the objective nature of things. Now it conversely means something like input of data into our subjective consciousness.

There is also a parallel to this reversal in natural philosophy. According to Aristotle, each thing desires to go home to its true place, the place that corresponds to its innate essence. Different things have so to speak different homes. A flame strives upwards because it wants to return to its true home, the *aithêr*, aether, the fiery heaven. A stone, by contrast, falls downwards, not, as we think since the days of Galileo and Newton, because of gravity, but because its home is the element of the earth. Things have here their own telos, dignity, center, meaning, their voice and claim, within themselves; we could perhaps even say they have a personality, individuality, a self of their own. With Galileo and Newton, this is totally different. Now there is a *universal* force, the force of gravitation which uniformly rules over everything in the world. The determining idea now is one of regular, rectilinear motion within a space conceived as a system of coordinates with one single center. Formerly, each thing, each person was a center of its own; it had its own gravity. Now gravity is all around them, and logically, psychologically, things have ultimately, figuratively speaking, been reduced to no more than point particles within its sphere of influence, or to positive facts. Their substantial individuality is gone. The theory of gravity is an egalitarian theory. The fact that subjectively, in what is called the lifeworld (*Lebenswelt*), in our personal experience, things still seem to have a dignity of their own is true only for the ego, not for the soul. What they are for *the soul* comes out most clearly only in our days, namely in the fact that they are commodities in the context of a throw-away and recycling society.

Gravitation and the one geometric space are correlates. The soul has left the level of individual phenomena, the level of things, persons, and in fact conquered a notion of *the systematic whole* for itself; it has risen to the level of the abstract universals of gravitation and space.

The soul's rise to a higher level as its coming down to earth

The rise to a notion of the whole in which all phenomena exist and can be seen entails the fact that the things that we can see have lost their soul, their weight and authority. All soul authority has moved from people and objects to gravitation and space as the abstract and invisible medium or container of all things. Things and people have been metaphysically foreshortened, *sublated*, in the double sense of this word. They have logically been negated, overcome, superseded, but as logically superseded ones they are empirically preserved as sublated moments within the newly conquered element of the abstract universal space and gravity.

This ontological devaluation of the visible world seems to be contradicted by the fact that it is precisely Renaissance painting that ostensibly concentrates devotedly on the visible world. It shows the holy figures as real people, as potential likenesses, and it situates the scene to be depicted in empirical-looking interiors, landscapes, or cityscapes (Fig. 15, Rogier van der Weyden,

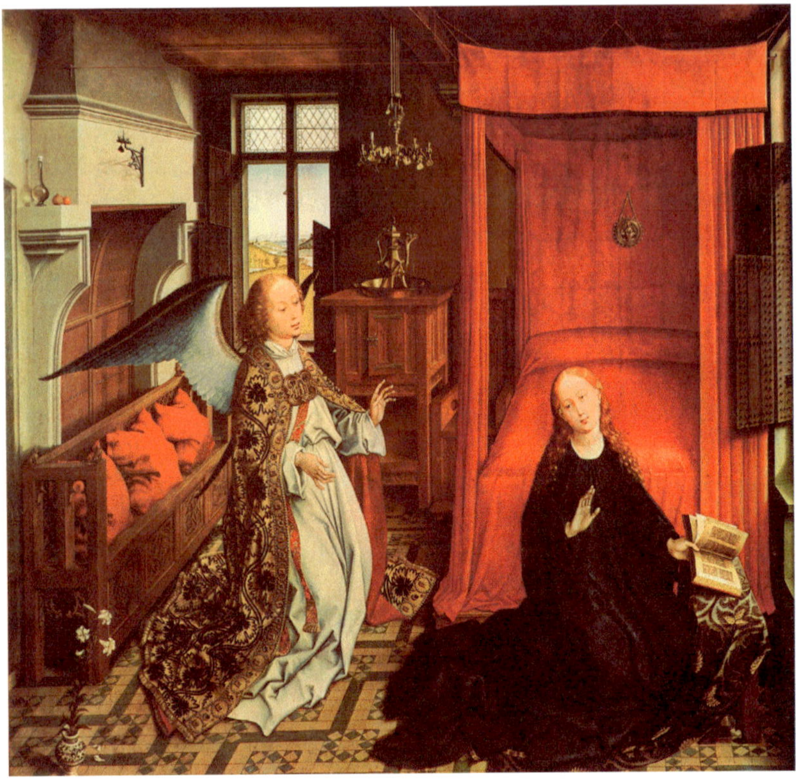

Fig. 15. Rogier van der Weyden, Annunciation, 1435, Paris, Louvre

Annunciation). Now there is all of sudden a real interest in the natural world as it really appears, and the painters struggle to do justice to all, even the most subtle aspects of the actual appearance of the natural world, such as the changes of the color of things in different light situations or in the far distance or through reflections of nearby differently-colored objects on a shiny surface. In addition, it is now the strong desire of the painters to show the world and everything in it as aesthetically beautiful. We can tell from their paintings as well as from many theoretical tracts written by them with how much devotion to nature and to every detail of the natural world these paintings were painted. In addition to its aesthetic task, painting also had an intellectual, almost scientific aspect, the search for the truth of nature and in nature. We can state that undoubtedly, all the artists' love and passion flowed towards the natural world in its appearance.

But now we have to realize that this is precisely the tell-tale sign for the psychological sublatedness and obsolescence of the things of this world. The dialectic of the situation is that while *ostensibly* and *explicitly* the human painters' whole attention and dedication went into the portrayal of the visible world and its phenomena (things as well as persons) in their beauty, *as far as the implicit logic is concerned* the soul's interest was precisely in the abstract truth of the invisible space that was the vessel for all phenomena. Implicitly, *an sich*, the soul is already on the higher level and has left beneath itself the level of things, the level also of the topics about which the paintings are.

And this is precisely why the artists now all of a sudden are *freed* to discover the natural world in its actual appearance. Only because the soul now has invested itself in space as the general container of whatever is and because the objects in that container have *ipso facto* become psychologically irrelevant or neutralized, can these objects become the explicit center of the artist's and the viewer's attention and love. But we must not forget that precisely in the explicit depiction of and arduous devotion to the visible natural world in its beauty, the artist and his work serve in truth, although unwittingly and only implicitly, the realization and rule of space as such. Linear perspective means: space is the actual topic, but it is the soul's, not the artist's topic.

What does the discovery of space mean psychologically? It means that the soul had become conscious of itself as the realm or space of consciousness as such, as the general space or "container" for all contents of consciousness, for all individual perceptions and ideas, all knowledge and all memories. Geometric space is the way consciousness itself can show itself in painting. Space is the symbolization of consciousness. If we call those contents—all possible contents—the semantics of consciousness, then the soul's having risen to the level of an awareness of consciousness itself could be called the soul's attainment to a consciousness of its own syntax. The I has become aware of itself as I.

But the other side of the rise to the fundamentally higher level of consciousness as such is the soul's descent from heaven, from being up in the clouds. *Now* the soul had come down to earth. And this is mirrored in its explicit concern with the natural world in its naturalness and actual empirical appearance. Man now had psychologically arrived in the empirical world. We see this, for example, in such paintings as that of Rogier van der Weyden (Fig. 15, Annunciation) that situates the sacred mystery in a concrete and very realistic domestic environment.

This change does not consist of two opposite movements, one up to the awareness of the abstract notion of consciousness and one down into empirical reality. *The soul only comes down to earth by rising to a higher level of consciousness.* It is one and the same movement, which we therefore might better have to comprehend as a differentiation, separation, bifurcation of what previously had been one single amalgamated soul condition. Let us look once more at this condition.

Medieval man had not been capable of deeming the actual likeness of people worthy of depiction or of devoting himself to the actual appearance of the natural world because on the one hand the sense of reality was entirely and exclusively absorbed by the universal, by the concept, the type. The universal concept was the possessor of the attribute of realness. On the other hand the universal concept during the Middle Ages was not anything totally abstract and purely syntactical like space as such. Space is just the *empty form* for everything, logically negative. No, the concept was absolutely concrete, it was the universals in the sense of the medieval realism regarding universals as well as the sacred mysteries of the Biblical stories and the stories of saints, or it was the numinously loaded ideas of "king," "emperor," "pope," "bishop," or holy relics and symbols, in other words, it was in itself semantic and imaged, a concrete universal. The sacred stories dealt with bodily figures and events and on top of it were quite concretistically thought to be historical, empirical.

This means that instead of a true transcendence and otherworldliness, instead of a duality of worlds, namely the empirical visible world here and the invisible transcendent world somewhere else, we find here a situation in which there is only one single theater or stage, one and the same world, so that in this world the concrete universal with its overwhelming impressiveness and authority absolutely outshines and obliterates all the personal, individual, empirical realities—both all the ordinary real individuals, the real common people, who in contrast to the saints, kings, popes, bishops were not the actual presence in this world of the universal, *and* the individual natural appearance and particular *features* of real kings, saints, etc. The empirical is overlaid with, and disappears behind, the concrete universal. Everything individual was not truly real at all so that the actual natural appearance of things and persons was of no interest whatsoever.

But in the new situation the concrete universal divides. The amalgamation of the universal with the semantic and imaged is dissolved. The universal is purified, distilled, evaporated, becomes logically negative, so that it turns into the empty, hollow form of space as such. At the same time the semantic and pictorial is *ipso facto* released from out of the former amalgamated or concrete universal. The universal lets go of it. What is in fact visible is now free to take on its own reality and significance over against the empty container of space, within which it now merely appears. Because container and content have become neatly separated from and independent of each other, the actual empirical appearance (looks) of individual things and persons has become something real in its own right.

We can illustrate this by looking, e.g., at Raphael's *Sistine Madonna* (Fig. 16). Semantically and ostensibly, the figures are on clouds, in other words, in heaven, removed from this empirical earth down here. But logically and psychologically, those very clouds are quite natural, empirical, very earthly clouds, and the persons shown, despite their idealization, look like very real people. They are no longer painted concepts, generic types, but real individuals. In fact we happen to know that although the male figure on the left represents Pope Sixtus II (who did in 258 A.D.), his head is an actual portrait, the real likeness, of Pope Julius II (who died at Raphael's time, 1513). *Semantically* what is depicted is, as before, the sacred mysteries, but the *style* is decidedly worldly, *naturalistic*. The implicit style or the logic now contradicts the explicit message. The message aims for piety, but what one sees is depicted and imagined as ordinary humans, real *individuals* in the ordinary physical world, which in turn has the consequence that piety has now been reduced to a subjective inner feeling, an emotion. The only difference to the customary ordinary reality is twofold, the idealized aesthetic beauty *and* the unnatural, miraculous character of some of the semantic details. It is miraculous that one can stand on clouds as if they were something solid. But the miracle is itself shown in absolutely realistic, natural terms. In a similar way, Rogier van der Weyden's *Annunciation* (Fig. 15) shows the angel naturalistically as a normal human individual, but with the added miraculous feature of having large wings. But the wings are in themselves again very natural like wings of natural large birds. Painting now wants to create an *illusion*, where the word illusion means the absolutely natural appearance of what is at the same time supposed to be the opposite of the natural, namely the reality of sacred, heavenly mysteries. Raphael creates the illusion as if we were immediate *eyewitnesses* of this scene, which in turn makes this *semantically* impossible scene *logically* in no way different from ordinary life events seen by us. Only the content and *suggested* meaning is different. The sacred transcendent mysteries have been brought down into empirical reality, removed from the *decidedly non-spatial soul space* that had so evidently displayed itself in the medieval gold background paintings.

In Stephan Lochner's *Madonna of the Rose Bower* (Fig. 12) we have before us an in-between stage between the 13th century Italian *Madonna on a Throne* (Fig. 11) on the one hand and Raphael's and Rogier van der Weyden's paintings on the other hand. With the older Madonna, Lochner's picture shares the other-worldly gold background, but its Madonna does no longer have the unapproachable austerity of the 13th century Italian Madonna, her still rather *conceptual* depiction, but comes much closer to the natural, real-people appearance of the Madonna's in the other two paintings. In Lochner's foreground we also already get a suggestion of three-dimensional space, which contradicts the gold screen in the background of the same picture, inasmuch as a gold background precisely depicts the *negation* of space and the natural world. Lochner's painting therefore lets us witness part of the historical process in action, that process in which the new perceptual mode with its commitment to real individual things and persons slowly frees itself, sets itself off, from the strictly conceptual and generic medieval mode.

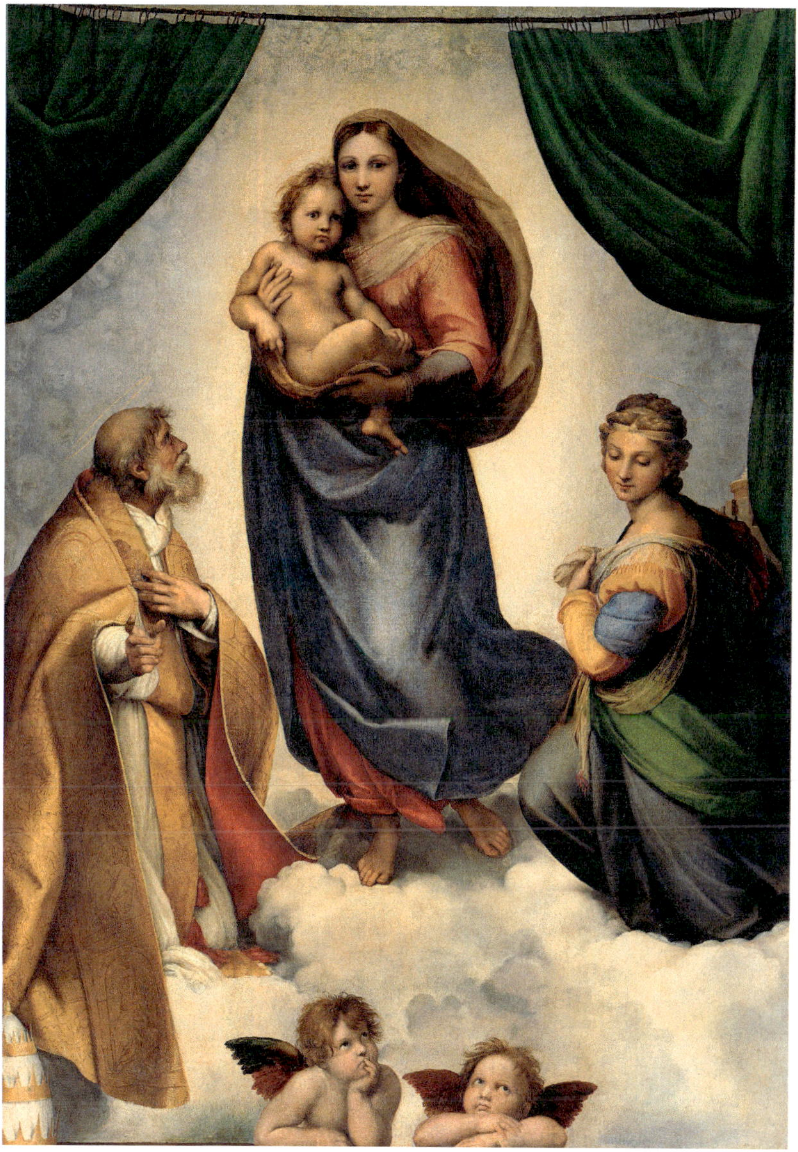

Fig. 16. Raphael, *Sistine Madonna* (Dresden).

The early-medieval saints, Madonnas, and divine figures were as depicted concepts shown as being eternal, transcendent.[94] The moment that the figures are fully individualized and natural-looking, they inevitably *appear* as mortals, even if semantically they are, like Rogier's angel, *supposed to be* eternal.

Raphael's painting also demonstrates the revolution of the gaze that I pointed to earlier. At first glance we notice that the Madonna seems to gaze at us. And so we could think that in this painting we have again the old medieval situation of our being hit by the gaze coming from the sacred figure(s). But first of all, the gaze depicted here is a *literal* gaze coming from biological *eyes* which see in the manner of sensory perception, not metaphysical, logical, psychological gaze, not a gaze through which the *truth* of the depicted sacred or metaphysical reality itself and as a whole penetrates us and pierces our very being. And then, the fact is that the Madonna does not really gaze at the viewer at all. The Pope depicted on the left side of the painting points with his hand to something outside the picture and the Madonna's gaze follows the direction of his pointing. To understand what it is that he points to we have to know that the painting had originally been placed opposite and facing a large Crucifix. Through the combination of the masterly composition of the painting and its original placement, it thus within itself referred to Christ's death on the cross.

But what for us as psychologists is most important to realize is that all these intricate relations have their place on the level of ingenious artistic refinement. They belong to the sphere of aesthetics, hermeneutic understanding, and subjective feeling, *above* the cold, objective, sober level of the soul's truth.

Another painting, now by Mantegna, *The Dead Christ* (Fig. 17), shows us the opposite, not the artful production of a convincing uplifting and heartwarming illusion of being eyewitnesses at a sacred event, but the absolute foreshortening of the Christian mysteries. Perspective always produces foreshortening. But here this foreshortening is carried to extremes and is applied to the central figure of faith, Christ himself. This dead Christ is therefore dead to the power of two. He is only a natural, human, all-

94 And thus as the property of the soul.

too-human corpse. His sacredness, his divinity is gone. Of course, the faithful Christian knows that Christ's divinity has precisely risen to heaven. But this painting does not show any trace of this, not even hint at it. So we could say that this painting displays the very separation itself of the medieval amalgamated or concrete universal that I have been talking about. In it the universal is present in its purified form, namely in the empty space as general container, space that becomes visual through perspective foreshortening. And conversely, the physical has been completely severed from the universal concept so that it appears in its naked naturalness.

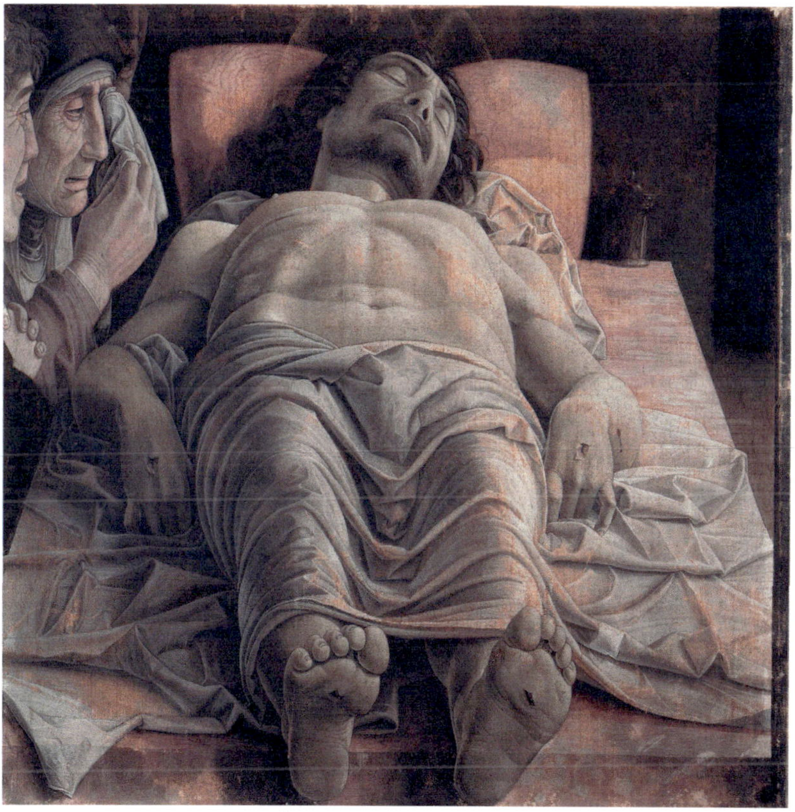

Fig. 17. Mantegna, Lamentation of the dead Christ. Milan (Brera)

The aesthetic beauty of the phenomenal world as evidence of the sublatedness of the phenomenal world

The condition of the possibility of aesthetic beauty is that the truth, the mythic, religious, or metaphysical authority, has gone out of the things and persons depicted, that those things and persons no longer of their own account gaze into the lives of people with a binding claim on them, as, for example, the pictures of Christ, Mary, and the saints did in earlier representations. The subject must have been released from them, emancipated from their demand to be devotedly acknowledged as events of truth. The subject must have gained a distance to them in order to now feel free to appreciate *aesthetically* what is shown in pictures. The obverse of the I's emancipation from the figures is the figures' fundamental sublatedness. The soul has no longer any stake in them. The *sublatedness* of what is seen as beautiful is the precondition of its beauty. What is seen as beautiful must have abdicated as psychologically relevant. What is experienced as beautiful is *ipso facto* beautiful *for the I*, for the subject and its feelings or judgment of taste, not for the soul, whose commitment is to truth and its very different (namely not aesthetic) sense of beauty. The things now represented are beautiful, beautiful in their external appearance, not ontologically in their being as the actual manifestation of truth.

In the (aesthetic) beauty of the depicted world it is the I that celebrates itself by giving the natural world a transfigured, idealized appearance on its, the I's, own authority. It is the I that in idealizing reality celebrates its own triumph of having fundamentally risen above the empirical manifold to the superior level of space as such, the space *in which* empirical things and people exist, while formerly it was the soul that found its full satisfaction in the figures themselves—even if from an aesthetic point of view they were by no means beautiful. During the Renaissance, the singular significance of beauty is also evident from the fact that in its name the fine arts, *le belle arti, les beaux arts, die schönen Künste*, managed to emancipate themselves from the spectrum of all the arts, which during the Middle Ages had included the liberal arts mathematics, logic, and grammar as well as the mechanical arts and crafts. The fine arts had managed to attain to the absolutely elevated, indeed divine, status that it had from then on.

The rule of aesthetic beauty in art lasted throughout the time of the I, even way into the 19th century, and only with the emergence of "the ego's" seizure of power, visible in the art of classical modernity (most notably cubism and expressionism), this principle of beauty had been once and for all overcome, if it was not much rather again and again and ever anew intentionally systematically violated.

In the world of beauty, all individual things are fundamentally relativized, which makes their sublatedness visible in the paintings themselves. The precise way they appear—how tall they are in the picture, what side and how much of them is visible, the particular hue of their color, whether they are in the light or in the shade, etc.—is dependent on contingent circumstances, on where they are placed in space, what is in front of them, what time of day it is, where the light source is, how high or low the eye-point is, etc. In addition to linear perspective, the artists, especially Leonardo da Vinci and the Venetians struggled to master aerial and color perspective, the fact that in the distance things slowly take on a bluish hue and that their outlines lose their sharpness. Formerly, the figures shown had their independent, we might even say absolute, form, size, color, just as much as they themselves determined from which side they had to be shown, because all these aspects were dependent on their intrinsic natures, their soul importance, on the concept of them.

In order to underline the fundamental sublatedness and reflectedness of what is shown in Renaissance paintings, I now turn to that goldsmith, architect, engineer, and artist who is considered the actual inventor of linear perspective.[95] At some time during the period 1402-1404, he traveled to Rome with his friend Donatello, who had received his training as a goldsmith in the same goldsmith shop as he, and started with the careful study of

95 In the following I rely mainly on the brief account by Stefan Winter, "Ruin der Repräsentation", in: *Reality strikes back II: Tod der Repräsentation?* Hg. Kathrin Tiedemann / Frank Raddatz, Berlin (Theater der Zeit) 2010, S. 24-31.

the Roman ruins of temples and theaters, a study which, so it seems, had never been done before. On the basis of exact measurements he reconstructed their ground plans and front views. And this work slowly enabled him to *picture in his mind* how ancient Rome must have looked prior to its destruction.

In this his picturing something in his mind we see something very new at work. It is what in philosophy will be called *repraesentatio*, representation, German *Vorstellung* (a "placing before the eyes of the mind"). It is what we do when we imagine something. Representation literally means the making present again (in and for the mind) of something that is not present of its own accord. This is exactly what Brunelleschi did and what was revolutionary: he gave a new presence in his mind to ancient Rome that in reality had been ruined for centuries. Through a mental image, Brunelleschi created the illusion of looking at Rome how it actually had been. He focused on the optical impression of how Rome must have looked. It was *as if* he saw ancient Rome despite the fact that he did not really see it.

What he produced was in itself contradictory. On the one hand, it was his free fantasizing (and thus utterly subjective, "inner"). On the other hand, this fantasizing was based on and bound by empirical evidence, on his exact mathematical surveying and reconstruction work, and as such it was an essentially disciplined fantasy. And the disciplining of his fantasy activity was required for, and had the purpose of, coming close to the actual empirical looks of what he imagined, the literal optical sight of ancient Rome, the historical sight of the city at the time of the Roman emperors. This new way of imagining showed something to the mind that was decidedly known by this mind to be, and even meant to be, obsolete, historical, the literal-factual truth of an irrevocably bygone past. Inherent in this mental picturing was thus an "as if," an unsurmountable distance, here the distance of 1,400 years. The prefix "re-" in "representation" gives expression to this fundamental distance, to the fact that inherent in this kind of picturing is an admitted irrevocable leave-taking from the very thing that is represented. Admittedly it is *logically*, *psychologically* dismissed and as such sublated, even while *empirically* and *psychically* it is precisely given a vivid, possibly even emotionally exciting presence in the mind. "Sublated" does not mean totally absent, forgotten, gone. It means precisely preserved and present, but present only as a subordinate moment, content, aspect within a new truth, not as a truth in its own right.

This kind of imagining or representation is totally different from what painters in the early Middle Ages did. The painter of the illumination of John, the Evangelist, in a Gospel of around 1150 did not *imagine* John; he was not interested in showing us how John might actually have looked. He was not at all interested in the optical appearance of his historically correct sight. Historical knowledge and archaeological studies would not have helped the painter. He did not *re*-present St. John, which means to create the vivid *illusion as if* we saw him how he actually might have looked in his own time. The latter's actual looks were absolutely uninteresting. The painting by our painter was not a pictorial reconstruction ("*re*-presentation") of a bygone past. Instead, it made Saint John immediately *present*. It confronted the viewer not with Saint John's looks, but directly with *him*, him as a religious or metaphysical truth, him with his claim on us, his claim on our faith and devotion. It showed him in his truth, his spiritual essence, him as concept.

The new type of re-presentation, the first occurrence of which we may have before us in Brunelleschi's imaginings, does not necessarily presuppose something that is historically bygone. The essential sublatedness of the very contents of what is represented, i.e., pictured in the imagination, can also be shown in something that is still a present reality. Here I turn again to Brunelleschi, namely to his famous experiment of 1415 or so which is often seen as the very beginning of linear perspective.

After his excursion to Rome, he had returned to Florence, where he continued and refined his mathematical surveying and measuring procedures, and opened the way for the application of mathematical construction to architecture and painting. The experiment I alluded to was described by his biographer, Antonio Manetti. Brunelleschi painted a small panel showing the Baptistery in Florence as seen from the central front gate of the as yet unfinished cathedral. The special thing was that at the vanishing point of the painted panel he drilled a hole. Now he determined that one should look through this hole from the back side, i.e., the unpainted side of the painting. And then one was supposed to hold, on the one hand, a mirror at the exact distance that proportionally corresponded to the distance between the Baptistery and the cathedral and the size of the painting, on the other hand. So the viewer saw the *reflection* of the painting in this mirror, and then, as his biographer says, the Baptistery appeared to the viewer "as if he would truly see it how it really is" (*che si videssi 'l proprio vero*). The experiment had the purpose of creating the absolutely convincing *illusion* of seeing the real thing. (It already points ahead to the *camera obscura*.) The aim of creating the illusion of seeing the real thing is tied to sensory perception, not to *imaginal* (or mythic) seeing.

This experiment is more than an isolated curiosity. Much rather, it again shows us the general logic of representation, *Vorstellung*, as such. Neither the real thing, the Baptistery, nor the painting is looked at directly, but is re-presented. You start out with the reverse side of the painting, in other words, with a negation of it. You turn away from it. But then you look at it indirectly through its reflection in the mirror, and you look at it as something sublated. Thereby you both *re*-presented it *after* having turned away from it and you explicitly placed the picture in front of yourself (*vor-stellen*).

From then on, all painting was to be implicitly what Brunelleschi's experiment made explicit. The painters had to paint the improved, idealized *illusion* of reality; the paintings had to have the mirror and the looking-at-the-reflection in its very style. Beyond what this means for the art of painting, the described procedure makes also explicit for us the logic of the so highly esteemed *image* in psychology. The modern psychological image is twice removed from the soul's truth. On top of the sublatedness that is anyway inherent in the image as it was established by Renaissance art, the psychological image is the sunken, sedimented form of the formerly great cultural heritage of the Renaissance. At a time when on the cultural level, the level of the so-called great artists, writers, inventors, and thinkers, representation has long been obsolete and superseded, it has finally seeped down to the level of the private felt experience of ordinary individuals.

In a way, Brunelleschi's whole experiment seems of course absolutely pointless, if not absurd. Why go to all this trouble if as a Florentine you can simply stand at the cathedral gate and see the real Baptistery right before your eyes? With this experiment, you not only turn away from the front side of the painting, but also from *what* the painting is the depiction of. At work in this whole move is a fundamental negation, *separatio*, a leave-taking or dismissal. What you see in the mirror is fundamentally sublated. One might perhaps think that this experiment is supposed to make this experience (of seeing the Baptistery as if it were absolutely real) accessible even to those who are not in Florence or for those times when one is not there. But I think it means much more.

The deeper psychological goal and function of this experiment is *the fundamental transformation of seeing as such* from immediate seeing and immediate presence to representation, reflected seeing. The immediate sight has to be rendered logically obsolete. From now on the sight *of the real* that the *painting* offers, i.e., the painted *illusion*, is the higher reality, higher and more true than the real thing itself. This is also why in the competition between the different arts for highest rank painting was from now on for a number of centuries indubitably considered the highest and most exemplary of the arts, higher than poetry (which is why Horace's *ut pictura poesis* remained the much discussed ideal for poetry during the Renaissance and the Enlightenment). And conversely, through this aimed-at transformation of seeing as such, and in the long run of all our seeing, even the immediate seeing of the real thing, was to become *representation*, seeing reality as "paintings", as what now, centuries later, in psychology is called images, as once and for all sublated.

In a way, this radically new type of seeing may already have occurred three quarters of a century prior to Brunelleschi, in April 1336, when Petrarch climbed Mont Ventoux for no other than aesthetic reasons. At that time it was absolutely unheard of that a person would climb a mountain unless there was a very strong practical reason for it, such as a strategic or administrative purpose. Petrarch may well have been the first mountaineer. At any rate, he climbed up this mountain out of idle curiosity, just for the pleasure of seeing and enjoying the impressive sight it offered. And immediately after his descent he in addition made *literary* use of his subjective experience by writing his famous letter about it to his fatherly friend Francesco Dionigi of Borgo San Sepolcro. His seeing was already fundamentally emancipated seeing, free-floating seeing just for the sake of personal enjoyment, and his turning it into a subjective experience worthy of being preserved beyond its own time in a piece of *literary writing* once more underlines the sublatedness of what was seen.[96]

The subject as *alter deus*

I have so far concentrated on the internal differentiation that happened within the image as it had been in medieval times, the differentiation between and separation of space as empty vessel, on the one hand, and object or content, on the other hand, which is in a way a vertical differentiation inasmuch as space is the superordinate form that contains the semantic contents as sublated elements within itself. Now I want to discuss a second distinction, one which goes in a horizontal direction, but not from left to right or vice versa, but from front to depth. One main point of perspective in art was the possibility to give the illusion of depth on a flat surface. The medieval depictions had optically been flat. (Of course, they did not need to show optical depth because they were deep in a psychological sense; they directly portrayed the revealed truth, the soul's highest truth.) Paintings in perspective, both those showing architectural sights or interiors and those with landscapes, pull the viewer's gaze into the far distance. We speak

96 The fact that James Hillman celebrated this event of Petrach's climbing Mont Ventoux in his fundamental book on psychology, *Re-Visioning Psychology* (1975), reveals much about the deeper sense and the inner reality of the concept of *image* in imaginal psychology and about imaginal psychology as a whole. (By the same token, he thought that the emergence during the Renaissance of perspective in painting, whose decidedly, if you wish, "monotheistic" and "I" character I have shown, could be interpreted as a sign of a new consciousness of the soul's depth dimension, a closer participation "in" the "reality" of the image, and a new awareness of the soul's multiplicity, its several points of view, and that it thus could be seen as a support for a polytheistic psychology. The topic of perspective and depth, namely, the illusion of depth, is discussed in the following chapter.)

of vanishing lines and vanishing points because it is inherent in the logic of perspective that it ultimately makes visible reality vanish in the distance, in infinity.

The counterpart to this vanishing of the objective world presented in paintings in the far distance is that the subject as viewer of the depicted world in front of the painting comes to stand fundamentally outside the picture and vis-à-vis it. Both the vanishing point and the eye point transcend the picture. By contrast, at the time of medieval paintings there was no subject that, as an I, faced the painting from outside, with the intent of aesthetic appreciation. No, what later would become a subject was conversely drawn into the world of the painting, absorbed into the sacred reality it depicted. Reality enveloped the soul completely. Man's in-ness in the painted revealed truth, in ritual, and also in the world as such prevailed. But now, with perspective, the subject emancipates from what is seen and gains a clear distance to it (we already discussed the sense of aesthetic beauty made possible by distance). The subject becomes something in its own right vis-à-vis both the painted reality and real nature itself.

Emancipation here means that in and via the process of developing seeing in terms of spatial perspective and in and via the ritual of again and again painting pictures with perspective, this emancipated subject is *produced* for the first time. Emancipation does not mean that there had always already been an existing subject which, however, had formerly merely not yet been emancipated, and that all the subject did now was to shake off its fetters. The emancipation I am speaking about is the first-time fabrication of that very thing which emancipates itself, a first time creation by means of the *ritual* of subjecting our seeing to linear perspective. Or the other way around: only in and through the act of its emancipation this (emancipating) I or "subject" is *made* in the first place. It is autogenetic. The act and the agent performing the act are equiprimordial. This is why the fabrication of the I happens in a ritual. The I is the product of the soul's *opus*, namely the *opus* of the soul's transformation and *further-development of its self-knowing* and of the corresponding self-manifestation.

The subject became the sovereign owner of the gaze. We already talked about this revolutionary shift. We also mentioned that it meant the expropriation of the gaze coming from the painted sacred figures or scenes and the appropriation of it by the subject. But it is even more. Ultimately this appropriation of the gaze amounted to a *theft of God's gaze*, which comes out most clearly in Leon Battista Alberti in the motif of the eye-emblem, which, originally the property of God, was now claimed by the near-divine artist for himself.

It also comes out in Alberti's interpretation of the myth of Narcissus. Narcissus was interpreted by him as the inventor of painting. As the new Narcissus, the artist appropriates the world in his own gaze. And Brunelleschi's experiment can serve us as the best illustration. The world (here pars pro toto represented by the Baptistery) appears *between* the picture of the Baptistery previously painted by Brunelleschi and the mirror. It is sandwiched between them, encased in a precursor of the *camera obscura*. The subject embraces it because it is in front and in the back of the visible world. The world as seen and depicted by the painter has logically become a priori completely interiorized, surrounded by the subject. It is the subject's own mental property. Illusion, a playful conjuring up of an impression! However illusion not in the negative sense, "nothing but illusion, i.e., deception," but rather illusion as the proof of the subject's having conquered the world, having made it its own object, a property of the mind.

We must understand both the Narcissus motif and Brunelleschi's experiment as *symbols* rather than taking them literally as self-sufficient individual ideas, events, or procedures. As symbolic for something larger than they, they express a whole mode of experiencing the world, an entire metaphysical stance towards the world and not only something particular imagined or performed *within* the world. Seen literally, Brunelleschi's experiment still has the real Baptistery outside itself. It seems now that we have two Baptisteries, the real one and the one experienced in the mirror reflection of the painted one. But in reality, what happens in the Renaissance is that the mirror-image of the painted Baptistery psychologically slowly *replaces* the real one. The painted-picture/mirror relation is now the sandwich around all reality. The world has really been "done in," interiorized or integrated into this superordinate relation. Or the other way around, this relation has become the embracing frame around all visible reality. This also underlines once more the sublatedness of the whole phenomenal world as well as the fact that the soul has indeed advanced to the standpoint of the surrounding container of everything.

This analysis would already be enough to show why the subject as artist experienced itself as *alter deus*, a second God (as the *Corpus Hermeticum* puts it). Whereas previously, artists were seen as simple craftsmen and usually remained anonymous, now the artist turned into something divine, a genius. Emperor Charles V even bent down to pick up Titian's brush when it had fallen down and handed it to the painter. Why divine? Because if early modern man as artist had indeed become the new Narcissus, his seeing the world was much like God's seeing the world. For God, the world is his own creation. It is not an external fact outside of him, but rather his own idea in his eternal mind.

The divine aspect of early modern man as artist becomes even stronger when we consider that the artist is now also considered *creative*. No medieval artist would have felt to be creative. Only God was creative. The artist was merely the recipient and pictorial recorder of God's revelation. But now art is all of a sudden seen as creative work. In philosophy, this insight into the work of the artist as being more excellent than a mere *mimesis*, a mere imitation of nature, was already expressed by Nicholas of Cusa. And Leonardo da Vinci wrote in his diary, "The fine art is of such excellence that it does not only turn to the phenomena of nature but *produces infinitely more phenomena* than nature produces."[97] And in his *Trattato della pittura*, he wrote, "If the painter wants to behold beautiful things that move him to love, then he has the power to *call them into being*, and if he wants to see monstrous and frightful things *he is lord and God over them*."[98] However, lord and God over them, we might need to add, only over them as their illusionistic representation. The work of the artist in the Middle Ages was merely religious *service*, the service on the part

97 Leonardo da Vinci, *Philosophische Tagebücher*, ed. by Guiseppe Zamboni, Hamburg 1958, S. 83. (My translation and emphasis.)

98 Leonardo da Vinci, *Trattato della pittura. Das Buch von der Malerei*, Vienna 1882, n. 13. (My translation and emphases.)

of a child of God. The work of the artist from the Renaissance onwards is in itself *semi-divine*.

God's world

One might conclude from our discussion that what happened here amounted to a terrible inflation, to man's identification with God, which in turn would imply an absolute godlessness inasmuch as then man would have taken the place that formerly had been God's. Analogously, my comment that Mantegna's picture of the dead Christ showed him as nothing but dead might induce one to think that the other side of such an identification with God is an utterly secularized stance. By the same token, if now the sacred figures are completely individualized and look like other mortals, only perhaps a little more beautiful, idealized, we could think that the soul's coming down to earth was tantamount to the loss of real transcendence, indeed, that deep down, logically, God was already dead, even if *semantically* he was still celebrated in words, paintings, and rituals.

I had also pointed out earlier that what is shown in the paintings of the Renaissance and thereafter belongs to the sphere of aesthetics, hermeneutic understanding, and subjective feeling, *above* the cold, objective, sober level of the soul's truth. Does this mean that the soul's truth had altogether been lost and that one was now only concerned with an empty semblance of truth, with mere words and subjective-semantic belief-systems?

To think so would be completely wrong.

God had not been dethroned. God was not yet dead. Man had not usurped His position. God remained the ground of nature and precisely also the very ground of the creativeness of the artists. The Renaissance, and the centuries that followed it, were by no means anti-religious or anti-Christian. The depictions of individualized figures, the merely semantic message, and the paintings' addressing primarily only our subjective feeling were still truly backed up and authenticated by the soul's truth; the knowledge that this earth and we ourselves were part of God's creation was unshaken; there was still the unchallenged fundamental difference between the sublunar world and the firmament above, which with its planets and fixed stars was *visible daily evidence* of the eternal; the Christian faith was indeed the "faith of the *world*" (Hegel) and not the private belief-system of certain individuals.

The idealization and sweet beauty for example of Raphael's Madonnas is not kitsch. The subjective feeling and the aesthetic appreciation were by no means already the modern ego's nihilistic feeling, driven by its greed to fill its essential vacuity with ever more momentary excitement, entertainment, and felt experience or with "meaning" and ideologies. We are here in the sphere of the I of the early-modern period and not in that of "the ego" of modernity. The I lived a truth and lived from within truth. Maybe it is easier for us than from paintings to see this, or rather: *hear* this, in such an example as the music of Johann Sebastian Bach. The texts of his cantatas and oratorios are often rather naive and sentimental, clearly appealing to a subjectivized feeling, to the I. But the strength and convincing power of his *music* shows that the soul's truth is here in full force and backs up and authenticates those naive feelings.

The discrepancy that we detect must therefore not be explained as the sign of a loss of truth, but much rather as the articulation of the further-development of Christian consciousness, which shows in a move in two opposite directions, (a) as an upwards move to the level of logical form or syntax, a move in the sense of an alchemical refinement, sublimation, of the soul's truth itself, and (b) as a coming down to earth of the soul's truth *in the spirit*, as part of the Spirit's realization, part of the *Incarnation*. That "God became man" and "the Word became flesh" shows in the fact that the sacred events are now depicted in concrete individualized (no longer generic-conceptual) form, in terms of our earthly perception.

We have to be aware of the dialectic of this move. It is the Incarnation, "God's coming down to earth, becoming man, becoming flesh," which allows God to lose all his human, all-too-human qualities (so characteristic of the Homeric gods as well as of the jealous Old Testament God) and to rise into the lofty height where he is Spirit and Love in an alchemically "distilled," no longer natural sense. He (and along with him the soul's truth as a whole) is not humanized, naturalized, secularized. And just as God is freed of his natural, all-too-human properties, the human being is conversely relieved of having to try to literally embody special higher mythic or sacred roles.[99]

The "becoming flesh" paradoxically can only happen as its seeming opposite: a logical ("distilled") transformation, not a natural(istic) change ("in the flesh"). The Incarnation is the realization (the becoming real) of the *Word*, the *Spirit* as the third person of the godhead, not the realization of the flesh. It is precisely a logical or form change, not a semantic change. The (b)-aspect of the move—the Incarnation—is in itself an alchemical transformation in the sense of (a). Figuratively speaking: Pentecost *is* the real Christmas; only through Pentecost and within it can there be Christmas (the birth of the Word in the world, its incarnation) in the first place; and only at Pentecost is the Incarnation complete. And historically ("in the flesh"), the emergence of the I during the early-modern period *is* the event of Pentecost, Pentecost as a *real event* in the *empirical history* of the soul, not merely as a quasi mythical, imaginal, or archetypal and thus timeless *story* or *image* (in the Holy Writ or in the creed of people).[100]

---

99 This became historically manifest through the Reformation which abolished the literal roles of monk or nun and the literal roles of priest and pope, while conversely comprehending every believer *tel quel* as "priest." Priesthood had become incarnated, had come down to earth, while simultaneously having become distilled, vaporized: an invisible *logical* status of (any) ordinary man instead of a social role of a few select consecrated persons.

100 This is a point where it becomes apparent that an *imaginal psychology*, in other words, a psychology that on principle defines the basic activity of the soul as (and thus restricts it to) imagining, is deficient. It excludes from its vision at least one whole half of psychic reality, the soul's need to "catch up with" its "pro-jected" imaginings, its myths and stories, in order to bring them home to itself, to integrate them into the very form or logical constitution of consciousness. This latter process is the soul's "alchemical" *opus*, an *opus* performed in and as the process of history. Imaginal psychology tends to see the images as the supreme result. But the myths and images are only the intuited prime matter in its initial physicalness (in the naturalism of the imagination), only the starting point for the soul's actual alchemical *Work* that only begins once there are "projected" images as its prime matter. Imaginal psychology does not only *deal* with images, but on top of it also tends to *conceive* them "platonistically" in imaginal terms (as abstract universals and as timeless) and to freeze them in their imaginality and timelessness. Showing too much of a soft spot for the innocence of the imaginal and being too narcissistically infatuated with the anima, it shuns the brutality of seeing them "alchemically" as matter (raw material) for the Work. The dialectic of the

A similar dialectic to the coming-down-to-earth move appears on the higher, abstract level of logical form or syntax itself (the (a)-aspect of the move), which in painting finds its own expression in linear perspective as the condition of the possibility of *representing* that superordinate, fundamentally invisible space which encompasses as well as permeates everything semantic.

Let us here return to the subject and its eye-point, which remains outside and vis-à-vis the painting. This eye-point has its correspondence in the vanishing points in the painting itself. The vanishing points are those points in which all visible, finite reality is sublated in infinity. The viewer of a painting looks into the vanishing depth of the portrayed scene. Correspondingly we could say that in the back, or from behind the back of the painted scene, infinity itself—God's infinite mind—gazes forward towards the viewer. The creation of the reality of everything to be seen in the painting was the work of God's creation. The visible things—the semantics—are sandwiched between and embraced by thc human subject here and the supreme ultimate subject over there. The human subject can comprehend itself as an *alter deus* because as intelligence it knows itself to be a spark of the divine intelligence. In this sense, man had by no means become inflated in a pathological sense, but rather truly "in-spired." And because it was ultimately the spark of God's intelligence that was at work in the artist, too, the world that the artist depicted and that he also experienced outside of his art in nature was guaranteed to be both a beautiful and an intelligible world. The beauty of the world came from this inspiration, from this certain knowledge and faith that it was God's own spirit that was at work in man's finite intellect.

Work is that while (and through) ruthlessly working off the physicalness of the matter and thus vaporizing the matter, making it fine and subtle enough to enter the *form* of consciousness itself (rather than crudely being the external object of consciousness to be venerated), it slowly takes the matter down from the abstract ideal heights of images entertained (envisioned, "dreamed of", entertained) in the mind and brings it into concrete historical reality, into the actual form of the culture, truly incarnating it. Once this work has been achieved and the message of the image has been distilled and integrated, the mythic image in its original form has necessarily become psychologically obsolete (cf. Jung's notion of the death of symbols in the course of time). It has done its job. It has no message any more, or a message that is old hat for the soul.

In this sense we must now realize that the work of the painter was a pious ritual, after all. It was religious service. The religious character of a painting, however, did precisely no longer consist in and depend on the *literal topic* of the painting, on its semantics, that is, on its being an explicitly religious topic depicting the birth, life, crucifixion, or ascension of Christ, the stories of saints, or the Last Judgment. No, the religious character was independent of the content. It now was in the logical *form* of the painting as such, (a) in the fact that as governed by perspective it represented the world as permeated by infinity and aiming for, ultimately becoming sublated in, and indeed logically vanishing in infinity, and (b) in the intelligent harmonious order and transfiguring beauty of the world in its true natural appearance, a beauty that in itself was witness to the presence of the divine spirit in the natural world.

For this reason it was not enough for art to be simply mimetic, to imitate nature. It precisely needed man's creative power; it needed what is divine in the human artist, namely the art-creating intellect. This is why the new illusionist depiction is higher than a veristic imitation of nature: because in it, it is the creative intellect that possessed the power to reveal the divine order and beauty which is inherent in factual nature, but also to a large extent concealed in factual nature.

And this is also why art and science went closely together in this whole early-modern period, why the artist was *ipso facto* also a student of nature. Art and science had to devotedly study nature because nature is, as Nicholas of Cusa said, the *explicatio dei*. God himself is infinite and thus invisible. Therefore one needs to look into nature because as His own creation it is where the absolute becomes *manifest*. However, the phenomenal world *as such* is not the divine. The divine is the intelligent order and beauty that through science and art, and only through them, can be revealed as being inherent, but also hidden, in nature. Nature, as long as it is not studied and revealed, is the *deus implicatus*, but science and art reveal the *deus explicatus*.

Already long before the Renaissance, as early as 1266–68, the Franciscan Roger Bacon had written in the introduction to the fourth part of his *Opus majus*:

> Oh, how inexpressibly beautiful would the divine wisdom shine if all the geometrically conceivable things contained in the Holy Writ would be presented to us in bodily shape! ... Everything reported in the Bible we would perceive as if it were present. ... Therefore I consider nothing worthier of a scholar of God's wisdom than the evident depiction of three-dimensional forms of this type.

Because God is infinite spirit and as such on principle invisible, man as artist and scientist had to turn to nature and to visible things to discover him there. Concerning the paintings in spatial perspective we can say that they absolutely needed the phenomenal, the semantic in order to make space-as-such visible, representable. Without the three-dimensional appearance of things in space and their being inescapably being foreshortened, the newly gained sense of space could not realize and concretize itself; without them space and thus the new level of self-consciousness, of the I, that had been reached could not be represented and articulate itself. It is precisely by showing people and things as being subject to the inescapable fate of becoming foreshortened, in other words, as being subject to the irresistible pull of the vanishing lines which ultimately vanish in infinity, that the soul celebrates infinity, celebrates God. The fundamental *foreshortening* and *sublatedness* of the depicted reality and the painters' *loss* of the medieval painters' immediate conceptual knowledge of the divine truth *are* a gain of a *concrete* awareness of infinity, an actual sense of infinity (no longer infinity only as a word that, to be sure, strikes a deep chord in *the soul* and gives profound satisfaction to it, but remains absolutely transcendent to *our* understanding).

This is also what connects linear perspective with *infinitesimal calculus*, which, just as linear perspective, is also a discovery and invention of the early-modern period (Leibniz and Newton).

Infinity itself, the powerful dynamic of infinity, has come down to earth, has become psychologically real, and its transcendent shine can be seen in the ideal beauty of the world shown in the paintings. The soul's enormously dynamic pull into infinity in conjunction with the visible idealized beauty comes out most evidently and impressively in such illusionistic (*trompe-l'œil*) paintings that seem to transport us directly into heaven (Fig. 18, Martin Knoller [1725–1804], *Heaven*, Neresheim Abbey).

Finite and infinite intelligence

Whereas in the medieval status of the soul, God and the sacred figures could directly, semantically, be depicted as substantiated, thing-like beings, although in the unapproachable austerity of generic types and concepts, the soul had now attained to a status in which the divine has become alchemically refined, distilled, sublimated, evaporated—pure invisible spirit, no longer semantic, but logical form. The soul is no longer in the depicted religious *themes* themselves, but in their depicted *beauty* and in the seeing-in-perspective which is the establishing, the confirmation, and the pictorial expression, of the in-itself invisible, strictly syntactical unity-and-difference between the finite and the infinite. The soul

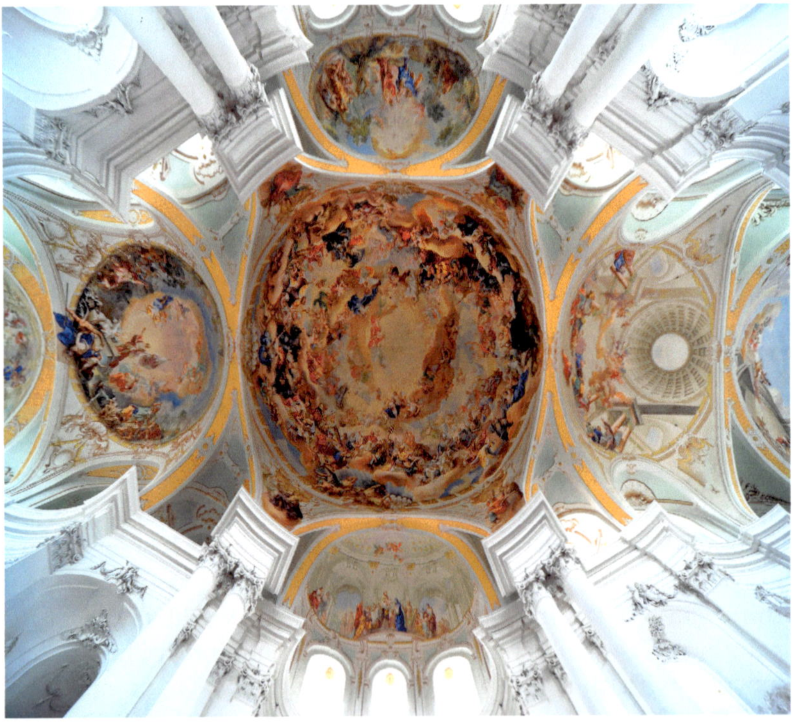

Fig. 18. Martin Knoller (1725–1804), ceiling fresco.
In the central cupola: Looking directly into heaven,
to the Trinity and the hierarchy of the Saints, 1770–75, Neresheim Abbey

has attained to this higher level. The I has become conscious of itself as I.

Whereas previously in the Middle Ages, the relation between God and soul was characterized by a fundamental hierarchical distance, a vertical gap between God and the children of God, now the difference, although it still exists, is no longer vertical and

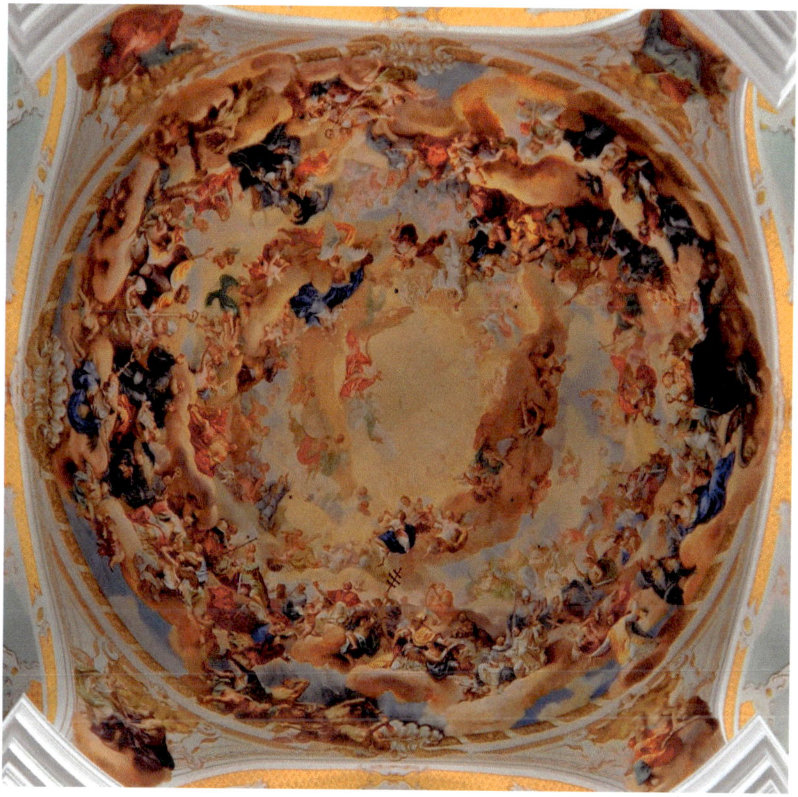

Fig. 18a. Enlargement of the central cupola fresco.

hierarchical, no longer qualitative and substantial, because on both sides it is the same spirit, the same intelligence, only different by degree. It is the difference of the visible semantic foreground and the disappearing horizontal depth, the difference of the eye-point in front of the painting and the vanishing point behind the painting, the difference of God and the second god, of the infinite intellect and the finite intellect. It is an infinite difference, but the finite mind and the infinite mind are connected by a seamless continuity and transition, as becomes visibly apparent from the undisrupted vanishing lines leading into infinity. God and the subject as *alter deus* are now, as it were, peers, despite their undisputed infinite difference, because they are on the same level, as we can see in the logic of perspective, and together they embrace the visible world between them.

Because on both sides it is the same intelligence, the soul has risen to an understanding of itself that is no longer characterized by total otherness. Now God and the subject are in a certain, limited sense peers. The soul has *begun* to comprehend that it is self-relation, that the infinity is its own internal infinity, and that it does not relate to a wholly Other, projected out and away as gods or God. And this is why it can now rightly comprehend itself as I, as subjectivity; it is why now the psychic I has also given itself the definition of I. The difference between the finite and the infinite has been seen through as a soul-internal one.

Being a child of God meant that there was a fundamental gap between God and man. But the counterpart of this situation was that the soul was in heaven, directly able to face the divine mysteries. Conversely, the realization that the soul is self-relation and as such "I" means that it has much more come down to earth, into empirical reality, although, we must not forget this, into a still *idealized, transfigured* empirical reality, but it has also lost its elevated, grandiose soul status of being in paradise.

Now it would be a grave mistake to confuse the subject as the second god with ourselves, with empirical man. The counterparts or correlates are *psychologically* the two intellects, not naturalistically a theologically imagined God and the anthropologically imagined human being. In the human artist it is "the genius," the divine spirit, at work in him who produces the works of art, not he, the empirical artist, himself. In the Middle Ages, the artist had been an ordinary human craftsman. It had been a human craft to paint. Now it required the presence of a genius, which was *logically* an element of the universal constitution of the I, but *empirically* showed itself only in certain select individuals and in them only at certain moments. Those select individuals were, as it were, the symbolic representatives of the logic of the I.

Whereas formerly God had still the essentially naturalistic and ontological form of an existing *being*, in antiquity the form of Father (Father Zeus) and in the Middle Ages predominantly the form of the Son (Christ), now this naturalism and semanticism had become impossible. Although in language the old substantiating word God continued to be used, the soul had at least implicitly, in principle, left its mode of ontologizing and advanced to the subtle mode of logic. God had become spirit instead of a being. The stage of the third person of the Trinity, the stage of the Spirit, had in principle, even if not explicitly, realized itself in the soul. This stage is the stage of logical form, of fluidity. It had realized itself as the I or the subjectivity that was the *spiritus rector* of the early-modern era, the era from about 1400–1800.

From the I to "the ego." A few hints by way of conclusion

Although the I is a historical *sine qua non* for the modern ego, this "the ego" is something else, something in its own right. Just as the I as a new *psychological* form of the *psychic* I came into being through a revolution of seeing, so also the ego presupposes another historical revolution, one that is even more radical than the previous one. But, in order to merely hint at this briefly, for understanding "the ego" it is necessary to describe its nature in two different steps.

(1) It is true that "the ego" is the psychological form of the psychic I that corresponds to a historical situation in which a completely new logic of being-in-the-world has come about. "The ego" belongs to the time of Industrial Modernity, to the time of a psychological situation in which God is irrevocably dead.

(2) But although this is true, what we call "the ego" in Jungian psychology does precisely not, like the early-modern I did for its time, represent the *truth* of this new mode of being-in-the-world. Rather it is its decidedly untrue form, a distorted, deficient form. It is an intrinsically neurotic idea. It came about because in it, the I, which is a universal concept, took itself absolutely literally, identifying itself with the positively existing individual. The semantic message "I" went to the individual person's head. The lat-

ter became inflated (now in a pathological sense) and thus autistic-personalistic. This shows in "the ego's" features, of which I will merely name a few. It is imperialistic, positivistic. It is sentimental, and deluded (calling itself "creative"). It is fundamentally nihilistic, trying to compensate its nihilism intellectually by ideologies and emotionally by vampirically feeding itself off the whole world by using it for its own felt experience, its fun, its entertain-

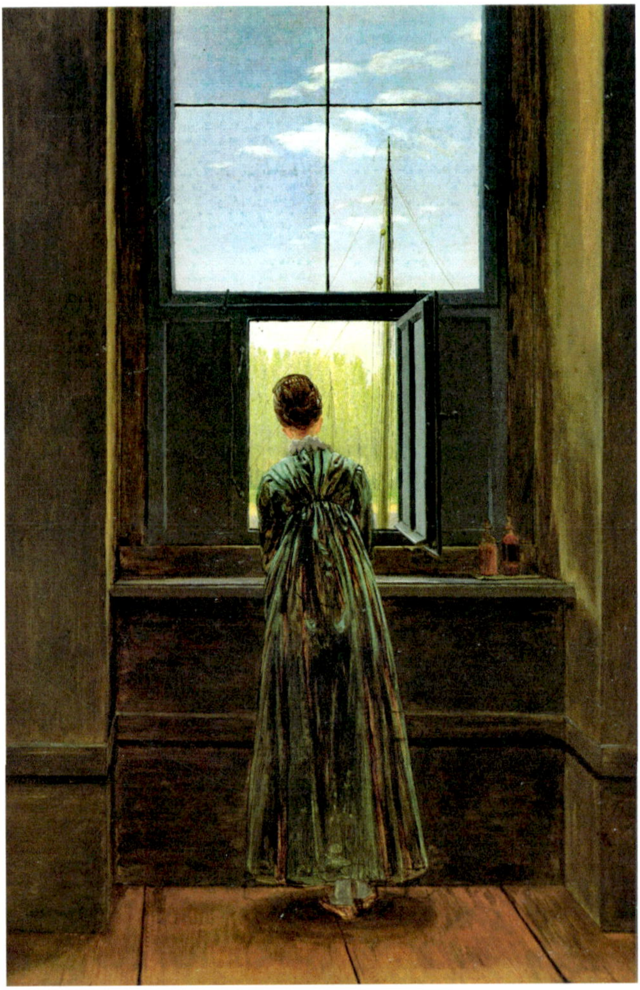

Fig. 19. Caspar David Friedrich, *Woman (the artist's wife) at a window*, 1822, Alte Nationalgalerie, Berlin.

ment, its fears and hopes.

We always have to remember that "the ego" is not a constituent part of the psyche. It is one of the self-definitions of the psychic I, and we would do well to liberate ourselves from this definition so that we can be "only that!"

Let me end by commenting on at least one painting from the time right around the first emergence of "the ego" that shows "the ego" in its truth. This painting by Caspar David Friedrich (Fig. 19, *Woman at a window* from the year 1822) shows that the subject now has become dispossessed of the gaze. The door to the soul and to what is important to the soul has been shut. Whereas the medieval painters let us directly see the sacred mysteries and with the gold-background paintings allowed us to look into heaven itself, and whereas the Renaissance painters spread out before us the ideal beauty of the world, we now only see the massive, impenetrable wall in its positivity and the completely covered back of a woman presumably looking out the window. No "aspect" in the sense of Brunner-Traut, no face. *What* the woman sees and if what *she* sees is worthy of being seen in the first place, or if it is not perhaps much rather just as positive-factual and boring as the walls that we see, is not to be known. It may be that the *woman* in the picture is still owner of the gaze. But at any rate we, the viewer, the subject, are not allowed to participate in her seeing. We see nothing of soul significance. We are blind, fundamentally unconscious concerning the soul's truth. This painting is the opposite of Knoller's *trompe l'œil*. It does not deceive the eye. It is honest. It forces the eye to see the bare and painful truth that there is nothing to be seen, but it makes this new truth that there simply is no soul truth to be seen any more all the more painful because through showing us a window and through a few suggestions of what might be outside, the picture tantalizes us by evoking a hope that it at the same time irrevocably disappoints.

Appendix:
A note on the needs of psychology

Friedrich's painting can also serve us as a wonderful illustration of Jung's intellectual starting point. Jung realized that if our direct gaze would try to go forward in the style of religion and metaphysics, it would inevitably run against an unsurmountable wall or at least a border to transgress which would amount to "the deadly sin of making metaphysical statements" (cf. *MDR* p. 70, *Erinn.* p. 75). But Jung wanted to rescue the gaze, the potential of our seeing the soul's mysteries, and so he turned around, away from the wall, of course not to the just-as-hopeless opposite wall, but to the one remaining new place between those two positivities: to our inner. He found a loophole, our dreams, which was supposed to be our salvation from the predicament, the salvation of the gaze. For through this loophole he believed we would be able to see the soul's truth encased in the *camera obscura* of the unconscious (or of its external replica, the *camera obscura* of the analytical consulting room) in its primordial form ("Urerfahrung"), much like Brunelleschi had made it possible for him who looked through the peephole in the back of his painting at the mirror reflection of the front side of his painting to see the Florence Baptistery "as if he would truly see it how it really is."

Because of Jung's clinging to the idea of "the inner" and the unconscious he could not fully prevent that his psychology remained or became psychologistic. Ultimately, his thinking could not overcome its naturalism because "the inner" forced him to give to the literal individual in his positivity downright metaphysical weight as the one essential and important factor.

Decades later, James Hillman realized that this turn to our inner, rather than providing direct access to the truth of the soul, was really only "the ego's" narcissistic self-mirroring. The real gaze into the soul was therefore precisely missed. His reaction to this insight was to turn back once more to the former orientation that had been systematically left by Jung, but now without any danger of thereby becoming metaphysical, because through his "re-visioning psychology" he had meanwhile made it intrinsic to the very form and definition of psychology as such that it did not believe and hypostatize ("literalize"), but only *imagined.* Instead of into our inner, Hillman wanted to look directly through "the window," in the hope of in this way restoring once more the Renaissance gaze into the divine beauty and soulfulness of the world.

His solution has, however, two problems. With his move he was able to save the gaze, but only for the price that it was no longer the gaze at the soul's truth. His move (away from both scientific or experiential knowing and from believing) to imagining amounted to the renunciation of truth as such. The second problem is that he ignored the fact that, as Friedrich's painting shows us, access to the window (in contrast to the loophole of dreams) was now explicitly blocked (something which had been clear to Jung), and that the view out through the window was now blocked precisely *by the anima herself* standing there and turning her back on us (something which Jung for his part had ignored, or else he would not have located the anima inside, in the unconscious, leaving the real world to the wolves, conceiving it as fundamentally soulless, as the world of ego-consciousness and its machinations). Hillman is right, the anima is in front of us. But he is wrong to think that the gaze could still go out through the window. It is the anima herself (and not only the hard walls of positivity, nor our forgetfulness of the soul) that obstructs the gaze.

In real life, we can push someone away or step beside the person so that we can both have a place at the window. Not so in dreams, in paintings, in the world of the soul. They give the complete and definitive picture. Therefore, all that was possible with Hillman's move was to *imagine* to be able to gaze directly into the world of the soul or at the soul of the world. What was possible was to imaginatively *identify* (become identical) with the anima at the window, which of course meant that this type of seeing was also only imaginal or imagined seeing, "as if"-seeing—the inwardized, sublimated, spiritualized, psychologized *trompe l'œil*, but now, in contrast to the *trompe l'œil* initiated by the Renaissance, a *trompe l'œil* no longer backed up by the soul's truth and by the logic of modern reality.

At the same time, the identification with the anima in her new position meant that unwittingly one got her turning her back to the subject into the bargain, to that modern subject that experienced the world of modernity and the *historical* changes brought by it. The awareness of the history of the soul was replaced by the idea of a timeless soul, and what in real life did not fit to this idea was categorized as part of a "fallen world" and as due to the fault of *our* forgetfulness of "the Gods."

Neither Jung nor Hillman dared to settle in the situation of the dispossessed gaze and to make themselves at home in the room with the massive walls. If the subject had left relentlessly behind the wish for the direct gaze into the soul's truth, without resentment and repressed longing, and had truly *settled* in this barren room, it could, figuratively speaking, fill the hard walls of positivistic fact with numerous pictures from our cultural past and with floor-to-ceiling bookshelves full of the treasures of literature, philosophy, theology, music scores, etc. In this way the subject could get authentic, vivid, inspiring access to the soul's truth, of course no longer direct access, but reflected access, an access in *Mnemosyne* which has a fundamental separation, a leave-taking within itself.

Jung wanted to rescue the direct gaze by interiorizing the *semantic substance* of the soul's truth (claiming, as it were, that the truth is in a literal inner, namely in our unconscious). Hillman wanted to rescue the direct gaze by interiorizing the aesthetic illusionistic *form* of the soul's truth ("imagining" in the sense and context of "the imaginal"; of beauty; image-sense, *aisthesis*; of "animal certainty"; of *anima mundi*), which meant that his interiorizing did no longer lead to a literal inner location ("the unconscious"), but to psychologizing as a style. Both saw the necessity of interiorization in our time. But both tried to get away with only a half-hearted or token one, namely with a literalized partial interiority, in order not to have to proceed all the way to the full inwardness demanded by the soul in that new status that it has reached in modernity.

Not only as long as the soul's truth had been ritual event, mythic epiphany, religious faith, or metaphysical knowledge, but also as long as modern psychology conceived it be it as inner experience or as imagining qua soul-making, the soul's truth remained fundamentally *exterior to itself* because it was event, epiphany, knowledge, inner experience, imagining always *for the human subject*. It was *facing* us, showing its front view, and it was what we would necessarily be upward-looking to. Both Jung and Hillman rescued the direct gaze of old by holding, each in his different way, the psychological down on the level of the contents, of the soul's semantics that faced us: *Urerfahrung* (Jung) and the image as the *ultimate* psychic reality, and therefore as *the* Ultimate, if not at times even as "Gods" (Hillman). They thus rescued the direct gaze not for the subject of the early-modern period, the I, but precisely only for "*the ego.*" *Malgré leur*, they feed "the modern ego" with what it craves for: the simulation of the experience of the gaze of old.

Jung, we could say, saw the back (of the anima), without seeing that it was (the back of) the *anima.* So he rescued the gaze by redirecting it inwards to look for the anima there. Hillman saw the anima standing at the window and looking out, but he did not see that it is her back that she turns on us. Each took only one half of the message. The message is both halves at once: yes, it is the anima, and yes, it is precisely her back.

Jung rightly realized that a turn-about was necessary. But he thought that the wall or the back means that the subject, that we, that our eyes have to turn around and now gaze into ourselves. But this is too easy, an ersatz for the psychologically required true bending back. It is a defense in the manner of acting out the rebound in our behavior instead of "remembering" it, or in the manner of literalizing instead of interiorizing it psychologically. This type of defense—letting the person (the human *being*), i.e., *ourselves*, bear the brunt and burdening it with the obligation to do what is needed, in order to spare our most precious *principle* or soul value, here the direct gaze, and protect *it* from having to change—is of course an all-too popular one. But that does not make it any better. Something ontological, a behavior on the part of the individual, has to take the place of something psychological, consciousness's awareness of the transformation of the soul's logic.

That it is the back that the anima turns on us means much rather that it is the *gaze itself* (not we or our eyes) that comes to a stop and is reflected into itself. The anima can no longer be gazed at and faced directly (for example, as the *anima mundi* in Hillman's sense). This is a logical, psychological change. It does not personalistically refer to a necessary behavior on our part. *We* do not have to do anything in this situation. We can stay where we are. *We* do not have turn around and from now on look into ourselves in order to reflect ourselves in the psychoanalytical mirror (as Hillman correctly realized). Rather, the gaze itself, the "objective" gaze at the anima, has to become a seeing from behind, a seeing that is in itself, in its logical form, negated, *in itself* turned away.

The real interiorization is thus (a) the interiorization *of* the gaze itself and (b) its interorization *into itself*. The soul's truth does not want to stay external to itself any longer: no longer the *object* of *our* seeing and upward-looking reverence or, conversely, the manifest depth of reality *facing* us. *It* wants to turn inwards. *It* wants to come home to itself, become interior to itself, which of course—for us, for the human subject—means the (logical, not literal) *departedness* of the soul's truth. What is departed no longer faces us. However, for the soul itself its interiorization into itself precisely means that it has become truly "objective" (truly "objective psyche"), now facing itself. For us it means the end of the direct gaze itself, the loss of immediacy and of the object of our upward-looking, or, to put it the other way around, for us it means that our access to it can only be a *second-hand* access. The fundamental departedness of the soul's truth—departedness as its logical character or mode, not as its literal absence, not as nihilism—*is* the realization and fulfillment of true interiority.

Psychology proper is the study of the *departed* soul, and the departed soul is the true soul. As long as there were ritual, myth, religion, or metaphysics, there was no need for and no possibility of psychology in our modern sense, as Jung had already clearly seen, and under these conditions the true home of the soul—the underworld, for example—had to remain *projected out* as an *imagined* place in the cosmos "out there", *somewhere* "under" the earth (or, in Christian times, up in Heaven, or metaphysically in "transcendence"), that is, in external reality and within a thinking in terms of spatial imagination (the difference between here and there). Now the underworldly, ancestral character of the soul—its departedness—is no longer projected and imagined. It has been absolute-negatively been inwardized into itself and thus come *home*, home *to itself*, to what it is in its truth.

The imagination was unable to *think* the departed soul. This has two consequences. The first consequence: It had to split what in truth is the one reality of the soul's absolute negativity into two, into form and content, logical departedness and substrate that is departed, negativity and positivity, and it thus literalized[101] or concretized both. It had to imagine an empty, containing *space* as the imaginal or literalized representative of the logical moment of negativity (departedness as such, absence), i.e., the underworld, Heavenly Jerusalem [or Hell, respectively], or more philosophically transcendence on the one hand and *entities* as representatives of the moment of positivity (literal dead souls dwelling *in* that space as negativity) on the other hand. This difference has disappeared on account of the interiorization. Each of the two have "died" into the other, because both have been deliteralized or alchemically distilled and "evaporated" into absolute negativity as such.

The second consequence of not being able to *think* the departed soul but staying stuck in the imagination is that it could not see the soul of and in the real, having to transfer the soul away from the here and now into the beyond of the ideal space of the imaginal. From the point of view of this ideal sphere, above all modernity appeared to psychology to be decidedly soulless, a Fallen World, both to Jung and to Hillman most of the time.

Having paid the full price demanded by the new status reached in the history of the soul, the stance of Mnemosyne does not try to escape modernity, nor does it need to wish to rescue or revive the externalized ("facing-us") soul in a curtailed form (namely as image deprived of its binding truth). This stance is not, and does not need, an anti-modern counter-program. Precisely by having paid the price this stance opened the door to true *psychology*, a psychology of true, namely logical, inwardness.

The access of the Mnemosyne stance to the soul's truth is—as the realized Incarnation—therefore again authentic, and at the same time very much down to earth and systematically uninflated,[102] because it is indirect, a priori distanced, reflected

101 For imaginal psychology, the imaginal or metaphorical and the literal are mutually exclusive opposites. But this is a superficial view. It overlooks that the imagination in itself necessarily literalizes. It logically or syntactically literalizes, while of course semantically expressly not taking its own images literally.

102 Even if both Jung and Hillman are not personally inflated, their psychologies are certainly systematically inflated (just think of certain of their essential

access—the simple study of the decidedly *this-worldly*, *empirically* accessible phenomena and treasures of concrete cultural history. This includes our ancestral past just as much as what is real in our present-day world. This is so because the latter can *psychologically* be viewed *as logically* being 'past': as in its *depth* and *inner essence* (in contrast to its pragmatic foreground aspect and from a utilitarian standpoint) being always already departed, not immediate.

An unpretentious awareness of the soul's truths, but an awareness with the power of the intellect and the depth of feeling. No mystification. No numinosity. No higher mission.

The other side of the soul's homecoming to itself and of its essential departedness for us is our human emancipation from the soul. We no longer have to, we cannot, ought not, wear mythic garments, cloak ourselves in some form of soul. We now have to be ourselves; we each have to stand on our own feet. Individuation. The soul set us free. The subject is relieved (or should I say cured) of its former pompous demand that it and its world ought to be *more* than "*only* that!" ❦

"categories," the heightened emotion of Jung's "numinous," the "myth of meaning," "the rescue of the world," etc.; Hillman's "Gods," "beauty," "*anima mundi*," for example).

Chapter Four

The Future Potential of the I

From *Psychic* Awareness to *Psychological* Consciousness

"Primitive 'awareness'" or the inferior state of being conscious

It was probably only through his intensive study of the writings of the medieval alchemists and the revolutionizing influence of the spirit, the hermetical logic, at work in the alchemical project that Jung was able to make the decisive move from his earlier still very much personalistic stance in psychology to the later psychology of the mature Jung based on the notion of the *objective, autonomous* (and thus no longer person-bound) soul. For psychology it was a crucial shift, because it is only through it that psychology could begin to come home to itself as psychology in the rigorous sense of the word. For alchemy itself, one of the first necessities was the dissolution of the *unio naturalis*. It happened in the alchemical opus through all kinds of *negative* operations or processes, such as *nigredo, putrefactio, fermentatio, corruptio, mortificatio*, but it is also at work in alchemy's self-interpretation, its theoretical idea of the very purpose of the Work. This idea is, for example, articulated in the alchemical statement: "*Quod natura relinquit imperfectum, ars perficit*". It not only talks of a pushing off from *natura*, the state of the givenness of the prime matter or whatever *is* (we could also say: from the state of its positivity and factualness), to *ars*, the state of producedness through the artful and thus artificial work of the *artifex*, the *adept*, his intervention in the natural process. The cited dictum also conceives this transition or transformation as one from imperfection to perfection. What is simply given, lacks something essential. It is incomplete. It needs the *ars*, the being processed, sublimated, distilled, for its own fulfillment and completion.[103]

Jung adduced this alchemical dictum, among other things, also for the description of the ultimate task of our working with dreams. "We have simply got to listen to what the psyche spontaneously says to us. What the dream, which is not manufactured by us, says is *just so*. Say it again as well as you can. *Quod Natura relinquit imperfectum, Ars perficit*" (*Letters 2*, p. 591, to Read, 2 September 1960). In my book *Working with Dreams* I have tried to elucidate the complex implications of Jung's statement and the alchemical dictum. But this dictum has not only consequences for our working with dreams. It implies something of general psychological validity, of crucial importance for the proper understanding of a (usually unseen) aspect of the very nature or definition of modern psychology in the Jungian sense, inasmuch as it teaches us about what the deeper *psychological* sense of "consciousness" is. The move from *Natura* to *Ars* implies on a first level the waking up from the sleep of the sleeping soul to waking consciousness. But on a second level it implies an even more radical shift relating to this waking consciousness itself, a fundamental differentiation within the very concept of consciousness itself, namely the distinction of ordinary, "*Natura*"-like (waking) consciousness from *psychological consciousness* in the strict sense.

In another passage, Jung performs this differentiation or distinction for us, even if in an entirely different context far away from our alchemical dictum and yet directly relevant to it, by distinguishing "consciousness" from "awareness". I have to turn here to the German original text, *GW* 11 § 638, and give my own translation, because the *CW* omits Jung's elucidations that are necessary for a German audience but not so much for the English reader. Jung speaks there of an "*inferiore Bewußtheit* [an inferior state of being conscious; this phrase is emphasized by Jung]", a

103 As the word "completion" indicates, "perfection" in this context must not be understood in the nowadays frequent utopian sense of supreme excellence or having reached an ideal state of absolute faultlessness. It means a phenomenon's state of having arrived at the full unfolding and realization of its potential.

Bewußtheit that "seems to be not much more than a primitive 'awareness'." Jung uses the English word "awareness", for which there is no German word. This is why he continues, "... We can circumscribe this term [awareness] with 'merely perceiving consciousness'". It is characterized by the fact that it lacks, as he adds, a "consciously reflected inclusion of the subject, whose individual existence is simply taken for granted [lit.: is unproblematic]", i.e., remains completely implicit or unconscious.

Examples of "awareness" in this specific sense of "merely perceiving consciousness" are such popular notions nowadays as gaining "body-awareness" (e.g., through Yoga or Feldenkrais, etc.), and the "higher awareness" gained through meditation.[104] A form of this psychic awareness, i.e., this "inferior state of being conscious", occurs even in animals, for example, as awareness of approaching enemies and natural threats, of the borders between their own and their rivals' territories. But animals lack consciousness, let alone "*psychological* consciousness". Another example is the mental state produced by so-called mind-expanding drugs, LSD, etc. These drugs are by no means what they have been said to be: *consciousness*-expanding! They only produce new (*psychic*) *awareness*, of whatever is experienced, together with the possible momentary feeling of intensive enchantment and intoxication.[105]

At another place (*GW* 11 § 272, again I have to use here the German edition and my translation), Jung likewise compares and contrasts "The unreflected, merely perceived state", on the one hand, with "the reflected and rational state of consciousness", on the other.[106]

104 Of course, meditation is also a highly cultured *artificial* method and thus *as method* or practice not a sign of *Natura*. It is an artificial method, but a method of preserving and expanding psychic *awareness* as perceiving consciousness, rather than producing *psychological consciousness*.

105 Drugs in primitive societies were different. In those societies the culture *as a whole* was on a level of the sleeping or dreaming soul, of (higher) psychic awareness, of "dreaming the myth". Certain drugs could successfully be used for enhancing in a deep and meaningful way this culturally established awareness as a *perdurable* personal possession, for example, in initiation processes. For the atomic individual in modern societies, by contrast, drug-induced experiences remain isolated, stray events, not backed up by collective knowledge, and thus truthless.

106 By no means the same, but nevertheless a similar insistence on the necessity of taking the "consciously reflected inclusion of the subject" into account and

So we have to make a fundamental difference between awareness and consciousness. But the crucial point here is that it is precisely the ordinary and hitherto prevailing concept of consciousness that is downgraded by Jung as not being true consciousness at all but in truth an "*inferior* state of being conscious" or mere "primitive 'awareness'", so that *his* concept of consciousness, namely consciousness in a psychological sense, is something completely different and new. It has its place on a logically higher level. We must beware of this equivocation and the ensuing danger of confusion.

The difference is not a matter of degree or quantity such as on a scale from dim to clear. It is a categorical difference involving a reversal (from ⟶ to ⟵). Awareness is *merely-perceiving consciousness*, merely *receiving* consciousness. It is passive (conditioned by impressions). It is "psychic", not "psychological". Jung calls it an inferior consciousness because it is not veritable consciousness at all. It is 'primitive' because it is a *natural* form of consciousness that lacks the "consciously reflected inclusion of the subject". Having acquired and now being in possession of, knowledge (knowledge in the sense of what we nowadays call "information" and "data") has nothing to do with psychological consciousness. It is merely an awareness. Much of the work even in the most advanced sciences happens on the level of what Jung named "inferior" or "primitive" consciousness.[107] With respect to it we could also speak of an "object (or content) consciousness". Psychological consciousness is something completely different.

The birth of a self-conscious subject

I will now try to prepare the ground for a better understanding of

the insistence on the in-itself reflective, polar (subject/object) structure of mental phenomena is contained in Jung's statement about the modern sciences, namely, that they "try to represent the results of their investigations as though these had come into existence without man's intervention, in such a way that the collaboration of the psyche—an indispensable factor—[*die unerläßliche Mitwirkung der Psyche*] remains invisible" (*CW* 10 § 498).

107 This means that "primitive" and "inferior" does not at all mean unintelligent or semi-consciousness. Jung's designations have to be understood in terms of a psychology with soul, not of academic psychology.

this difference and of its fundamental significance for psychology by pointing out some exemplary events in Western intellectual history in which the dissolution of the *unio naturalis* and along with it the birth of the self-conscious subject took place, which is the precondition for the possibility of the emergence of such a thing as a truly psychological consciousness.

Let us first take a look at Socrates, who took a radical step away from, or rather beyond, mere psychic awareness. By deliberately taking the completely artificial position of not-knowing ("I know that I know nothing"), Socrates has once and for all broken with the *unio naturalis*, his *natural* identity with all the knowledge that he had. It was not that he literally knew nothing. He knew thousands of things, the streets, the agora, the Acropolis of Athens; he knew his fellow-citizens, the difference between day and night, what wine and bread are, what 2 times 2 is, recent events in history, the myths and cults of the Athenian gods, etc. But all this knowing is now disqualified by him as not being veritable knowledge because it had naturally come to him of its own accord in the course of his living life. It was knowledge, we could say with our modern term, as awareness of "information" and in the status of givenness and passive receptivity.

His statement about not knowing is not a sudden insight, an idea that came to him. It is not a perception. It is a radical *act*, a doing, a deliberate artificial intervention: the total clearing away at one sweep of all tacitly assumed possession of knowledge. Socrates MADE *tabula rasa* and, disrupting the natural continuity of the mind, positioned himself on a zero point as the standpoint from which to proceed, one that does not exist *naturally* at all. This is a perfect example of an act of reflection born of human freedom.[108]

108 We may be reminded here of a centuries older parallel to this radical negation to a kind of zero point, but a negation not with respect to the topic of knowing, but of selfhood, that is recorded in the Odyssey. Held captive with some of his men in the cave of the giant Polyphemus, clever Odysseus answered, when asked by the drunk and drowsy giant what his name was: "Nobody". Apart from the fact that this witty answer afterwards proved helpful for Odysseus' escape, psychologically it shows the subject's capability to totally abstract from itself, to withdraw to the point of being nobody. This is a *determinate* negation in contrast to a total annihilation: Odysseus keeps his existence ("*being* nobody"), but in his self-relation and self-understanding actively sweeps away

With these comments I have only characterized Socrates' *act*. Now we need to look at what this act achieved or produced. More closely translated, his famous dictum reads, "I *know myself as* knowing nothing". Socrates' sweeping away all given knowledge led to a fundamental separation within knowledge between "the knower" of knowledge (the self-knowing Socrates), on the one hand, and the contents that are (allegedly) known (which in his case is of course precisely "nothing"), on the other. The knowing subject has become explicit as the place of knowing and as distinct from what is to be known. Prior to this, the knower had only been implicit; he had been completely submerged in, and had thus disappeared in, his knowledge itself as a simple fact, a compacted reality. It (I cannot really refer to this submerged knower as "he") had been totally dormant in all the specific instances of knowledge, all the ideas, images, feelings it contained. And therefore the knowledge, all these contents, ideas, notions, convictions, had not distinctly been felt as residing in the knower, but were tacitly assumed to have their actual place *in the reality out there itself that was known* in this knowledge. The mind was *in* the things and events of which it knew. Socrates' act pulled the knowing subject out of its submersion in and identity with its contents of consciousness and stripped it of all contamination with anything like content, thereby freeing it to *itself*, which means to being nothing else than the very zero point of knowledge. It is not itself a content, another known idea, but it is only an abstract logical form, an empty point. We could perhaps even say it is nothing but the concept of the "origin" of a system of coordinates for all possible concrete knowledge.[109]

The second and concomitant achievement of Socrates' act naturally happens on the other side of this separation within knowledge. This achievement is that it redefined the very notion of veritable knowledge once and for all as something that has to be artfully (methodically) *established* through the human mind's intervention. From then on it is something that is dependent on the

---

all his concrete real features and attributes and presents himself as a clean slate ("being *nobody*").

109 Jung tried to define the I, with his rather pictorial thinking, as the center of consciousness and depicted it graphically in diagrams as the center point of a circle.

human mind's jurisdiction (its *lógon didónai*, its "accounting for") and only because its rational soundness has been established IS it real knowledge in the first place. Even if Socrates was far away from *modern* subjectivity, he has nevertheless adopted a logical stance equivalent to the one that later in alchemy was called *Ars*. We could almost say he was an "*artifex*" avant la lettre: a philosophical one.

About two millennia later Descartes performed[110] a comparable radical clearing away of all naturally given certainty by subjecting *everything* on principle to (methodic) doubt: *De omnibus dubitandum*. And in his thought we witness again, but in even more pronounced form, the "consciously reflected inclusion of the subject". The radical negation that takes place in the Cartesian doubt establishes (or is the expression of) the early-modern "I" as self-consciousness. I said that what Descartes performed was an act comparable to the one performed by Socrates, but its being "comparable" applies only to the abstract form of this act. In what it does and achieves, however, it is the first act on a fundamentally higher level, this act to the power of two.

In the Socratic move the knower as the zero-point emerged as distinct from the known contents. But the knower did not experience himself (or set himself up) as an independent reality. He was still completely dedicated to the knowing, and as zero-point functioned only as the agent of *reason* who had to examine whether a particular content indeed qualified as true knowledge or not. The knowing subject remained imbedded in and dependent on the cosmos, which means that it was, notwithstanding its truly critical function, still essentially receptive. When Socrates said, "I know myself as knowing nothing", what counts is the establishment of the human mind per se as rational judge, not the I. So with respect to Socrates we cannot rightly speak of "self-consciousness". It was much rather an *awareness* of the subject. What he had become indeed *conscious* of was the inner complexity of what *knowledge* or *knowing is*, not of the I as such. The I as such still re-

110 We must not view Descartes as the true author who produced, and is solely responsible for, the development of modern subjectivity. It is more reasonable to see in Descartes the place at which, and the person through whom, a movement in the history of the soul's life crystallized and expressed itself.

mained implicit, submerged in the now complex reality of "knowledge" as the relation between the knowing subject and the known content.

With Descartes, however, the I as such has become fully explicit. From his stance what is at stake is no longer merely the rationality of human knowledge (which would for Socrates have guaranteed truth). No, what has now become crucial is much rather the I's own *certainty* concerning that which it assumes to be true (its rationality by now being a prerequisite as a matter of course). The fact that the I is concerned about its certainty shows that it now takes *itself* absolutely seriously as the *punctum saliens.* Instead of a mere awareness of the subject we thus now have here true self-consciousness.

But this is not all. For it is not merely so that this I is from then on the zero-point of knowledge and as such the prerequisite that underlies all knowledge that in modernity wants to be accepted as true knowledge about reality. And it is not merely so that its striving for knowledge about the cosmos as a whole no longer has the sense of pure receptivity (mere awareness). Rather, this I is also, as above all Kant showed later, what itself actively *constitutes* that which there *is* to be known: namely, no less than the whole world or 'objective reality' as such. True knowing is now ipso facto the way this *construction* of objective reality takes place; it is the human mind's translation of sense experience into the objectivity (objectual form) of the world. Reality is no longer the *angeschaute* (intuited, perceived) world, but the result of a *making*, a positing by the self-conscious Concept. A logical net now lies over the world and has, for this stance, always already set it up as a homogenous whole and organized it as the locus of rational *Gegen-ständlichkeit* (form of objectivity, objectual character).

It is clear that with the insight into the I's own *constituting* empirical reality, the form of what Jung called "merely perceiving consciousness" is objectively once and for all left behind, even if, as we already heard Jung complain, the style of the modern sciences is still such that they "try to represent the results of their investigations as though these had come into existence without man's intervention, in such a way that the collaboration of the psyche—an indispensable factor—[*die unerläßliche Mitwirkung der Psyche*] remains invisible" (*CW* 10 § 498).

Kant, as we know, made it clear that the I that constitutes the objective world is not the empirical I, the empirical subject, but the transcendental subject. And this organization of *the world as the locus of rational ob-jectivity*[111] *under the principle of unity* is of course also not the result of an empirical doing on the part of the I, but itself a transcendental and a priori act (which is why the sciences, working on the empirical-practical level, can so easily remain totally unconscious of "man's intervention"). With the distinction between empirical and transcendental subjectivity, another negation, separation, and distancing takes place, now not within knowledge (as with Socrates), but within the I itself that was formerly naively held to be a uniform entity. The I as empirical I has to humble itself. It is still the I to whom the (now objective) world comes as an absolute given. It is a perceiving consciousness. But it can also (and must) get a distance to itself in order to rise to the level of the transcendental subject, above all by turning veritable scientist, and, by in this way taking the standpoint of the transcendental I, advance and confirm the constitution of the objectualized form of reality as a single unitary and on principle totally and uninterruptedly determined world.

Here now, with the keyword "constitution", we have already touched on the previously deferred topic of what modernity involves. Heidegger had pointed out that within the Western tradition it is only during modernity (*Neuzeit*[112]) that a "subject" originates that REPRESENTS (from Lat. *re-praesentare*) its objects or the world, that is to say, "*vor sich hin stellt und zu sich her stellt*" ("places" [the objects as well as the world at large] "in front of it-

111 Lat. *objicere* from *ob* (toward, against) and *jacere* (to throw) means originally what is 'thrown or put or held before'. The hyphen in "ob-jectivity" is supposed to emphasize the radical externality and vis-à-vis character of objectified reality.

112 In German we can distinguish between the *Neuzeit* or *neuere Zeit* as the period from the Renaissance or even the late Middle Ages up to the time of the French Revolution/Napoleon, the beginning of the Industrial Revolution, and the end of metaphysics with Hegel and Schelling, on the one hand, and *die Moderne*, on the other, which is inaugurated by the Industrial Revolution and is the age of positivistic thinking governed by the modern logic of the "function" in Frege's sense. In English the term modernity can cover both periods or be reserved only for the latter.

self and towards itself").[113] We note the act, the intervention. Things are not just *found* by this subject as phenomena that *come* to it, are not simply there and *present themselves*, make *themselves* present. No, they are "artificially" positioned and *re*-presented: given a *new*, *secondary* presence to the viewing subject *by the subject's grace*, one might perhaps even venture to say: as the subject's "projection". (What the subject projects is of course only the rational objectual *form* of reality, whereas the material aspects of reality are given to the subject by sense experience). Conversely, it is this *re*-presentation that establishes the modern subject, the I, in this respect. Both are equiprimordial.

In this shift from natural presence (self-presentation) to this new secondary re-presentation of the world we recognize of course again the reversal from $\longrightarrow$ to $\longleftarrow$. All science in the modern sense starts out from the zero point of (transcendental) subjectivity, and the scientifically seen world is a fundamentally new, artificially re-constructed world, not an immediate, direct experience of the world. A wonderful illustration of this "re-presentation" of reality and at the same time of the "projection"[114] (from the zero-point of subjectivity) implied by it is the invention of central perspective by artists during the Renaissance,[115] about two centuries before Descartes. Central perspective is mathematically constructed. What is crucial about it is that it mentally subjugates everything in the painting (and by implication in the mind) to one single vanishing point (which, however, is actually the viewer's eye point as the "origin" of the re-presented world. As such it is the visual presence of the "I" in the painting, its presence *as the syntax*, the logical organization of the world as such, not as a semantic entity in the world).

Modernity in general, on a cultural level, is in this sense characterized by the fact that the *representation* of the contents and aspects of the world *in subjectivity* (transcendental, not empirical subjectivity) has become the ultimate *hypokeimenon* (substratum,

113 Martin Heidegger, "Die Zeit des Weltbildes", in: *idem*, *Holzwege*, Frankfurt a.M. (Klostermann) ^{5}1972, p. 85.

114 "Projection" not understood (as in depth psychology) as one's attributing certain of one's own unconscious images, ideas, feelings to others, but as the term is used in geometry or in the phrase "map projection", etc.

115 See chapters 2 and 3 above.

subiectum, 'that which underlies') of reality as such. This is the reversal of the pre-modern situation, in which it was the innermost nature of the cosmos itself that used to be the *hypokeimenon*—originally in the last analysis the nature spirits and the gods (or, later, God) embodied, or at work in, the cosmos. This interiorization or integration from out there into subjectivity, or this subjugation to subjectivity, does not show only in the theoretical conception of 'objective reality' (that is, in the field of knowledge [in science] as well as, more popularized, in the 'scientific world view'). It shows in two different ways or areas, namely, in addition to the theoretical sphere (the rationally *known* world) also in the lifeworld (*Lebenswelt*, Husserl), and there in the form of *Erleben* (felt experience).

Concerning the former way we have to realize that all statements the sciences make about "objective reality" are *primarily* NOT statements about the world itself (or aspects of and things in the world), but about *how* the world can be *re-presented in transcendental subjectivity*[116] in such a way that the principle of non-contradiction (or of abstract identity[117]) remains the absolute ruler. Knowledge no longer means "merely perceiving" and "receiving", also no longer seeing things, entertaining ideas and images, let alone having had visions. Knowledge means *the (transcendental) subject's* knowing, and this requires that it be systematically and methodically produced and established by the subject and *for* or *towards itself*. It cannot simply and innocently be *found*, nor can it be something that happens as a natural event to a person of its own accord, such as in the form of revelations or illumination or culturally inherited images and conceptions (no matter how archetypal, numinous, sublime, deep, intellectually sophisticated and elaborated, precious and time-honored they may be). It requires the explicit self-consciousness of the transcendental subject (*in* the empirical subject) as the knower of what is known and the subject's sense of responsibility for the knowing, and thus a method.

Concerning the second way, we can state that *Erleben* is really

116 Even if *through* an empirical subjectivity, that is, a particular individual (an empirically existing scientist).

117 Identity that has difference radically outside of itself.

a form of consumerism. Through *Erleben* the subject uses the impressions that come from things in the world as stimulants for emotionally heightening its sense of self, for its self-representation, its self-indulgence. Here, too, it is of course the empirical subject in and by whom this act is performed, but it nevertheless really serves the purpose of the edification of an experiential equivalent of (epistemic) *transcendental subjectivity*, namely the general logic of "I". The *personal* benefit for the empirical individual (the "high" feeling) is no more than the bait that seduces the empirical subject to crave for more *Erleben* and thereby unwittingly serves the objective psyche, the abstract, transpersonal logic of the I as an experiential reality.

Jung and modernity and his critique of the *natura* status

Jung was certainly a severe critic of much that is specific to modernity. And he also upheld as a matter of course the importance of dreams, visions, revelations, symbols and archetypal images—of all phenomena which came to the subject of their own accord and in principle come to the "primitive 'awareness'" of a merely perceiving consciousness. But all this must not blind us to the realization that

- according to him psychology is itself a decidedly modern discipline, radically divorced from the times of myth and traditional religions, and in this sense inevitably based on modern subjectivity (I will come back to this topic later). Significantly, Jung frequently refers to it expressly as "modern psychology", thereby not merely placing it in an external sense at a particularly historical time, but rather indicating that modernity, being modern, is inherent in its nature. It is the unique difficulty of psychology that it is in itself the conflict between its task to study psychic phenomena that present themselves of their own accord ("what the psyche spontaneously says to us", "*Natura*") and its having to study them as a modern discipline and as such inevitably from the point of view of modern subjectivity.

- and that he disparaged mere psychic "awareness" and the *Natura* state which comes with the attributes of givenness and with the modes of perceiving and receiving and that in the spirit of alchemy he decidedly opts for *Ars* and the violent human intervention necessary for psychological *consciousness* proper.

I want to present two passages in which this basic orientation of Jung's comes out clearly.

The first comes from his discussion of the "Spirit in the Bottle" fairy tale (in his "The Spirit Mercurius"). Concerning the fact that the Spirit had been enclosed in the bottle at some time prior to the beginning of the story, Jung points out that "the mercurial essence, the *principium individuationis*, would have developed freely under natural conditions, but was robbed of its freedom by deliberate intervention from outside, and was artfully confined ...". Here Jung introduces the clear opposition between the natural conditions that come with undisturbed innocence of a freely unfolding spontaneous life, on the one hand, and the act of violence intruding from outside and deliberately disrupting this free life, as well as the artfulness of the spirit's confinement in the bottle, on the other hand. Instead of condemning this brutal and almost "criminal" (he says "robbed") interference, Jung states, "Sheer instinctuality and naïve unconsciousness ... would prevail if the Master had not interrupted the free development of the natural being...". And thus he comes to the conclusion that "... we must concede that the strange intervention of the master of souls was absolutely necessary for the development of any kind of consciousness...", because, as Jung had said a few sentences earlier, "... if [man] should develop in the natural way the result would be a product not essentially different from an animal" (*CW* 13 § 244).

The last idea ("not essentially different from an animal"[118]) shows *what* Jung ultimately thinks of a merely perceiving consciousness.

It needs no stressing that Jung was very interested in the semantic contents, the images, symbols of alchemy, in the *lapis philosophorum*, the *aurum nostrum*, *Rex* and *Regina*, the *aurora*

118 I had already pointed out above that psychic awareness occurs even in animals.

consurgens, the *unus mundus*, etc. On this level the alchemical imaginal world was, among other things, also precious to him because he believed that it provided a compensation to Christianity. But his still deeper fascination with alchemy and the real motivation for him to study it and to claim it for modern psychology as an implicit precursor, was based on the fact that it introduced Jung to something that previously, in his pre-alchemy time, he had not been clearly aware of, namely a new spirit and logic: the logic of the *artifex* as the modern subject who through deliberate human intervention and negation brought about the overcoming of the *Natura* state, thereby preparing the way for psychological consciousness. This deeper ground for his interest in alchemy has not really been seen and appreciated by his followers and interpreters.

That alchemy lends itself nicely to the wish of seeing this modern logic of the subject at work in it[119] and that this is also what is important for Jung about alchemy comes out quite clearly when Jung in the next paragraph of his "The Spirit Mercurius" essay says about a central aspect of the alchemical opus: "The bottle is an artificial human product and thus signifies the intellectual purposefulness and artificiality of the procedure... As the *vas Hermeticum* of alchemy, it was 'hermetically' sealed (i.e., sealed with the sign of Hermes)" (*CW* 13 § 245). Jung consentingly emphasizes the *artificiality*, *deliberateness*, and the *intellectual* nature of the alchemical operation: according to his description it is clearly the work of subjectivity in the modern sense. And of course, we can admit that alchemy, by putting the prime matter into the retort, pulls it out of its natural context, absolutely isolates it (puts it so to speak under 'laboratory conditions') and thus presents (re-presents) it *to* itself (to the artifex) from a zero point. It does not cultivate a "primitive 'awareness'", an inferior (because "merely perceiving") consciousness and not a pure receptivity towards what is simply given.

Quite obviously, the project of alchemy provided a way for Jung to appreciate the logic of modernity and to introduce into psychology the idea of the necessary disruption of the natural process through artful intervention by the subject (that thereby first

119 Or into it?

established itself explicitly). However, the paradoxical thing is that precisely for this, Jung felt he *had to rely on* the *givenness* of empirical material as the soul's spontaneous self-expression, such as it was presented by medieval alchemy. The notion of the artful intervention into *Natura* had to be *nature's* speaking, *not* Jung's own; he himself stayed innocent: just an empiricist—and thus he did not himself have to appear as intervening *artifex* and modern subject thinking on his own responsibility. This amounts to a contradiction: semantically he insists on the necessity of *Ars*, while syntactically he himself put the whole burden of responsibility for his insights on the "empirical facts" of the soul's phenomenology (such as the "Spirit in the Bottle" fairy tale).

Now I turn to my second Jung passage, a very different text (*CW* 11 §§ 955ff.) reacting to Shri Ramana's writings. It is crucial as a clear description and critique of what from Jung's and the alchemical point of view is the *Natura* status or "primitive 'awareness'" (where, as explained above, "primitive" does not at all mean the opposite of, nor exclude, "highly cultured", "differentiated", and possibly even "sublime").

> Shri Ramana's thoughts are beautiful to read. What we find here is purest India, the breath of eternity, scorning and scorned by the world. It is the song of the ages, resounding, like the shrilling of crickets on a summer's night, from a million beings. This melody is built up on the one great theme, which, veiling its monotony under a thousand colourful reflections, tirelessly and everlastingly rejuvenates itself in the Indian spirit, whose youngest incarnation is Shri Ramana himself. It is the drama of *ahamkāra* (of the "I-making"[120] or of ego-consciousness), in opposition and indissoluble bondage to the atman, the self or non-ego. The Maharshi also calls the atman the "ego-ego"[121]— significantly enough, for the self is indeed experienced as the subject of the subject, as the true source and controller of the ego, whose (mistaken) strivings are continually directed towards appropriating the very autonomy which is intimated to it by the self.
>
> This conflict is not unknown to the Westerner: for him it is the relationship of man to God. The modern Indian, as I can testify from my own experience, has largely adopted European habits of language, "self" or "atman" being essentially synonymous with "God." But, in contradistinction to the Western "man and God," the Indian posits the opposition (or correspondence) between "ego and self." "Ego," as contrasted with "man,"

120 I corrected the *CW* mistranslation here ("the 'I-maker'").

121 Throughout in this quote Jung uses "I" (German *Ich*) and not "Ego", thus here: "*Ich-Ich*" ("I-I").

> is a distinctly *psychological*[122] concept, and so is "self"—to *our* way of thinking. We might therefore be inclined to assume that in India the metaphysical problem "man and God" has been shifted on to the psychological plane. On closer inspection it is clear that this is not so, for the Indian concept of "ego" and "self" is not really psychological but—one could well say—just as metaphysical as our "man and God." The Indian lacks the epistemological standpoint just as much as our own religious language does. He is still "pre-Kantian." This complication is unknown in India and it is still largely unknown with us. In India there is no psychology in our sense of the word. India is "pre-psychological": when it speaks of the "self," it *posits* such a thing as existing. Psychology does *not*[123] do this. It does not in any sense deny the existence of the dramatic conflict, but reserves the right to the poverty, or the riches, of *not* knowing about the self. Though very well acquainted with the self's peculiar and paradoxical phenomenology, we remain conscious of the fact that we are discerning, with the limited means at our disposal, something essentially unknown and expressing it in terms of psychic structures which may not be adequate to the nature of what is to be known.
>
> This epistemological limitation keeps us at a remove from what we term "self" or "God." The equation self = God is shocking to the European. As Shri Ramana's statements and many others show, it is a specifically Eastern insight, to which psychology has nothing further to say except that it is not within its competence to differentiate between the two. ..."

In our context the only thing of interest is the *internal logical structure itself* of the one spirit (together with it the corresponding reported ideas discussed here by Jung) in contrast to the other mental stance described by him. The fact that what Jung focuses on happens to be *India's* and *a particular Indian's*, Shri Ramana's, thinking is of no concern to us. This is why we must not worry about the question whether Jung's analysis truly applies to India and Shri Ramana. Even if Jung's description amounted in some ways to a misunderstanding or misrepresentation, even if Jung might have projected something upon India, the distinction itself that Jung makes between the two states of consciousness remains and shows which categories are at work in Jung's mind and determine his own conception of psychology proper.

The first paragraph of the quoted text describes Shri Ramana's thought as not only cocooned within itself and perpetuating itself, but also as absorbing into itself the human subject who believes in and expresses this thought in his writings, making it its own

122 Jung's italics in *GW*.
123 Jung's italics in *GW*.

mouthpiece or new embodiment (new "incarnation"). Concerning my word "mouthpiece" we can recall Jung's having subsumed Shri Ramana under "[t]he carrier[s] of mythological and philosophical wisdom in India" (§ 951). Concerning the idea of Shri Ramana's being absorbed into what he portrayed in his writings, it is noteworthy that in § 958 Jung himself finds it evident that Shri Ramana "has either really been absorbed by the self, or has at least struggled earnestly all his life to extinguish his ego in it". (But Jung's "or" is probably misleading. The two possibilities he mentions are not alternatives. It is rather so that "absorption" describes Shri Ramana's psychology, the real logical constitution of his soul condition, whereas his earnest struggle merely takes place on the *psychic* level. For he naturally also wants to bring his ego-personality in line with his deeper truth.)

The cocoonment in the soul becomes also clear from Jung's further description. Although, according to Jung, there is endless variety within Shri Ramana's thought, this variety only "veils" the "monotony" of its one theme, a theme that in itself has the enchanting, if not downright entrancing musical quality of a "melody" and is therefore even referred to by Jung as "the song of the ages". The *Natura* aspect (in a more literal rather than psychological sense) also comes out in the comparison of this "song of the ages" with the shrilling of crickets on a summer's night.[124] Nothing disrupts the magic circle. Even though this song of the ages is *about* "a *drama*", telling the tale of the *opposition between* I and self or non-ego, the song itself is static ("breath of eternity") and remains safely intact, self-contained—"tirelessly and everlastingly" returning into its beginning like the uroboros, the snake biting its tail. Thus it is complete, has everything it needs within

124 On a different psychological level and without the nature aspect, the idea of the "song of the Ages" and the "shrilling of crickets on a summer's night" is comparable to what Jung had to say about certain religious statements in the West when they remain *unthought* because one is solely given over to the emotional impression (*Gefühlseindruck*) that they evoke: they sound "so solemn", "so religious, so splendidly religious" and the mind remains in a state "in which we do not think anything any more and just succumb to absolute suggestion. One becomes suggestible when one does not have conscious thoughts, but only unconscious ones" (see his *Über Gefühle und den Schatten.* Winterthurer Fragestunden. Textbuch, Zürich and Düsseldorf 1999, pp. 22 and 24 f. My translation or paraphrase, respectively).

itself—while having the real world outside of itself ("scorning the world"). In fact, more than that, it has even any outside ("outsideness" as such, the very concept of "outside") outside of itself and therefore is *absolute interiority*.

After describing its character, Jung makes it very clear that this whole stance is definitely *not* compatible with the other stance, that of psychology. "In India there is no psychology in our sense of the word. India is 'pre-psychological'". Now the question is what that is that makes it pre-psychological. Jung's answer is: it lacks something, namely an essential radical move. So far we can easily agree with Jung's assessment.

The problems with Jung's argument of "the lacking epistemological standpoint"

However, concerning the particular *description* or *analysis* of this move that it allegedly lacks I disagree with Jung. Jung says: it "lacks the epistemological standpoint". It "is still 'pre-Kantian'". Now it goes without saying that what Jung described as the Indian stance (whether correctly so or not does not interest us here, as I said) is pre-Kantian as well as pre-psychological.[125] But who

125 Apropos Jung's keyword "pre-Kantian" we have to realize that it is deplorably well possible to be able to recount Kant's argument correctly (in the sense of "merely receiving awareness"), that is, merely as one's *contents* of consciousness, while consciousness itself in its own stance remains unaffected by and immune to *what* contents it entertains. There are many examples of this, also in Jungian circles (in so far as they have taken note of Kant in the first place). — The same applies to the alchemical psychology inaugurated by Jung. One can be well versed in alchemy's wild imagery and know all about its operations, processes, and substances and also be able to apply the alchemical images of the *mysterium coniunctionis*, the pleroma, and the subtle body to the transference between patient and analyst—and one may nevertheless not have dissolved the *unio naturalis* and *participation mystique* with the contents one is dealing with, which dissolution alone would put oneself into the stance of veritable *artifex* and modern subject clearly vis-à-vis the prime matter as a one that is hermetically sealed in the glass bottle. Even Hillman's decidedly imaginal stance, despite its much higher level of intellectual sophistication and differentiation, may in some way be a case in point. (In his case, it is probably not so much a lack of "consciously reflected inclusion of the subject" as the fully conscious subject's deliberate, let us say for want of a better word, *nostalgic* decision to establish the sphere of the imaginal as the ultimate.)

says that it *should be* psychological, *should be* on the level of the Kantian position? Why does Jung expect, nay, demand that it respects the epistemological standpoint? Why does Jung not treat it simply as one of "the *documents* of the soul", documents that can become the *subject* of psychological study while themselves clearly being "pre-psychological", the same way we interpret religious documents, myths, fairy tales, dreams, symbols, and fantasies as the soul's speaking about itself at different moments in the history of its logical life? Myths and dreams also lack the epistemological standpoint and are also pre-Kantian. They are possible "prime matters" *for* psychology, but of course not themselves psychology. It does not make sense to say of Indian thought that it "lacks" something that it is not and does not want to be. This is a simple misunderstanding, a category mistake.

Another aspect of this problem is that Jung's charge of the lack of the epistemological standpoint and of being "pre-Kantian" (which factually, as I indicated, is well taken) also implies something concerning psychology itself that does not make sense. It suggests that what makes psychology is the presence of the epistemological standpoint, the step from a pre-Kantian position to that of Kant. It sounds as if one's adopting the Kantian stance and one's making a fundamental distinction between the "appearance" and "the thing in itself", or between empirical science and metaphysics, were the turning point from "pre-psychological" to "psychology in our sense of the word". Here I have to make it very clear that the modern development from Descartes to Kant that I briefly discussed above does *not* lead to psychology nor to a psychological consciousness in the strict sense. On the contrary, it not only leads ultimately to the positivistic sciences, to technology, and the scientific world view that is today's ruling metaphysic,[126] but as such also directly excludes psychology. Being concerned with the construction of the *total* positivization of the world and everything in it, the modern positivistic stance has to classify and reject dreams, myths, rituals, symbols, and other imaginal products as nothing but illusions, or as early erroneous attempts to explain the world, or as primitive superstitions and thus as non-

126 Although in the depths it has meanwhile, in the age of *medial modernity* (in contrast to *industrial* modernity), already become obsolete.

sense. (That this modern development was nevertheless in a particular way important for the possibility of psychology, which is why I discussed it in the first place, will be shown later.)

Psychology does not need the epistemological barrier. More than that: it has no use for it, indeed, the epistemological issue is even incompatible with psychology. I want to explain this by discussing a little more closely Jung's statement that psychology "reserves the right to the poverty, or the riches, of *not* knowing about" the self.

I think Jung is right, but I also think he does not take this insight about "*not* knowing" far enough. He has in mind no more than a *relative* or *qualified* "*not* knowing", whereas it needs to be understood absolutely. The "*not* knowing" has to be seen not only as a formal, but a *constitutive* determination of psychology. By speaking of "*not* knowing *about* the self", Jung, however, restricted the reach or validity of his insight to the semantic sphere, to the field of contents, issues, topics, when it would much rather have been necessary for psychology to cancel the "about" altogether in order to arrive at an all-comprehensive plain and simple "*not* knowing": at a point beyond the wish or need to *know* altogether, beyond *epistemology* as such. This would have been the real "poverty or the riches", namely the poverty or riches of absolute negativity as that dimension in which the psychological has its sphere.

The "about" is the problem. With the about, i.e., a specific qualification, Jung divided the whole semantic field into two by drawing "a barrier across the mental world" (*CW* 18 § 1734); we could also say: a barrier across the semantic field, so that on one side of it there is the range of topics that are in principle capable of being known by us (empirical facts) and on the other side there is what cannot possibly be known (such as the question of God and transcendence in general). The "epistemological limitation keeps us at a remove from what we term 'self' or 'God'" (where the "epistemological limitation" corresponds to the "barrier" referred to). What we need to understand is that by reserving the "*not* knowing" for one part of the *semantic field* (his "about the self"), Jung unwittingly precisely *upholds and defends the syntax or logic of knowing as such*, and, to be sure, of "knowing" in the specific modern sense: positivistic knowledge guaranteed by the transcendental I and kept under the absolute dictates of the principle of non-contradiction, total inner consistency of the world, and of the demand for certainty (reliability).

Psychology, however, *is* psychology because its topics are *nichts Wissensmäßiges*: not possible candidates for knowing in this modern sense, inasmuch as what psychology is dealing with is in the status of *absolute negativity*. Its only subject is the soul's speaking, is soul phenomena. And all of them are just ideas, images, feelings, fantasies *without any referent*. They refer exclusively to themselves. Late Jung himself insisted, as we know, that the image has everything it needs (*omne quo indiget*) within itself (*CW* 14 § 749). With respect to images it simply does not make any sense to draw a barrier across the semantic field. *Every* topic has (and has to have) fantasy or soul character in order for it to be a psychological topic, regardless of whether it is considered an empirical reality or as something transcendent. Psychology is concerned with the mother image, not with real mothers, with the motif of the virgin birth, not with virgins who give birth, with the fairy tale dragons, not with whether dragons exist, with the myths of the underworld, not with a real underworld, with the God idea, not with an objectively existing (or not existing) God. So the question of knowing in Jung's modern positivistic *epistemological* sense does not enter into the constitution of psychology one way or another (just as it does not enter poetry or the arts).

With his epistemological concern Jung is barking up the wrong tree. He goes off on a tangent. Psychology is an *Ars*, a methodology, an *opus*, a doing—a particular style of looking at and working with psychological phenomena in their absolute negativity. If the image contains everything it needs within itself, how can there be any doubt whether what "we are discerning, with the limited means at our disposal," "and expressing it in terms of psychic structures" (e.g., "the self") "may not be adequate to the nature of what is to be known"? The self-image, just as the God-image, are only adequate to themselves. There is nothing to compare them with. The question whether the self is God or whether it is not much rather "something essentially unknown"[127] IS paradoxically

127 Jung's statement that the "epistemological limitation keeps us at a remove

even the very overstepping of those epistemological limits that Jung so desperately wants to avoid because *syntactically* this question is *malgré lui* sold on *that* very "knowing about" that semantically he said to be off limits. But worse than that: it is the betrayal of psychology as such, in favor of the ego's and civilian man's fundamentally *external* standpoint of positivity as well as in favor of the idea that psychic images must have a (be it known or unknown) referent outside themselves. All this means for us: Properly understood, psychology's reserving "the right to the poverty, or the riches, of *not* knowing" requires our *altogether leaving behind* the whole question of knowing in this epistemological sense.

What was that which landed Jung in the epistemological trap? What was the reason, nay, not reason, but the powerful personal need that forced him to set it up for himself? And why is there this trap at all? The answer is because Jung mingled a religious ego concern—the individual's becoming self—into the psychological opus. We have to be very clear about it. The desire to become self (in Jung's high sense, namely, in terms of what he calls the "individuation process") is a human, all-too-human longing. Whether you are in the grip of the desire to get rich, to become President, a famous movie star or in the grip of the desire to attain the self or to experience mystic union with God is certainly in each case *practically* fundamentally different, but *psychologically* the same; they are so many different goals that people, civilian man, the ego are possibly striving for. The soul has no stake in all that. Psychology's interest is only in the development of a *truly psychological consciousness* on the level of the objective soul, and not in our personal development. Semantically, becoming self and overcoming the ego may look like a soul topic. But syntactically, and this is what counts psychologically, it is not. It is an ego concern.

Because Jung, as decidedly modern man, smuggled his personal

---

from what we term 'self' or 'God'" and above all from the "equation self = God" amounts to a mere quibbling about *words* or *names* and not about reals. If the self is "something essentially unknown", the word "the self" is simply synonymous with the word "God", inasmuch as God is by definition also defined as "essentially unknown" (and vice versa), while in psychology both are specific psychological ideas or images, as precise and well-circumscribed as any other psychological images.

religious desire to rescue God for himself (and for decidedly modern man in general) into *psychology* (in the psychologistic form of his "becoming self" program), and used the notion of "the unconscious" as a way to surreptitiously catch modern man from behind, he created a duplicity and contradiction. It was crucial for his project that "the self" was unmistakably presented as nothing but a strictly empirical psychological fact coming as "pure nature" from man's *own* unconscious. Yet at the same time it would nevertheless covertly *function* as the felt presence of God (*despite* its claimed empirical-scientific factualness). So Jung had to wage a war on two fronts. On the one hand he had to prohibit us from saying "the self = God" (in order to rescue his empiricism), and on the other hand he had to fight against the *wholesale denial* of this identification,[128] insisting that the "*not*" refers exclusively to our *knowing*, but *by no means* to the equal sign or to the whole "the self = God" statement itself. The truth of the equal sign was supposed to be left open. And the other way around: It was thus also possible for him to answer at once the question about the equation with "Yes" *and* "No". He could *suggest* the possibility of the ultimate identity while personally pleading innocent and hiding behind the idea of an epistemological curtain that shields us from the ultimate truth. This is why Jung needed the epistemological barrier. Kant, the way he understood him, came in handy. Jung *used* him for his sleight of hand.

Jung's famous answer to an interview question, whether he believes in God or not: "I do not believe, I know" is remarkable on two counts. First, Jung violates here his own epistemological principle, his "*not* knowing about" God, and in this sense becomes himself "pre-Kantian" and "pre-psychological".[129] That he would violate this adamant principle in turn reveals, secondly, the

128 Just before the statement about "*not* knowing" Jung says about psychology: "It does *not in any sense deny* the existence of the dramatic conflict" (my emphasis). With "the dramatic conflict" Jung refers to the question of the relation between man and God or self and God.

129 That the concept of "knowing" in his "I do not believe, I know" remark is fundamentally different (based on the idea of the real experience of a *collision* with God as a *counter-will*) from the epistemic or scientific concept of knowledge does not contradict this analysis. The fact remains that Jung does not rely here on "the right to the poverty, or the riches, of *not* knowing about the self" or God.

urgency that a defense of the reality of God in the modern world had for him personally.

In addition to the question of knowing or *not* knowing there is in Jung's reaction to "India" and Shri Ramana also the issue of "positing". Jung says: When India "speaks of the 'self,' it *posits* such a thing as existing. Psychology does *not* do this." As with his "pre-Kantian" charge, Jung is of course right, but again also completely unfair to India. For it is not really "India" at all that *posits* "such a thing as the self" or God as existing. Rather, it is the soul that does this: every dream *posits* the figures and events occurring in it as existing, no matter whether it is the incubus that literally oppresses a dream-I in a nightmare, or the burglar that is about to intrude into my home, or the dead baby I find hidden in a dark corner of the cellar, figures that may haunt me throughout the day. The soul *posits* as existing fairies, goblins, centaurs, dragons, witches, ghosts, demons, muses, heroes, gods, the Christian God, Buddha, the Virgin Mary, and so on. This is the very point of myths, fantasies, delusions, religions, poems and novels: to posit their content. How could a dream impress us if it did not posit as existing whatever it presents? How could religion produce devotion if it did not do the same thing? The soul's fantasy activity is, after all, nothing else than its speaking, inventing, producing (and this means positing, asserting) something. If you think that this kind of positing is wrong, illegitimate, off limits for us, then you turn against the soul's fantasy activity as such.

But it is far from Jung's intent to turn against the soul's fantasy activity. With his attack upon "positing such a thing as existing", he succumbs to an error and confuses something. His error is twofold. It is, first, that he does not see the equivocation in his use of "positing as existing" or, to put it another way, that he applies the modern positivistic *epistemological* sense to the *soul* sense of "positing" (the latter being one within absolute negativity), as if they were the same or at least commensurable. This is due to the second aspect of his error, namely to a category mistake, as I described above, or to a faulty comparison: Jung does not allow for "the historical difference"[130], but leaps across it and therefore

130 Wolfgang Giegerich, "The simultaneity of the non-simultaneous. Or: The historical difference", the second chapter of *idem*, *Pitfalls in Comparing*

treats positions that belong to completely different logical and historical statuses of consciousness as if they were on the same logical and historical level. This is the reason for his unfair judgement, for his *blaming* the work of the Indian sage for *lacking something*, instead of appreciating the fact that what *he* (Jung) as modern psychologist misses *does not belong there* in the first place[131] and that psychology in its turn is simply not comparable, not compatible with that Indian thought. Psychology is separated from it by a historical as well as logical divide.

The indispensability of the dissolution of the *unio naturalis*.

It is astonishing that Jung did not see this, or rather, that he did not draw the consequences from what he saw. For his own description of the world conjured up in Shri Ramana's writing makes it obvious that the human subject speaking here is just the mouthpiece of the soul's thoughts. It is "absorbed by the self", as Jung suggested, enwrapped in the soul, dreaming the Indian soul's dream. But as long as you stay *in* the dream, *in* the story of a fairy tale, then as a matter of course everything appearing in them is ipso facto posited, and rightly so, necessarily so. The point of the insight that Jung had but did not allow to come home to him, interpreting it instead as a shortcoming, is that in Shri Ramana's work he was confronted with an earlier stage in the historical development of the soul: with a situation in which the subject is floating and bathing in the Imaginal, in the archetypal or metaphysical sphere. It has not emancipated itself from the soul, not been born out of the soul. It is really just *dreaming* the Indian "song of the ages" onwards, where "dreaming" refers to a particular form or style of the thinking of the *waking* mind and not to processes during one's literal sleep. The *unio naturalis* is

Buddhist and Western Psychology: A contribution to psychology's self-clarification, ISPDI Monograph Series, vol. 2, CreateSpace Independent Publishing Platform, 2018.

131 Just as invertebrate animals do not *lack* a backbone. They are just fine the way they are. Nothing is *missing*. The primitives prior to their contact with modern people did not *lack* guns, atom bombs, television, or literate culture.

undissolved. This is the initial status that Pseudo-Democritus' axiom on nature described as "Nature rejoices in nature".[132]

When Jung demands of this world the application of the "epistemological limitation" he is confronting it with the result of European soul development from Descartes to Kant and to 19th century positivism. This development is the main process in which the *objective* and *collective* emancipation from the soul took place that in reality transported the Western soul away from itself, into externality and alienation. It amounts to the birth of man. By reaching this stage in the soul's historical development, the soul in the form of modern subjectivity, we can say, has *awakened* from its own, the soul's, dream that it used to dream or in which it used to be enveloped all the time before. This new stage is the situation described in Pseudo-Democritus' axiom as "Nature conquers [or subdues] nature". Here it is crucial to understand that on both sides of this alchemical formula of subjugation there is one and the same, namely "nature", "the soul". The subjugation is not an imperialist or colonialist conquest. What subjects nature to its rule is again this same nature. It is "nature's" own self-relation: self-differentiation. What is born out of the soul is the soul itself in its new form as modern subjectivity. In other words, that which is born out of it, truly out of it, nevertheless remains still encompassed by it.

Psychology cannot base itself on the first-mentioned status of containment in the soul. Psychology does not have the task of staying in, and is not permitted to regress to, the dream-mode. It cannot allow itself to merely "dream the myth onwards" and "say again" what the soul has spoken and in this sense remain nothing but the soul's mouthpiece. There is no room in it for this kind of "primitive 'awareness'" and "inferior state of being conscious". No archetypes-and-myth-mongering, no indulging in the ideology of "the gods in every man and every woman", or in a cult of

132 According to the alchemist Democritus "nature", for us this means: "the soul", is not fixed and set. There is an inherent dynamic in it. It passes through a dialectical development of three stages expressed in his "axiom on nature", which is mentioned repeatedly by Jung (e.g., *CW* 9i § 234, *CW* 16 § 469). This axiom about the three phases of nature's, the soul's, self-overcoming reads: "Nature rejoices in nature, nature subdues [or: conquers] nature, nature rules over nature."

synchronicity and "experiences of 'the sacred'". Psychology, in order to *be* psychology (and not merely the production of psychic material or one's bathing in it) has to have irrevocably awakened from the soul's dream, from the "song of the ages". Our task as psychologists is, as Nietzsche once said, "the being-awake as such".[133]

What in Shri Ramana's thinking seems to be *really* lacking from this point of view is that his ideas are, so to speak, put into a retort, firmly enclosed there and rigorously separated by the vessel's glass wall from the human being and thus kept vis-à-vis. This putting the ideas into a retort would be the act (the "human intervention") through which the difference would be established[134] between the intellectual or imaginal material, on the one hand, and the person entertaining these ideas, on the other, and, furthermore, through which this person would ipso facto have established himself as true subject, *artifex*, modern psychologist, and his consciousness as "the reflected and rational state of consciousness". While devoted to "the song of the ages" as his *object* of study (in the retort), he nevertheless would "keep himself at a remove from" this "song of the ages" and only in this way become able to *study* it and *work* with it psychologically in the first place. Psychology requires the explicit de-identification of the subject from its contents of consciousness and the disruption of the unconscious enchantment with them, the subject's being the soul's mouthpiece. Shri Ramana's problem, the way it is described by Jung, is not the specific "scientific" one that he was pre-Kantian and did not abide by the epistemological limitation. It is the fundamental psychological one that he stopped before the birth of man from out of the soul—before becoming modern man.

Jung very clearly saw that *psychology* is a decidedly *modern* undertaking.[135] It owes the possibility of its existence to the loss of

133 "... wir, *deren Aufgabe das Wachsein selbst ist*." Friedrich Nietzsche, „Vorrede" (1885) of *Jenseits von Gut und Böse*. Nietzsche is not speaking, as I do, about psychologists.

134 This is not the "psychological difference". It is another psychology-constituting difference. We could call it the "alchemical difference".

135 "But no culture before ours felt compelled to take the psychic background [*Seelenhintergrund*] as such seriously. The soul was always merely part of a metaphysical system. Modern consciousness, however, can no longer ward off the knowledge of the soul, despite the most intensive and desperate defensive

soul. It must have ruthlessly emancipated itself from the soul. There is no way back for it to a state *before* consciousness's having been born out of the soul. The logical status reached through the historical development of modern subjectivity from Descartes to Kant is one cornerstone of its very constitution.

For Jung this meant that psychology had to be conceived as a natural science devoted to establishing nothing but facts; it was with great satisfaction that Jung, in his answer to Martin Buber, quoted the statement from an article in the *British Medical Journal*: "Facts first and theories later is the key-note of Jung's work. He is an empiricist first and last" (*CW* 18 § 1502). This is the wrong conclusion. Psychology cannot base itself on a standpoint of scientific, empiricist knowledge nor on the "epistemological limitation" either. No way leads from there, from the positivism of the scientific stance, to the soul. As far as psychological contents are concerned, this stance with its commitment to "legitimate knowing" must inevitably, as I pointed out, disregard all soul products, all dreams, fantasies, myths, metaphysical and religious ideas as illusions, primitive superstitions, or as proof of the ignorance of former ages, or as ideas of merely subjective entertainment value, or as pathological, in short, as nonsense.

But it does not, nay, more than that, it *cannot* lead to psychological consciousness! Indeed, it does not even lead to consciousness at all, let alone truly psychological consciousness. Jung himself had, as we heard before, once blamed the modern sciences, these mighty exponents of this historical-logical stage in the soul's logical life, that they "try to represent the results of their investigations as though these had come into existence without man's intervention, in such a way that the collaboration of the psyche—an indispensable factor—[*die unerläßliche Mitwirkung der Psyche*] remains invisible" (*CW* 10 § 498). In other words, they have to be unconscious, purblind, on systematic grounds qua science, qua enterprises of empirical, positivistic knowing. In the structure of the sciences we find realized what Jung elsewhere

efforts. This distinguishes our time from all others" (*CW* 10 §161, transl. modif.); "This situation is new. All ages before us still believed in gods in some form or other" (*GW* 9/I § 50, my transl.). "It needed the *soul predicament* of our time, to cause us to discover psychology" (*CW* 10 § 159, transl. modif.).

called "consciousness's becoming unconscious". To be sure, it is a consciousness, but only a consciousness of technical *knowledge*, of facts, and thus an historically entirely new systematically narrowed-down *tunnel-vision* version of the most primitive form of "awareness", namely awareness of what today we call abstract "information".

To sum up the result of this issue: The logical constitution of consciousness inaugurated by such thinkers as Descartes and Kant, which is tantamount to the realization of the second stage of Pseudo-Democritus' axiom of nature as well as to the birth of man, is a prerequisite for the possibility of modern psychology. But this birth of man is not its *sufficient reason*. More and something else is needed in addition.

Although this stage of emancipation from the soul or of the birth of man represented the now in fact reached and *objectively* prevailing logical constitution of consciousness, it was, historically speaking, at first and for a long time limited to the strictly *intellectual* realm and to the tiny group of great scientific minds, and in the latter even only to the extent that they were actually engaged in strict thought and scientific study, but not as far as their private life and religious beliefs were concerned. A new stage of consciousness always seems to begin, in its first immediacy, by getting hold of only a selected few isolated minds and only in a special area. In the course of the centuries and decades it will have sunken down and permeated the lifeworld and have taken hold of the general mode of being-in-the-world of people (civilian man) and society at large. Then it will have practically become what it *logically* had been from the outset, the new truth, the new definition of consciousness, in which man inevitably and for the most part unwittingly lives.

Psychological consciousness requires movement beyond the second stage to a third stage. In order to reach it, psychology has to push off from the modern "science" stage (with its commitment to positivism) to a higher level. It has to push off from it in such a way that on this higher level it regains an access to the very opposite of the focus on positivistic fact, namely access to the dimension of absolute negativity. In a certain sense this amounts to a return to the first stage, but *on a fundamentally higher level*; we could also say that the movement at long last comes back to its starting-point, uroborically returning into itself, *but* with a surplus.

For it is not a regression. That it is not a regression is due to two facts, first, that the new stage is reached only on the basis of emancipation from soul and awakening from its dream. This stage is not revoked and cannot be revoked. Secondly, that the return to absolute negativity and thus to soul is a *methodological* (not a literal, existential) return. As methodological it is dependent on an artificial procedure (and thus on *Ars*) and reserved for those particular moments or times when this *Ars* is actually practiced. There must not be an attempt to nostalgically *simulate* an in-ness in soul (comparable to the status that Jung described in his passage about Shri Ramana), because *for us* (in contrast, for example, to Shri Ramana himself) this absolute interiority of the *unio naturalis* is no longer borne out by the now prevailing status of the objective psyche. As I showed, the birth of man is irrevocable.

Now we can see even more clearly why it was necessary to reject Jung's sense of "*not* knowing" reductively qualified as a mere "not knowing *about*" and to insist on the *absolute* sense of it as psychology's simply not being in the business of knowing (establishing knowledge) at all. By resorting to the barrier between semantic topics that could legitimately be known and others that had to remain strictly off limits, Jung entrenched himself in the second stage.

Having said this, we must immediately qualify this statement about Jung by adding that he entrenched himself in the second stage *only as theoretician*, while in his concrete work with soul phenomena he had the most amazing access to the soul's absolute negativity, that negativity the road to which as a theoretician he blocked by rescuing the syntax of *epistemic knowing* precisely through his reserving "the right to the poverty, or the riches, of *not* knowing about" the self, that is, through his staying fixated on the "barrier across the mental world". This split between the logical form of his work as interpreter of concrete soul phenomena and the logical form adamantly defended by him as theoretician, and above all the fact that he seems to have remained unconscious of this split, are of course in themselves remarkable.

* * *

But now I have to admit that the move I presented as leading to the third stage and to psychological consciousness does not at all truly go beyond the second stage, as suggested. Inasmuch as I characterized it as a *methodological* return to the dimension of absolute negativity and insisted that it is not an existential one, that is to say, one that is lived by the whole person as the self-evident objective truth of his existence, it reveals itself as a practice that, even if its semantic orientation is directly contrary to the positivistic stance, nevertheless itself occurs on the basis and within the context of the second stage. It is merely one of the things one can do within the framework of the modern world. As a methodological approach it is a matter of our choosing and thus it is contingent.

A "stage of consciousness", however, means that we have no choice. *Vocatus atque non vocatus*, willingly or unwillingly, wittingly or unwittingly, the logical form of consciousness that it implies envelops us and determines our sense of reality, the form of our experiences, and the values that prevail for us. So choosing an altogether different or even opposite orientation does not mean that the real level of consciousness that prevails over us has been surpassed. And the other way around, being firmly rooted in the second stage does not at all mean that modern people must exclusively do science or think positivistically 24 hours a day. They can also go hiking or swimming, practice yoga, enjoy novels and movies; they can go in for mysticism or Buddhist meditation and by the same token they can also practice psychology as a discipline of interiority—and yet they do not thereby leave the standpoint of the second stage. As a logical stage of consciousness, it is not solely committed to one single practice, orientation, or method. The second stage is much rather defined by a certain a priori definition of objective reality, by an unshakeable experience of the world at large as "objective reality". No particular (ontic) practice or behavior, no semantic belief or methodological orientation can bring about a breakthrough to a new syntactical, logical or ontological status. For example, a hermeneutic approach in many humanities, and one's regaining a sense of soul and absolute negativity in psychology are methodological enterprises, and precisely for this reason they do not in any way change, let alone revolutionize, the generally ruling syntax of the *real* world experience and world definition that represent the inner truth of the second stage, namely, the world as unitary and, on principle, totally and uninterruptedly determined objective reality.

Also, if we take into account how psychology works above all with dreams in therapy we must admit that dreams are ultimately mostly used for getting *information* about the patient (diagnostic knowledge as well as knowledge about ongoing inner processes or potential developments) and for enabling the patient to gain self-knowledge. In other words, what it aims for is an increase in psychic awareness; the form of consciousness that determines this work is still a merely perceiving one. Trying to *understand* a patient, a dream, symbols and symptoms, is just a kind of *knowing*, not of psychological *consciousness*!

So we have to ask: How does psychological consciousness arise? And what is psychological consciousness in the first place?

What could "psychological consciousness" possibly mean?

This question is a great challenge for us, for the simple reason that the third stage and this consciousness have not been reached, not been realized culturally. There can be little doubt that the prevailing consciousness in analytical psychology is largely "prepsychological" in Jung's sense. Its ordinary consciousness is mostly in the *Natura* state of "psychic awareness" and therefore may not even have an inkling of what Jung is talking about when he speaks about the "consciously reflected inclusion of the subject" and the establishment, through a ruthless intervention, of the separation of the psychologist as *artifex* from psychological phenomenology enclosed in the retort. As far as our reality is concerned, psychological consciousness lies still very much ahead of us. It is beyond ourselves. All that we can hope for as maybe being possible is to get some anticipatory idea of it. Jung indeed had an inkling of it, and some hints contained in Jung's thinking can show us the direction in which our thoughts about this topic must proceed.

The first hint comes from a surprising claim of Jung's concerning the ordinarily prevailing great difficulty of becoming conscious of one's feelings. In the casual oral talk on feelings and the shadow[136] that I already referred to above, an impromptu talk two years before his death, Jung observed that

> ... it is the great regrettable problem in our culture that we are strangely incapable of realizing our own feelings, that is, to notice [*spüren*, sense] the things that are of concern to us. One sees often that people pass over events or experiences without noticing [*merken*] what actually has happened to them. Because they do not realize at all that they have a feeling [*Gefühlsreaktion*]. Most of the time they merely notice what one calls an affect, an emotion, which goes along with physiological effects. Such as: an intensified activity of the heart, accelerated breathing, phenomena with regard to motor functions; this is what they notice. But when it is a feeling [*Gefühlsreaktion*] they often do not notice it at all because the feeling [*Gefühlsreaktion*] is not accompanied by psycho-physical phenomena. (*op. cit.* p. 12)

By way of example Jung mentions an experience he had in his young years when he performed his word association experiment studies. When investigating the question of how feelings and affects differ, he learned from a particular experience with one test subject, to whom something embarrassing had happened, that

> When he is alone with himself, he does not know what value this affair has for him, or how much it bothers him. But when he knows that someone else knows about it, then he gets the actual affect. (*ibid.* p. 13)

To become really conscious of a feeling requires, this is Jung's thesis, that it is not merely one's own private, personal knowledge. "If you experience [something] alone, it is as if it had not really arrived" (p. 15). It has not come home to you. Mere *awareness* is not enough, or to say it the other way around: consciousness is more than one's awareness of what one has done or what has happened to oneself. The knowledge of the *"fact that"* as well as of the *"what"* of the behavior or event, is completely insufficient, as far as consciousness is concerned. What the embarrassing deed or event psychologically *amounts to*, what it *means* to oneself, that is to say, to the soul, needs two things, first, a duplication of the knowledge. In addition to my simple knowing of the issue it also

136 C.G. Jung, *Über Gefühle und den Schatten.* Winterthurer Fragestunden. Textbuch, Zürich and Düsseldorf 1999. The following quotations are my translations.

needs *my* knowing that the issue *is* known (and that I *am* known). And, secondly, it needs that its and my being known refers to a truly alien knowledge, a knowledge by others, and that means that it is a knowledge which, in contrast to my own subjective knowing of the issue, is inexorable, inasmuch as it is once and for all out of my hands and reach. It means my own *being* known from outside (passive voice!): I have become the object, the victim of an alien gaze. In this sense there is a moment of violence and being intruded in this external *being* seen. It shatters the innocence of subjectivity, the intactness of my privacy and interiority.

Consciousness of "the things that are of concern to us", of "what actually happened to" us, cannot be had without this objective destruction of my innocence, the innocence of my own *(mere) awareness*. Even if I know that I committed a terrible crime or a truly shameful act—as long as it is only that I am aware of it, the innocence of my subjectivity is preserved intact. It needs the intrusive nature of seenness by others, my having to *suffer* my *being* known, to make my (at first merely subjective) "primitive" awareness *objective* and to only thereby turn it into more than awareness, into consciousness. Only then do we become "capable of *realizing* our own feelings". (This is the deeper reason behind the institution of "confession" in Christianity, especially Roman Catholicism, just as it is an important factor for the efficacy of psychotherapy. The analyst is the Other by whom the innermost secrets of the patient become known.)

My second example that can be taken as a hint about what psychological consciousness involves has nothing to do with "realizing one's feelings" about embarrassing facts. Instead it shows that deep down Jung had an intuitive premonition of the future necessity of what I called the moment of "seenness". I am referring to two dreams Jung had late in life. He tells us:

> In one dream, which I had in October 1958, I caught sight from my house of two lens-shaped metallically gleaming disks, which hurtled in a narrow arc over the house and down to the lake. They were two UFOs (Unidentified Flying Objects). Then another body came flying directly toward me. It was a perfectly circular lens, like the objective of a telescope. At a distance of four or five hundred yards it stood still for a moment, and then flew off. Immediately afterward, another came speeding through the air: a lens with a metallic extension which led to a box—a magic lantern. At a distance of sixty or seventy yards it stood still in the

> air, pointing straight at me. I awoke with a feeling of astonishment. Still half in the dream, the thought passed through my head: "We always think that the UFOs are projections of ours. Now it turns out that we are their projections. I am projected by the magic lantern as C. G. Jung. But who manipulates the apparatus?"
>
> I had dreamed once before of the problem of the self and the ego. In that earlier dream I was on a hiking trip. I was walking along a little road through a hilly landscape; the sun was shining and I had a wide view in all directions. Then I came to a small wayside chapel. The door was ajar, and I went in. To my surprise there was no image of the Virgin on the altar, and no crucifix either, but only a wonderful flower arrangement. But then I saw that on the floor in front of the altar, facing me, sat a yogi— in lotus posture, in deep meditation. When I looked at him more closely, I realized that he had my face. I started in profound fright, and awoke with the thought: "Aha, so he is the one who is meditating me. He has a dream, and I am it." I knew that when he awakened, I would no longer be. (*MDR* p. 323)

There is first an aggressive approach of a kind of telescope aiming straight at the dream-I and later one of a magic lantern likewise pointing directly at the dream-I. Whether what they do is to "project" Jung or whether they are merely focusing on him does not make much of a difference in our context. Crucial for us is this external gaze coming to him and depriving him of his own subjectivity by turning him into the object of their seeing or projection. We can also note the passive voice implied in Jung's own reflection about it: "Now it turns out that we are their projections." What the second dream about the meditating yogi adds to this whole experience of a reversal from subject to object and of *being* seen or projected/meditated is above all the sameness of the face (personality) on both sides. This is especially revealing with respect to the topic of consciousness. The Other who meditates C.G. Jung is Jung himself as his own Other. There is real otherness, something fundamentally alien, but the whole relation between the two is nevertheless a *self-relation*.

A third important topic that has a bearing on the question what psychological consciousness may involve is Jung's theoretical as well as therapeutic insistence on the necessity of our gaining a distance to ourselves. In a late letter Jung lamented: "They [Jung is speaking about modern creative artists, but what he says applies all the more to modern man in general] have not yet learned to discriminate between their wilful mind and the objective manifestation of the psyche. They have not yet learned to be objective with their own psyche, i.e., [to discriminate] between the thing which you do and the thing that happens to you. ... We are still in a shockingly primitive state of mind, and this is the main reason why we cannot become objective in psychic matters" (*Letters 2*, p. 590 f., to Read, 2 September 1960). Similarly he wrote another time two weeks later: "... at present man seems to be quite incapable of realizing that under a certain aspect he is a stranger to himself" (*Letters 2*, p. 595, to Serrano, 14 September 1960). To this we must add a third quotation, also from his last years, in which Jung, talking about the "childlike naïveté" of modern man, says: "He has no objectivity toward himself and cannot yet regard himself as a phenomenon which he finds in existence and with which, for better or worse, he is identical" (*MDR* p. 341).

By the way, Jung's unsparing or even brutal diagnosis that "We are still in a shockingly primitive state of mind" confirms the fact that my thesis expressed above, namely, that psychological consciousness lies still very much ahead of us in the future, is also Jung's assessment. Furthermore, we see at work here an anticipation of the future. With his judgement about the present age (our "shockingly primitive" state of mind) Jung is, as it were, 'looking backwards' from the expected or demanded future at our time and his own present. Jung's verdict does not just refer to ordinary people outside of psychology. It is comprehensive and thus includes, or is probably even mainly directed at, the prevailing consciousness in analytical psychology, for as a psychologist's "We" it must first and foremost refer to psychologists. As I suggested, analytical psychology's own consciousness seems to be largely "pre-psychological" in Jung's sense.

To become conscious means to have learned to distinguish oneself from oneself, to see oneself soberly, detachedly, as if from outside. It means to have become de-identified from oneself. The original *participation mystique* or *unio naturalis* with oneself has to be disrupted. One has to become to oneself just an objective fact, a given (given *to* ourselves), in the same sense that all the other facts of our world around us are objective facts and givens. One has to take an empirical, almost scientific, attitude towards oneself, maybe like a zoologist towards the animals he observes. This also implies that one has to know oneself as contingent and thoroughly relative (in contrast to the inevitable *"childlike-naïve"* sense of ourselves qua inalienable subjectivity, as being the center of our world as well as of our invariable identity with ourselves).

After these three hints coming from Jung that point to an anticipated future on the level of the *opus magnum* I now want to add an ancient traditional idea of the Christian West of greatest relevance to our present topic of seenness. It is the idea of the all-seeing eye of God. In Proverbs 15:3 we read: "The eyes of the LORD are in every place, beholding the evil and the good." In the past (this is now no longer true) people in the West grew up with the knowledge and feeling that everything they do is inevitably seen by God. Psychologically this is a most important idea because it adds to the sense and awareness of the subjective I the real feeling of an objective, absolute witness, a knowing that is not my own knowing. The most powerful expression is to be found in the Old Testament, Psalm 139, lines 1-16, which I will quote in the *New Jerusalem Bible* translation.

> Yahweh, you examine me and know me, / you know when I sit, when I rise, you understand my thoughts from afar. / You watch when I walk or lie down, you know every detail of my conduct. / A word is not yet on my tongue before you, Yahweh, know all about it. / You fence me in, behind and in front, you have laid your hand upon me. / ... / Where shall I go to escape your spirit? Where shall I flee from your presence? / If I scale the heavens you are there, if I lie flat in Sheol [the place of the dead], there you are. / If I speed away on the wings of the dawn, if I dwell beyond the ocean, / even there your hand will be guiding me, your right hand holding me fast. / I will say, 'Let the darkness cover me, and the night wrap itself around me,' / even darkness to you is not dark, and night is as clear as the day. / You created my inmost self, knit me together in my mother's womb. / ... You knew me through and through, / my being held no secrets from you, when I was being formed in secret, textured in the depths of the earth. / Your eyes could see my embryo. In your book all my days were inscribed, every one that was fixed is there.

The inexorable seenness is total and all-comprehensive. The I is surrounded on all sides by God's seeing, even "fenced in" by it: inescapably imprisoned in it, spatially as well as in temporal regards (past and future).

Usually, the Christian idea of the "Last Judgement" is imagined in terms of eschatology. The Last Judgement is conceived (imagined pictorially) as a particular, one-time event in the distant future, postponed to the end of the world and the end of time. But one's constant and inescapable seenness by the all-seeing eye of God in its pressing presence is already, we could say, the continually ongoing Last Judgement. To be sure, in Psalm 139 God is not shown as judge, whether damning or saving. He is presented exclusively as the one who *sees* and *knows* me through and through: as my relentless seenness and knownness. But the point here is precisely that we need to understand that psychologically my inexorably *being* seen and known IS in itself already the very judgement! A literal judgement with a threatening hell versus an eternal salvation is not needed (it may have its place in the "childlike naïveté" of the picture-and-story thinking of civilian man or ego-consciousness). In my being seen I am unsparingly confronted with my truth. This, the moment of truth, *is* the terrible judgement. There is a quality of violence in truth. Truth breaks through and shatters the protective shell of the innocence and warmth of my *just being*, my cocoonment in myself, in my subjectivity, and pulls me out of my concealment in it into the open, turning me, my being-so, inside out into the exposedness that we call truth. This movement is the revolutionary change from unconscious *being* (cocoonedness in simple being and living) to *consciousness*, and psychologically Psalm 139 could be called the articulation of the first immediacy (no more) of *explicit* consciousness.

At the same time we see that consciousness has nothing whatsoever to do with an "*awareness* of facts", the simple awareness of what I have done, what my character and nature, my shortcomings and "shadow" or what my virtues are. "Consciousness" is not concerned with "information about ..." in the modern sense, with contents, details, the semantic. All it means is my ruthlessly having been turned inside out and become defenselessly exposed to an *objective* unamenable seeing and knowing. Consciousness is the accomplished transition from "just being" to knownness, and in this sense, metaphorically speaking, from "ontology" to "logos", to the noetic, to the dimension of truth, just as, conversely, unconsciousness does not mean ignorance, but "just being", simply being the way one is. Unconsciousness is not beyond, but on this side of the whole opposition of knowledge and ignorance, and indifferent to it.[137]

Requirements for "psychological consciousness"?

In our attempt to clarify what "psychological consciousness" as a future possibility intuited by Jung could mean we have looked at four examples, three presented by Jung and one stemming from our cultural history, that might serve as hints giving us some anticipatory idea of it. Two examples (the one about conscious "feeling" and the other one about one's gaining "objectivity towards oneself") were rather personalistic and subjective, whereas the other two (Jung's UFO and yogi dreams as well as the all-seeing eye of God) showed the spontaneous objective appearance or, respectively, the a priori existence of an external Other gazing at, projecting, or knowing the subject. The first group bemoaned a deficiency on the part of us or of modern man and thus at least indirectly suggested an ought: "We are still in a shockingly primitive state of mind" and so we *should* become able to realize that we are strangers to ourselves and develop objectivity in psychic matters; we *should* de-identify ourselves from ourselves so as to learn to see ourselves as if from outside; we *should* become able to be truly conscious of our feelings, of what value events truly have in the depths. A self-othering is needed, i.e., demanded. In other words, here Jung appeals at least indirectly to the ego. Nothing of the sort is the case in the other two examples. They merely report what in fact happened or always is. There is no need to do anything, no need for an effort or striving, not even for a longing. In these latter two examples, what is reported is objectively already simply the case.

In addition to this difference between the indirect suggestion of a moral appeal and an objective description of a fact there is a second important difference between the examples. Two of them, the same two that were concerned with our deficiency and incapability, stay within a *narrowly* defined sense of psychology, the

137 Knowing your "shadow" does not in itself imply (partial) consciousness!

intra-personal sphere. They refer to our personal self-relation. The other two, by contrast, present the subject in an external relation to a literal other, the one even coming from outer space, the other one being God, the extramundane creator of the world. Just as Psalm 139 is obviously a religious or theological and not a psychological text, so are also Jung's two dreams not really about something psychological, but cosmological or "metaphysical". From a psychological point of view we have to say that in both examples "the psychological other" is projected out of the human and intra-personal sphere into literal outer space in the one case and into or rather beyond the universe in the other. It is still *imagined.*

The UFO and the yogi dreams paradoxically lead *semantically* to Jung's conclusion that *he* is the one who is projected or meditated by the UFO or the yogi, respectively, while *syntactically* of course the UFO and the yogi are themselves projections by Jung's dream thought out of the psyche into a literal external reality. They as well as the all-seeing God are, within those fantasies, *hypostatized* as literal beings or entities and imagined as literally soul-*transcendent.*

The result of this analysis shows why Jung could not *think* the idea of a full-fledged "psychological consciousness", an idea that he nevertheless certainly intuited. There are two central problems.

In those two examples in which there is a literal transcendence and an hypostatizing, the—for a psychological consciousness—indispensable objective seenness from outside is fully realized, but does not become psychological. It remains literally soul-external. The objective seenness or knownness by some real Other is not *thought,* but merely imagined, a reifying or personifying picture thinking. The seeing Other is projected into the dimensions of space and time. The seenness is doubtless the semantic content of the experience. For the ego-personality it is perhaps, as in Psalm 139, even an extremely pressing experience, but it does not and cannot come home to the soul itself as *its own reality.* Keeping in mind the wording of Jung's lament about "the great regrettable problem in our culture that we are strangely incapable of realizing our own feelings" as well as the other sigh that "man seems to be quite incapable of realizing that under a certain aspect he is a stranger to himself", we have to say that the seenness is not *realized* as an aspect of *the soul's own* interiority. It remains something that is done to it or happens to it, much like one may be hit by a car; it is a kind of intrusion from an extraterrestrial source. Jung's UFO and yogi dreams certainly had a marked emotional effect on Jung (in the second case even one of "profound fright") and also produced an intellectual effect (a conclusion or new idea). But emotions belong to the ego-personality; they are psychic, not psychological. Jung comes up with the startlingly novel conclusion "that we are their projections. "I am projected by the magic lantern as C. G. Jung" only means that he now has a fascinating (Jung spoke of his "astonishment") new idea, a new theory *about* himself, but he himself and the inner constitution of his consciousness remain the same as before. To be sure, there is a new "awareness" or an awareness *of* something new, but not the realization of psychological consciousness.

In the other two examples the standpoint is entirely intra-psychic, if not personalistic. What I just said was missing in the former two cases seems to be provided here. But the price for its being present in these conceptions is that a real transcendence is missing. Even if there is the idea of a *real* Other (another person who knows of my embarrassing secret), it is the I's subjective knowledge of the knowing Other that makes the difference, not the external Other himself. In the case of "objectivity towards oneself", there is not even an Other at all. It is the subject itself that is demanded to actively take, within itself and merely mentally, an external position vis-à-vis itself so as to become able to see itself as if from outside. I spoke of a self-othering. But inasmuch as this self-othering would be the subject's own doing, it would be only a methodological shift of standpoint from which *the same old subject* would now look at itself. As a methodological performance it is a willful act, a subjective doing by the ego-personality taking place in time. As I pointed out already above, the change of one's methodological orientation is not capable of transforming the inner constitution of consciousness into that of "psychological consciousness". This is also why Jung's discussion of it gets stuck on the level of bemoaning a lack, on the one hand, and wishful thinking or a moral demand (an ought), on the other. He is so to speak in the position of Moses anticipating but being on principle excluded from the Promised Land. Fulfillment is projected into the no-man's-land of the future.

"Psychological consciousness" needs all four ingredients:

1. The external, transcendent otherness of one's *being* seen and known, and also

2. the true interiority of this external otherness in the subject, which excludes any hypostatization and literalization of the Other, any literal externality such as something coming from outer space or observing from outside the universe.

3. The required interiority must, in turn, not itself be a personalistically, ego-psychologically conceived one; it must have the full objectivity of having its place *not* on the level of the ego-personality or "civilian man", but solely on the background-level of the objective psyche, and

4. it can neither be the result of a literal doing (act or acts of behavior) nor be the *experience* of a happening (something that befalls us) in space and time, but must simply be the prevailing truth, the unquestioned syntax of lived life and experiencing the world. "Consciousness" in "psychological consciousness" can therefore no longer be seen as a kind of psychic "organ" in the personality, a part, realm, or agency of what has been called the "psychic apparatus". It does not belong to the human organism, to man as animal. It must be understood as a logical form, a particular *structure*. From this it follows that, in order to acquire an anticipatory notion of "psychological consciousness", we must leave behind all picture thinking, all concentration on semantic contents, in fact the entire "thing"-ontology, and advance to thought proper, to truly conceptual comprehension.

The soul's way into the future through its self-overcoming: projecting its future goal as "God" into heaven and then slowly realizing the projected idea

An external, transcendent Other and true interiority contradict each other. These two opposites can be reconciled only through the inwardization, integration of the transcendent Other into the logical form of consciousness. But it must be an inwardization that precisely preserves the transcendent otherness. This inwardization cannot be an appropriation by, assimilation to, or absorption into the subject in its old form, for the transcendence aspect is indispensable. Thus the contradiction must not be altogether removed, it has to be transformed. It appears in the structure of the I or subjectivity itself as an internal tension, or cleft, between the empirical subject and the transcendent subject. With this cleft we see that there is a real self-othering, which, however, would not be the result of "our" doing, but the I's own internal logical form.

This makes it analogous to the Kantian concept of subjectivity as the difference between the empirical subject and the transcendental subject. The difference between the subjectivity structure of "psychological consciousness" and the Kantian subjectivity structure is that between "transcendental" in the one case and "transcendent" in the other. We can show the analogy schematically (see diagrams, left and right).

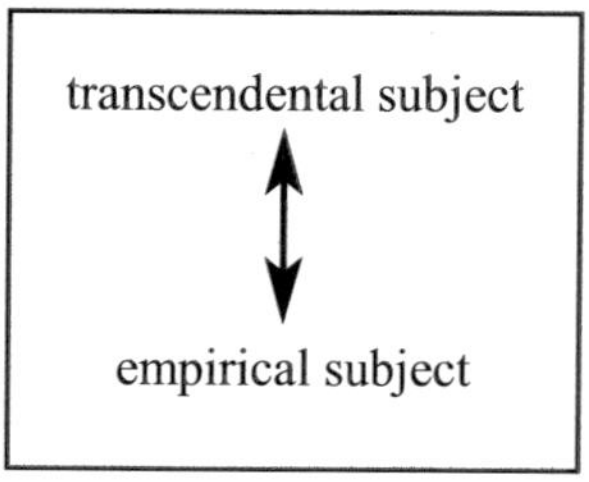

The logical structure of the Kantian subjectivity

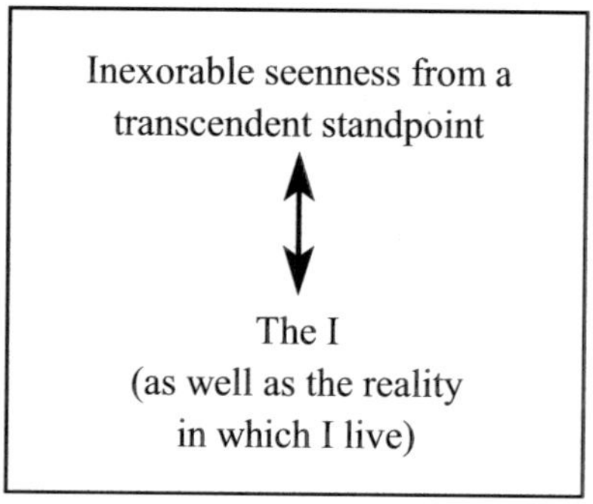

The logical structure of psychological consciousness

But we also have to understand the difference between them and the particular reason for the difference. In order to get a handle on this issue, let me refer back to a thesis I advanced decades ago in my Eranos lecture of 1983, "Das Begräbnis der Seele in die technische Zivilisation".[138] I tried to show that technology can be

138 In: *Eranos 52-1983*, Frankfurt/M. (Insel) 1985, pp. 211-276. In English translation: "The Burial of the Soul in Technological Civilization", in: W.G., *Technology and the Soul. From the Nuclear Bomb to the World Wide Web.* (=

understood *psychologically* as the Western project of the technical fabrication of God, and thus his *Wahr-machung* ("veri-fication" in the literal sense), so to speak, in "the flesh" (that is, in concrete material reality).[139] Whereas previously thinkers had to struggle to establish *intellectual* proofs of the existence of God, the early modern soul made man (unconsciously, unwittingly) establish the existence of "God" by (of course only in approximation[140]) *producing* the attributes of God down here, on earth, in empirical reality, which above all in recent developments, such as in the areas of Artificial Intelligence and genetic engineering, becomes more and more evident.[141]

The general idea behind this thesis is that the emergence of Great Ideas, such as that of the Judeo-Christian God or of Plato's doctrine of the soul's ascent to the Ideas as well as of the highest Idea, that of the Good[142] must *psychologically* not primarily be taken at face value, for what they are *meant* to be, namely religious or philosophical ideas, a cognition about cosmic, or ontological factors or aspects of the world, as well as, possibly, objects of worship. They are soul-stuff, inventions by the soul. Psychologically, the appearance of the Creator God (to stay with this idea) is the projection into super-celestial height of the human mind's first (as yet completely unconscious) intuition or vision of a future possibility and task. What appears to the imagination reified and personified as an always already existing divine being who before all time created and since then rules the world has covertly in itself

W.G., *Collected English Papers*, vol. 2) New Orleans (Spring Journal Books) 2007, pp. 155–211.

139 The observation of the empirical facts underlying this view are usually discussed and interpreted under the completely different label and theory of "secularization".

140 It is the approximation character, that is, the impossibility of the full realization, that is responsible for the "unending project" character of this project.

141 The aspect of God as Sustainer of the world and modern man's (unwitting) identification with that God can also be seen at work behind the present-day zealous concerns about "preserving the Creation" and "saving the world from 'climate catastrophe'". (By contrast, Heidegger still thought that "Only a God can save us"!)

142 I also discussed Plato's parable of the cave from the indicated point of view in my "The Occidental Soul's Self-Immurement in Plato's Cave", in: W.G., *Technology and the Soul. From the Nuclear Bomb to the World Wide Web.* (= W.G., CEP 2) New Orleans (Spring Journal Books) 2007, pp. 213–279.

the character of a project, an assignment. The projection *into the vertical height* is actually (implicitly), but without being recognized, the projection of a distant *destination* set for man *into the horizontal historical future.* The Great Idea is not just a concept or truth resting within itself. It is in truth a psychological *motor* with its own inherent dynamic, momentum, and motivating power. Being at first utterly out of reach and beyond all feasibility (considering the real practical-technical capabilities, powers of comprehension, and psychological constitution of consciousness of the people in whom this Idea appeared), a Great Idea needs ages of being venerated (and even feared) as a wondrous ideal or numinous superhuman object up there. In this way it can slowly take roots in human consciousness and man's inner feeling, come closer to its own intellectual comprehension, until it can at long last surreptitiously (from behind) unfold its powerful influence over the human mind *in a practical way.* Then, what originally had been absolutely out of reach can be taken by man into his own hands as a concrete project, which of course at the same time means that the former numinous Creator God becomes obsolete; he or this idea has done its job; it has nothing to do any more and therefore can also no longer fascinate the soul.

The historical development in the soul's logical life thus proceeds in three steps: unconscious projection of the initial vague and not understood idea or hunch that is exalted to the skies; man's psychological and intellectual slowly catching up with this idea and his thus becoming psychically on a par with it; his taking charge of it as a project to be practically realized.

Seen in this light we can say that the soul's idea of the Creator God was the deeper meaning and driving force behind the whole project of the age of *Neuzeit* (the early-modern period), what I called the second stage according to the axiom on nature by Pseudo-Democritus. As the stage of the (soul's) emancipation from the soul, its overcoming of the *unio naturalis*, and its having awakened from its former blessed dream, it was also the time of the formation of the modern I. The modern I established itself as the center of the *logical constituting* of the experience of all reality, which in turn expressed itself in the modern sciences and the step-by-step transformation of the given natural world into technological civilization. With the thesis of the verification of God in mind, that is, the thesis of the translation of the metaphysical idea of God in the beyond into positive-factual technical reality, we can recognize that also in the second stage's new philosophical conception of "knowing" and subjectivity there is a logical movement. It brings God as the Maker of the world down from his transcendence and back from having been projected out, by inwardizing him into the very concept of subjectivity, as the Kantian "transcendental I". Conversely, the idea of the divine Creator of the world can in retrospect be comprehended as the soul's first dim vision of the possibility of establishing itself in the form of an I, a subject that knows the world as *objective reality*, a world that is logically *constituted* by the transcendental subject itself and no longer a "thing in itself". As "appearance" it is irrevocably known to be the product of the human mind's own formation.

Owing to its integration the transcendental I is inherent in the structure of both human subjectivity and (indirectly) in the world itself qua "objective reality"; it is no longer *transcendent*. But because it is fundamentally different from and alien to the empirical I and because it is its unchangeable a priori background, it is nevertheless at least, as Kant put it, "transcendental".

So far, I spoke of the integration or inwardization of God, but this is not quite accurate. We should rather speak of the inwardization of the whole traditional *relation between man and God*. This relation reappears in completely altered form in the depicted logical structure of Kantian subjectivity (and of the second stage as a whole).

As an aside I have to point out that my thesis of "God" being brought down from Heaven and, psychologically as well as practically, realized on earth, on the one hand in the constitution of man as subjectivity and on the other *in* or *as* science and technology, is incompatible with Jung's view concerning the God idea or the archetypes in general and concerning Nietzsche's idea that "God is dead". The latter is of course a catchy slogan, a stark, popularized expression of the much quieter and larger historical process of "the birth of man" (which is tantamount to the psychological integration of the God idea into the constitution of consciousness). At any rate, Jung repeatedly suggested that by declaring God dead, man would become unconsciously identified with God, that is, *inflated* by the God archetype and in this sense endangered by psychosis. This means that the moment the God topic was concerned, Jung was not capable or willing to allow for the possibility of a true *integration* of a psychological projection and a corresponding downward movement of the projected content. For him God inevitably stayed up there, and if you dared to deny Him (note the capitalization!), you did not pull Him *down* at all, but, conversely, He unawares sucked you mentally up so that you psychologically lost the ground under your feet. Inflation versus integration. For Jung "God must not die!", and God does not die. But this position makes Jung, in this one regard, malgré lui think and speak as a theologian or religious man, and desert his status as psychologist: as a student, observer, and an analyst, who, without an agenda of his own, studies the soul's logical life as it *really* develops.

Now the important thing to realize is that this interiorized former God is only one aspect of him, his being the Creator and Sustainer of all things, the aspect of the Maker, in other words, (from our modern point of view) the aspect of technology. This restriction is the limitation of the second phase (or stage) in its factual historical realization. The second stage makes absolutely amazing progress in knowing the world and bringing about technological innovations, but it pays for this progress by narrowing its world experience (and even its own very concept of knowing itself) to the terribly restricted sense of 'getting to know how things work, the way they function, and how they can be manipulated'. What it allows for is what we call an "awareness". It completely excludes consciousness.

But psychological consciousness is the issue of the third stage, and in order for it to come about—if it should ever come about—an analogous integration of the God idea into the structure of consciousness would be required. But it must be the integration and interiorization of an entirely different God concept, namely that of the all-seeing God. We can say that this idea is the soul's projected, reified, and personified initial hunch of its own potential to become a "psychological consciousness".

Again as an aside, let me mention that there is a third aspect of God that, if inwardized and integrated, could lead to a fourth stage. It is the idea of God as Love. Such a stage remains for us at an even greater distance, namely in utter darkness, than that of the possible stage of psychological consciousness. We have not even an inkling what "Love" could mean in this context. For the time being it is only an empty word, liable to be misconstrued in terms of the all-too-human senses that love has for us now. About psychological consciousness we can at least already form a concept.

Whereas inwardization and integration of the Creator God led to the change from "transcendent" to "transcendental" (in Kant's sense), the integration of the all-knowing God into the logical structure of consciousness must preserve his transcendence. The very point of it is the seenness from outside, by a real unamenable Other. However, this real Other, once it is no longer projected out, but interiorized, must be the contradiction of an "inner real other", an "*internal* 'from outside'". Such a consciousness must *as* active *subjectivity* nevertheless have within its own structure its own being "passively" *subjected* to an objective, inexorable seenness and knownness. The second stage in Pseudo-Democritus' scheme overcomes nature by "conquering", "subduing" it. It can remain consistent, syntonic with itself. The third stage, however, allows *the contradiction* into its own logical form, and only by virtue of this *endured* contradiction is psychological consciousness possible. According to Pseudo-Democritus, on the third stage "Nature enjoys its mastery over nature": it is no longer the one side of the conflict, one of the conflicting parties. It has the very conflict or contradiction within itself and is not threatened by it. It maintains itself in it. This is the step beyond mere "awareness".

This is why de-identification with itself/oneself is indispensable for psychological consciousness. The subject has to freely *release* itself into its factual being-so. It cannot, as far as its nature or behavior is concerned, try to protect itself in its childlike-naive innocence and original unity with itself; it cannot try to escape into *feelings* of shame or guilt, these fundamental defense mechanisms. The inexorable seenness by the internal transcendent other means the release of what *is* (whatever it is and however it may be) into its truth. It could almost be said to be a brutal releasement, perhaps similar to that releasement with which, according to the concept of Creation, God at Creation *freely released* the world out of the blessed containment in the ideality of His thought into the earthly reality of its being-so, with all its greatness, shortcomings, faults, miseries, sufferings, terrors, its finiteness. Just letting it be, leaving it to its own devices and fate—so to speak without flinching.

Now it would be easy to draw the wrong conclusion from these last remarks, namely, that WE, the subject should perform this kind of releasing. Psychological consciousness can of course not be something that I or you have to bring about. It is not the result of a doing, an effort. If it were our achievement, or if its coming into existence would be something we *experience* (such as a happening, an event), it would precisely still be an event within the present logical status of the second stage: an artificial construct, a willed pose, in the one case, or a particular empirical occurrence within the world as "objective reality", in the other case. The subject of the second stage would remain supreme.

* * *

Psychological consciousness must not be thought to be a *subjective* attitude or private form of thinking. Real consciousness is always something general, common, objective, not personal. It cannot be "in us". It is all around us. If "psychological consciousness" should ever be realized, it would exist simply as a general *objective structure*, as the prevailing form of man's world experience: as the unquestionable *truth* in which mankind objectively lives, so to speak as the character of reality. It would be much as in the second stage, in which it was or rather is the positivistic character of the world as "objective reality" that was and still is the prevailing truth in which we all inevitably live (even if it should be the case that subjectively some of us have our reservations, be they moral, emotional or intellectual objections. Such objections would be the ego's private entertainment, but would make no *real* difference). Already the consciousness of the second stage is not a subjective or personal way of looking at the world. But for "psychological consciousness" this objectivity character is all the more necessary inasmuch as in it the subject is subjected to the inexorable seenness from a transcendent (and as such superior) standpoint. It is reduced to an "object" of this external seeing.

If we wanted to describe *what* the character or inner logical constitution of reality under the prevailing truth of "psychological consciousness" would be, we would probably have to assume that it would mean that as empirical subject I would see myself from the standpoint of the transcendent subject and thus indeed, as Jung had demanded, as if from outside. I would "under a certain aspect" have become a stranger to myself. I would look at myself as if I were an Other, a 'prime matter' firmly enclosed in the hermetically sealed retort, an ongoing dream dreamed by the "yogi who has my own face". I would exist as my own internal Last Judgment. "Last Judgment" of course not in a childlike-naive moralizing sense with ideas of "heaven and hell" inspired by wishful thinking and the dream of impeccable perfection, but as my sober being *logically* and *objectively* de-identified from myself and my ruthless consciousness of my finite-deficient being-so as my inexorable truth.

What this "psychological consciousness" would mean for me (and for all human individuals in general) is not all. As a general *structure* of consciousness it would also impart itself to our entire world experience. Then the new character of everything in the world would be that it, too, has its objective seenness from a transcendent point of view, its "Last Judgment", *within itself* as its own always already prevailing logic and inexorable truth.

This, we must assume in anticipation, would be the realized "psychological consciousness", of which Jung had the first vague and partial intuition. What this would concretely feel like and how precisely it would affect human being-in-the-world and man's world-relation cannot be anticipated. But one thing is certain, it would be a world experience and world-relation fundamentally different from the present second-stage one, which is the logic behind our technological civilization and in which every piece of, and every thing in, the world is by definition and on principle constituted as irrevocably possessing its rigid self-identity and seamlessly fitting into the construction of the world as an absolutely consistent, uniform whole. ❦

Image Sources

The following pictures were accessed December 15, 2019. They are public domain and have been identified as being free of known restrictions under copyright law, including all related and neighboring rights:

Unnumbered picture by Johann Erdmann Hummel in Chapter 1. Source: https://commons.wikimedia.org/wiki/File:Zimmerbild_78.jpg

Fig. 4. Source: https://en.wikipedia.org/wiki/Gardens_of_ancient_Egypt.

Fig. 7. Source: https://upload.wikimedia.org/wikipedia/commons/4/46/Jacopo_Tintoretto_-_The_Last_Supper_-_WGA22649.jpg.

Fig. 8. Source: https://upload.wikimedia.org/wikipedia/commons/f/f8/St._James_led_to_his_execution.jpg.

Fig. 9. Source: https://de.wikipedia.org/wiki/Datei:Friedrich-barbarossa-und-soehne-welfenchronik_1-1000x1540.jpg.

Fig. 15. Source: https://commons.wikimedia.org/wiki/Main_Page.

Fig. 16. Source: https://en.wikipedia.org/wiki/Sistine_Madonna.

Fig. 17 Source: https://en.wikipedia.org/wiki/Lamentation_of_Christ_(Mantegna)

Fig. 18. Source: https://commons.wikimedia.org/wiki/Category:Frescos_of_Abteikirche_Neresheim?uselang=de#/media/File:Kloster_Neresheim._12.jpg. Photo by Holger Uwe Schmitt. Creative Commons licence CC BY-SA 4.0. Fig. 18a is a detail of this photo.

Fig. 19. Source: https://en.wikipedia.org/wiki/Woman_at_a_Window. The work of art depicted in this image and the reproduction thereof are in the public domain worldwide.

Fig. 10. Source: https://www.britannica.com/art/tempera-painting#/media/1/586515/149442. Photograph by KaDeWeGirl. The Metropolitan Museum of Art, New York City, The Cloisters Collection, 1961 (61.200.1) Creative Commons Legal Code

Fig. 11. Source: https://images.nga.gov/?service=asset&action=show_zoom_window_popup&language=en&asset=149434&location=grid&asset_list=149434&basket_item_id=undefined

A16760.jpg Open access

The following three reproductions are part of a collection of reproductions compiled by The Yorck Project. The compilation copyright is held by

Zenodot Verlagsgesellschaft mbH *and licensed under the GNU Free Documentation License*:

Fig. 12. Source:
https://en.wikipedia.org/wiki/Madonna_of_the_Rose_Bower.

Fig. 13. Source:
www.zeno.org/Kunstwerke/B/Dürer,+Albrecht%3A+Der+Zeichner+des+liegenden+Weibes.

Fig. 14. Source:
www.zeno.org/Kunstwerke/B/Dürer,+Albrecht%3A+Der+Zeichner+der+Laute.

Fig. 1 and **2** are my redrawings.

Made in United States
Troutdale, OR
10/07/2026

55376491R00197